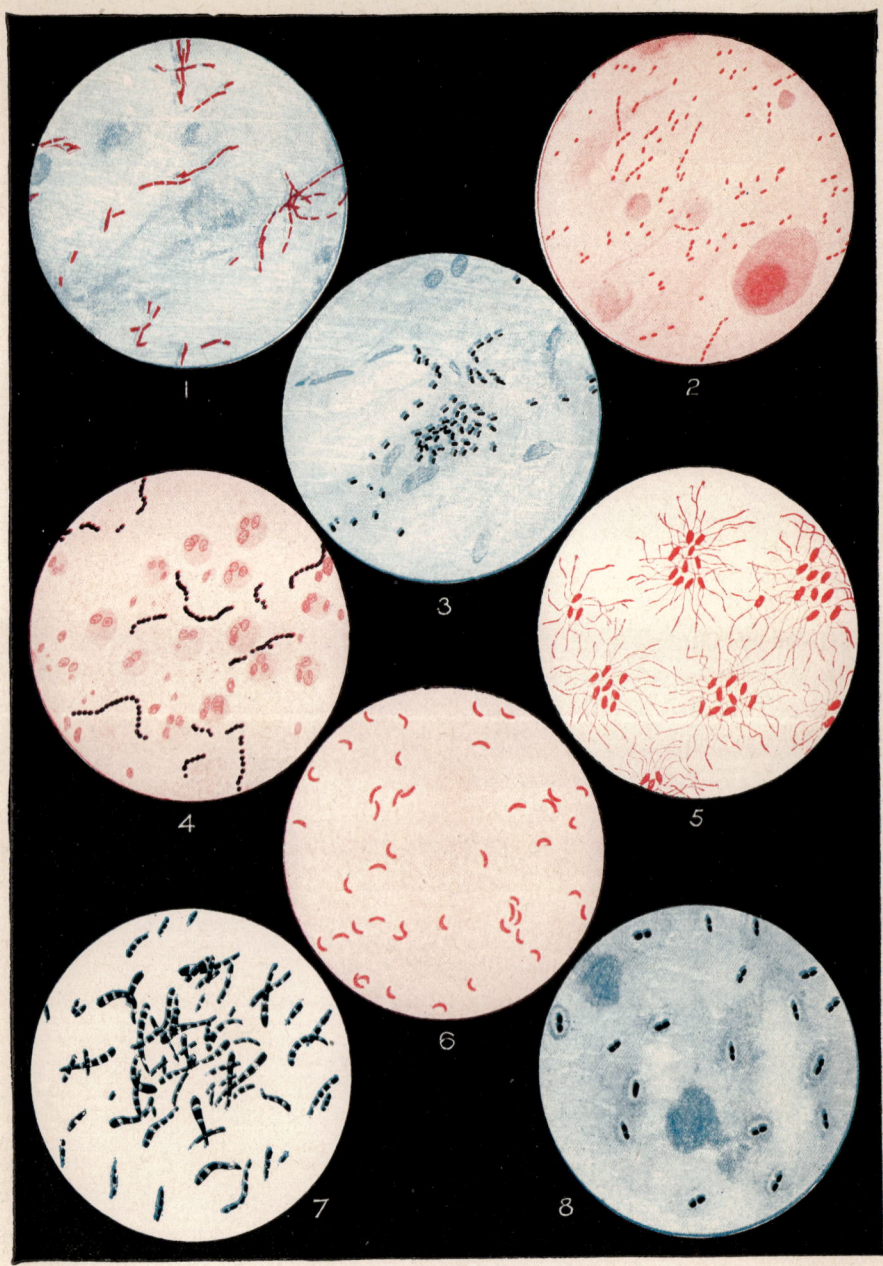

PLATE X.   BACTERIA OF COMMON DISEASES

1. Bacillus of tuberculosis of the lungs. 2. Bacillus of influenza. 3. Micrococcus found in cases of acute rheumatism. 4. Streptococcus of erysipelas. 5. Bacillus of typhoid fever. 6. Bacillus of cholera. 7. Bacillus of diphtheria. 8. Diplococcus of pneumonia.

The
NEW PEOPLE'S PHYSICIAN

THE CONCISE ENCYCLOPEDIA OF HEALTH

edited by
VICTOR ROBINSON, Ph.C., M.D.

PROFESSOR OF HISTORY OF MEDICINE, TEMPLE UNIVERSTY.
EDITOR IN CHIEF: MEDICAL REVIEW OF REVIEWS, THE MODERN
HOME PHYSICIAN. AUTHOR: THE STORY OF MEDICINE, et al.

In Eight Volumes

VOLUME FIVE

New York
WM. H. WISE & CO., INC.
1942

Copyright, 1941
Wm. H. Wise & Co., Inc.
Printed in the United States of America

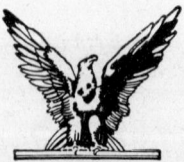

The publishers are wholeheartedly cooperating in the effort to conserve vital materials and manpower by manufacturing this book in full conformity with War Production Board Ruling L-245, curtailing the use of paper by book publishers, and all other United States Government regulations.

This has been accomplished without abbreviating the book in any way. It is absolutely complete and unabridged. Not a word, not a paragraph, not a comma has been omitted.

All procedures and formulas printed in this work have been carefully drawn up by the contributors responsible for the text in which they occur; these have been examined and verified. But, while the utmost care has thus been taken to insure accuracy, the publishers cannot accept responsibility in cases of error of any kind. No prescriptions are given for specific disease where the treatment must be determined by the personal diagnosis of a physician.

CONTENTS OF VOLUME FIVE

Section XII — Constitutional Diseases (continued)

CHAPTER	PAGE
93. General Constitutional Diseases	1255
94. Diseases Due to Disordered Metabolism	1278
95. Deficiency Diseases	1299
96. Disorders of the Endocrine System	1304

Section XIII — Infectious Diseases

97. Inflammation and Fever	1321
98. Diseases Caused by Known Germs: Various	1337
99. Diseases Caused by Known Germs: Tuberculosis	1380
100. Diseases Caused by Other Known Organisms	1393
101. Virus Diseases and Rheumatic Fever	1403

Section XIV — Blood and Circulatory Diseases

102. Diseases of the Blood and Associated Organs	1417
103. Common Signs of Circulatory Failure	1431
104. Diseases of the Heart	1439
105. Disorders of the Blood Vessels	1461

Section XV — Diseases of the Respiratory System

106. Disorders of the Nose and Nasopharynx	1481
107. Disorders of the Throat	1493
108. Disorders of the Larynx	1503
109. Diseases of the Bronchial Tubes	1511
110. Diseases of the Lungs	1525
111. Diseases of the Pleura	1563

COLOR PLATES IN VOLUME FIVE

PLATE NO.

X. Bacteria of Common Diseases..Frontispiece

XI. Rash in Infectious and Other Disorders..............................Facing page 1345

XII. HEART: Various Aspects Showing How It Is Constructed and How It Works..Facing page 1425

CHAPTER 93

GENERAL CONSTITUTIONAL DISEASES

Cancer—Varieties of Growth—Manner of Spread—Cause — Symptoms and Progress — Diagnosis — Prevention and Treatment — Rheumatism — Chronic Rheumatism.

AS medical knowledge progresses, the mystery of disease continues to become less profound. Nowadays, in the absence of definite knowledge of the origin of cancer, that disease is left almost alone and uncharted, and, owing to its widely scattered influences is put in a class by itself. It is true also that rheumatic fever still has some ties which bind it to the category of general constitutional diseases, and for that reason it is included in this chapter; but it seems not unlikely that in the near future all the manifestations of what is known as the "rheumatic diathesis" will be satisfactorily explained, and that rheumatism will be classified with the infectious diseases. There is increasing evidence, though as yet no adequate proof, that a hemolytic streptococcus is the causative agent.

Cancer. We shall deal first then with cancer, one of the scourges of civilization.

Cancer is the general term applied to malignant new growths which develop in the body as a result of perverted growth of the body cells, and which may ultimately lead to the death of the person in whom they develop, unless corrective procedure is employed.

Cancer occurs in the lower animals as well as human beings. Dogs, cats, horses, and cows are all subject to the disease, and it is stated also to occur (rarely) in birds and fishes.

Cancer is found in every country, climate, race, and occupation, though the death rate from it varies considerably from country to country. It is undoubtedly less common among primitive people than in civilized communities. Doctors who have long practised among some primitive races, notably those living under very healthy conditions as to diet and general habits, state that they have never encountered any cases of cancer among their patients.

There is evidence to show that cancer is on the increase. While some weight must be given to the greater accuracy in diagnosis made possible by improved methods, there is no doubt that as a cause of death cancer is becoming more frequent. The increased expectation of life in modern times is also partly responsible, since cancer is essentially a disease of advanced age.

As is well understood, the unit of living substance is the cell. In every individual there are millions of microscopic cells, all of which are derived, by successive divisions, from the original fertilized ovum or egg cell. As the di-

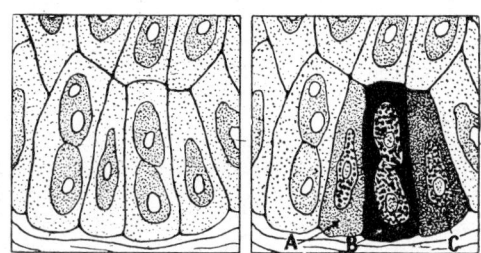

NORMAL AND CANCEROUS CELLS
Left: diagram of normal epithelial cells in section of skin. Right: same group showing stages of cancer development; cell B, definitely cancerous; cells A and C, in precancerous state. Probably a healthy cell does not become a cancer cell, but increasing change to cancer type occurs in successive generations of cells.

(1255)

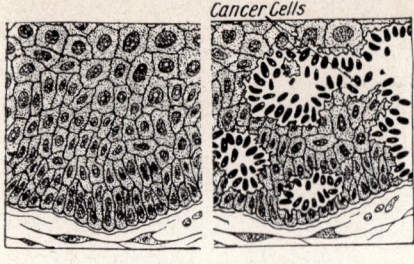

GROWTH OF CANCER

A carcinoma of the skin shown in semi-diagrammatic form. There is progressive destruction of adjoining healthy cells, but also isolated collections of cancer cells within the healthy epithelium.

visions take place the resulting cells assume two main types: one variety covering the outer surface of the body and lining the inner surface of the mouth, stomach and intestines, and the glands which open on to the one or other surface; and the other developing into the general framework of the body (muscle, bone, connective tissue). In the body at any period of its development there is a certain regular adjustment of growth and multiplication as between the two classes of cells and among the cells of either class. Each cell is kept in its place and prevented from undue multiplication by some regulating force which is as yet not understood by biologists and medical men.

But it happens occasionally that one local group of cells shows the capacity to exceed its appointed limits, to encroach on and supplant its neighbors, to appropriate the nourishment which belongs by right to them, and thus to destroy parts which are necessary to life. Such a predatory group of cells is termed a cancer. When this process occurs among the connective-tissue cells the formation is termed a sarcoma, while a similar change in the type of cells which line the intestines or glands and cover the skin is called a carcinoma.

Every kind of cell in the body is capable of starting a cancer, and the growth will consist only of that especial type of cell. The first small changes are on so small a scale that they escape notice. The presence of symptoms will depend on the position of the growth and the effect of metastases (areas of cancerous tissue which develop as a result of spread, either through the lymphatics or the blood stream, from the original growth). A cancer of the surface of the body will be more quickly detected than one deeply seated.

It is readily understood that the earliest stages in the development of cancer can only be detected by the microscope. The same instrument has been the means of revealing conditions in which cells are taking on slightly abnormal activities which have not yet reached the invading characters of cancer; such a state is termed precancerous and is interesting as showing that the transition into cancer is a gradual change.

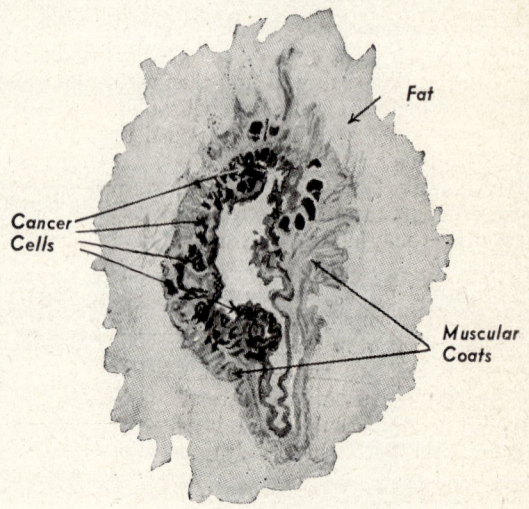

INVASION OF MUCOUS MEMBRANE

Transverse section of rectum in which the greater part of the mucous membrane has been replaced by cancer cells. The cancer has spread into the muscular coats.

GENERAL CONSTITUTIONAL DISEASES 1257

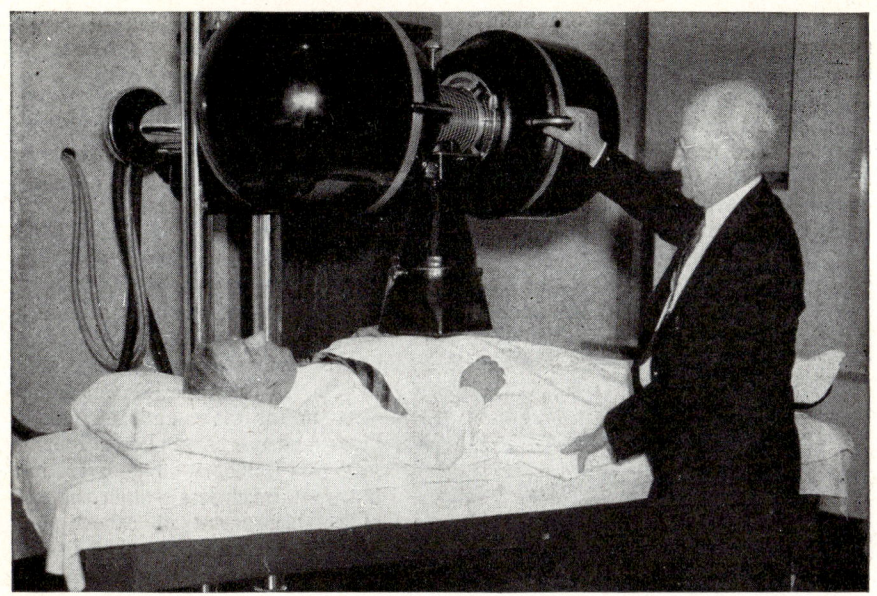

CANCER TREATMENT BY X-RAY

This modern apparatus in the Allegheny General Hospital, Pittsburgh, is typical of the developing effort to improve X-rays as an alternative to radium for cancer therapy. X-rays have the disadvantages of bulky apparatus but they can be controlled as radium cannot be, for its radiation is continuous.

© *Harris & Ewing*

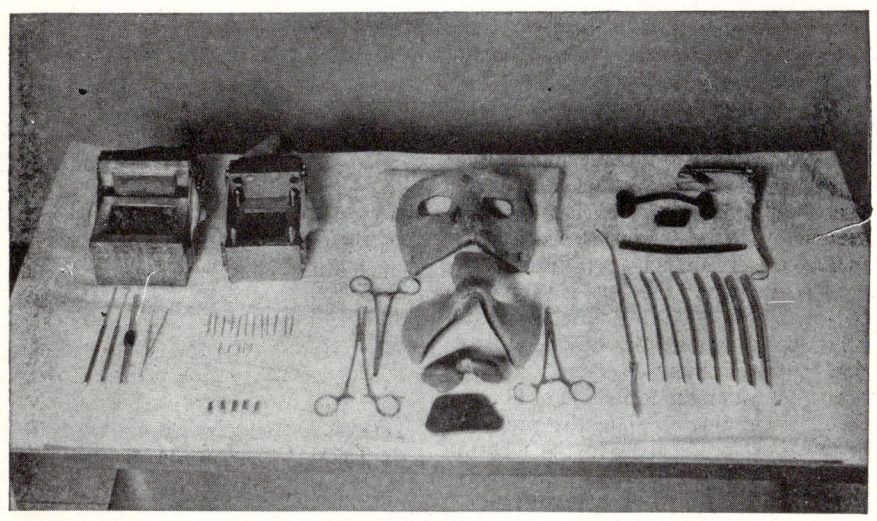

TO ADMINISTER SMALL DOSES OF RADIUM

Small quantities of radium in platinum cells, gold and platinum sheath needles and platinum capsules, wax molds, uterine sounds, Hegar dilators, etc., at St. Vincent's Hospital, West New Brighton, N. Y. *Courtesy of the New York City Cancer Committee*

A benign tumor differs from a malignant tumor in that the cells of which it is composed have no tendency to invade any of the neighboring parts, but remain limited and circumscribed. When once a cancer has begun it undergoes a steady growth, which is resisted to a certain extent by the normal cells adjoining. The characteristic invasion of

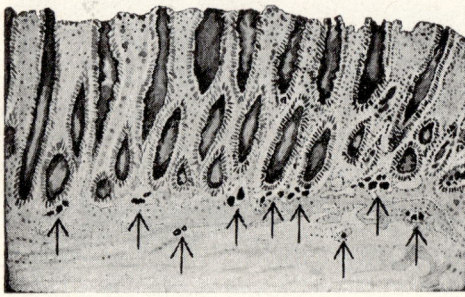

INVASION OF MUCOUS MEMBRANE
Section of mucous membrane of bowel with groups of cancer cells, each group being indicated by an arrow. The seeds have been carried in the lymphatic stream from a growth which is situated farther along the gut.

normal tissue by malignant growths results in destruction and spread.

Varieties of Growth. Many different terms are applied to cancers, according to the type of cells of which they are composed. An epithelioma is a cancer which develops in the epithelium of the skin or a mucous membrane. An adenocarcinoma is one that develops from a secreting gland. A rodent ulcer is a squamous-cell carcinoma which develops most commonly in the face, is very slow in its progress, and is not usually threatening to life; a scirrhous carcinoma is a slow-growing cancer (common in the breast) in which the formation of fibrous tissue attempting to stem the progress of the cancer cells gives to the mass a very hard consistency. Similarly, sarcomata developing from connective tissues are frequently named according to the tissue from which they are derived, e.g. osteosarcoma derived from bone, myosarcoma from muscle, etc. One variety which has black pigment in the cells is called melanotic sarcoma or melanoma.

Carcinoma seldom attacks young people and is quite uncommon before the age of thirty. Sarcoma is found at any time from early childhood to extreme old age. Speaking generally, malignant growths in youth and early middle age grow more rapidly than those which begin in later life.

Some parts of the body are much more prone than others to the cancerous change. The stomach and rectum, in both sexes, but more often in the male, and the female breast and uterus, are specially subject to carcinoma. The liver and lungs are much less seldom the site of commencement of cancer, but both are frequently affected secondarily to cancer developing elsewhere in the body.

Manner of Spread. The course of a carcinoma is somewhat different from that of a sarcoma. Carcinomata usually grow very gradually, and encroach steadily on the normal parts around. They tend to ulcerate onto a neighboring surface, and then it is not long before the ulcer becomes infected

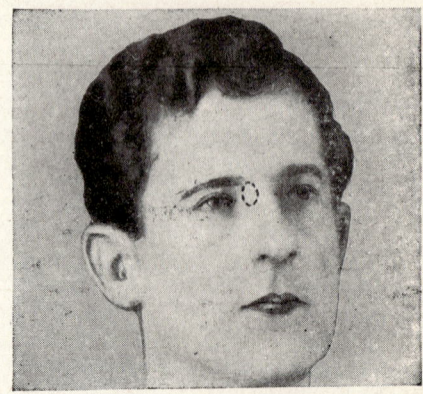

SITE OF RODENT ULCER
The face and scalp are the commonest sites for the appearance of a rodent ulcer, and especially the skin around the eyes and at the root of the nose. It begins as a swelling.

and results in an increasing discharge of foul matter and débris. Some of this is absorbed into the system and poisons the patient. The constant drain on the body fluids added to the septic absorption saps the strength. Sometimes the ulceration extends to some large blood vessel, and serious or fatal hemorrhage may occur.

After a time, which varies with the type of cell and the part affected, the cancer cells do not remain localized to the site of their first appearance. Some cells grow into the lymph channels and by a gradual extension, known as permeation, they advance in different directions. These outgrowing cells sooner or later reach the nearest group of lymph glands, where they proceed to grow and cause enlargement of the glands.

It also happens not infrequently that some cancer cells pass into a vein, and are carried by the blood direct to the lungs or other organ. It is common for the lungs and liver to be thus affected. Each transplanted colony begins to grow and to reproduce its own type of cells in the new soil. These secondary growths are usually the cause of death when surgical removal of the primary cancer has been delayed. A sarcoma is dangerous to life because it grows, spreads into surrounding parts, and may disseminate over the body to such an extent that vital organs are interfered with and the body nutriment diverted to the useless tumor.

The growth of a sarcoma is usually more rapid than that of a carcinoma. The neighboring tissues are invaded, though for a time they put up a limited resistance, but at the same time there is a tendency for portions of the growth to get into the blood stream and be carried to a remote part of the body, where the transplanted cells begin to multiply and form a subsidiary growth. These secondary colonies depend upon the site and nature of the primary growths. This method of dissemination by the circulation is much more common with sarcoma than with carcinoma, and con-

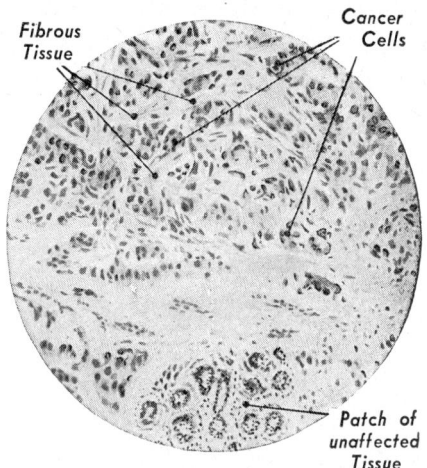

SCIRRHOUS: VARIETY OF CARCINOMA
In this section of a tumor of the breast a small area of normal tissue below is contrasted with tumor tissue above, notable about the latter being thick strands of fibrous tissue separating clumps of cancer cells.

stitutes a constant danger while sarcoma remains in or attached to the body. A sarcoma may also send cells along the lymphatics and settle colonies in the neighboring lymphatic glands, but this is not such a constant feature as it is with carcinomata. Dissemination by the blood stream is not so common with those tumors which have more highly differentiated cells.

Cause. As to the real cause of cancer, the answer will be found when we know what starts the vicious growth. Many theories have been advanced to answer this question, but none is as yet capable of proof.

One school believes that there is an actual living organism called a filter-passing virus which invades the body and causes the disease in the same way as other germs cause other diseases. This organism is called a virus to distinguish it from bacteria because it is so tiny that it cannot be seen by the microscope and passes through any filter. Its existence, therefore, can only be surmised at present, and it is the aim of the members of this school of thought to develop some means of isolating and studying this virus, which they postulate to be present in every case of cancer and to cause the disease. It is in connection with this point of view that the researches of Gye and Barnard are of such importance, although their discoveries have not been of such value as was at one time thought likely they would be. It was in the summer of 1925 that W. E. Gye, a pathologist, and J. E. Barnard, a very skillful amateur microscopist, who worked together, published results of their joint investigations which justified a hopeful view. They discovered in malignant tumors—both cancers and sarcomas—a living organism which they believed to be one factor in the production of such growths, and although it was so minute as to be invisible by the microscopic methods generally used in bacteriology, Mr. Barnard succeeded not only in rendering it visible, but even in photographing it. Their experiments tended to show that the organism was harmless in itself, but that, brought into contact with a chemical substance produced by the cells of a mouse, chicken, or other animal as the result, perhaps, of chronic irritation, it was capable of giving rise to a malignant tumor. This chemical substance seemed, therefore, an accessory factor in the causation of some cases of malignant disease, if not all cases.

The results thus obtained had the great merit of harmonizing the discordant results of earlier investigators, and at the time they were published it was thought that the central problem of cancer causation was about to be solved, and that with its solution some means for conferring immunity against cancer by some process of inoculation would speedily be devised. The matter was not as simple of solution as all that, however, and eleven years later the position with regard to both the cause and the treatment of cancer is still obscure, and Gye and other workers on the same ground continue their researches.

Another theory regarding the origin of cancer is that it is due to some non-living cause, either chemical or physical, or a combination of the two. This is the theory today which has the largest number of supporters, but the nature of the causative substance and the irritating substances are still an absolute mystery as this book is written.

It is generally allowed, however, that chronic irritation has an important influence in producing cancer, though this only applies to certain tissues. The natives in Kashmir, who keep themselves warm by carrying a basket containing burning charcoal against the skin of the abdomen, are prone to develop cancer in that situation (known as Kaugri cancer).

Unless the operator of X-rays wears protective covering, cancer is apt to develop as the result of repeated exposures to the rays.

Cancer of the tongue usually occurs opposite an irritating tooth. Another example is afforded by the sus-

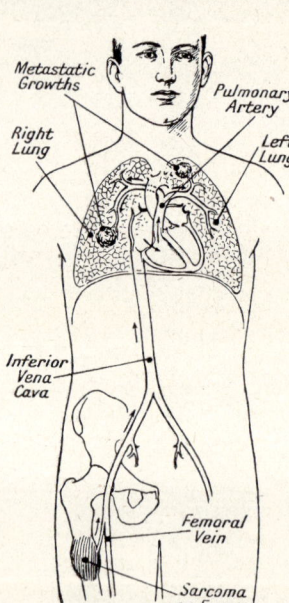

SARCOMA: METASTASES IN THE LUNGS

In this schema the route by which sarcomatous cells from a tumor in the thigh may reach the lungs is indicated by arrows. Fresh tumors arising in this way are described as metastases.

GENERAL CONSTITUTIONAL DISEASES

ceptibility to cancer of workers in some occupations as, for instance, mule spinners and workers in tar and aniline dyes, or English chimney sweeps.

It is held by many authorities that cancer never occurs in a tissue that has not undergone some previous degenerative change. This change may be due to mechanical irritation or to the influence of long-standing general poisoning of the body, or it may be due to local ulceration from septic infection.

As a result of breeding experiments in mice there is increasing belief that genetic factors play an important role in human cancer. The evidence points to the transmission of the susceptibility to cancer and not of the causes. The susceptibility may be general or specific, e.g. organ susceptibility.

As to these or other theories much work remains to be done before any clear light is thrown on this mysterious process.

Every hospital and body dealing with cancer research is constantly being importuned to test this or that cure or method which is supported by little or no evidence of scientific value. The public may rest assured that every suggested line of treatment or diagnosis which has any real likelihood of being useful is given a testing by one or another of the scholarly bodies which deal with cancer research.

In cases such as those of Gye and of Bendien in Holland, lines of investigation are opened up which, though apparently not fulfilling at this stage the claims made on their behalf by their more enthusiastic adherents, may lead to very valuable discoveries.

A word of warning is appropriate here. Many people talk as if cancer could be banished speedily from the world if only the cause of it were known. This is not likely to be so. It is not even likely that an infallible cure will result. What will result will probably be the discovery of more efficient means of prevention. This was the case with that other scourge of humanity, tuberculosis. The discovery of the bacillus causing the disease led to the adoption of methods of prevention of the spread of the disease and its recognition in stages early enough for it to be cured in a large number of cases by the means already known.

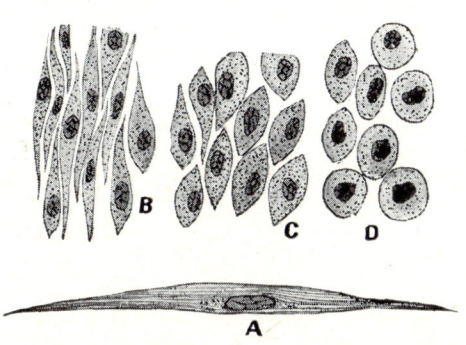

NORMAL AND ABNORMAL SPINDLE CELLS
(A) Plain muscle cell, a normal spindle, or fusiform cell. (B) Units of a spindle-cell sarcoma; in a tumor these may be replaced by (C), oat-shaped cells, and later by (D), round cells.

Symptoms and Progress. The actual beginning of a cancer is painless and it does not immediately cause any noticeable change in the condition of the patient. When it has advanced to a certain stage, however, it inevitably causes symptoms which are always among the following five groups: (1) A tumor or swelling; (2) pain; (3) discharge; (4) interference with the function of some organ; (5) general weakness or loss of weight. It must be clearly understood that only in the last stage of cancer are all these symptoms present; in early stages only one symptom may be present, and early diagnosis of cancer depends, therefore, upon careful investigation of slight symptoms often neglected by patients.

A tumor or swelling is the first symptom with cancers of the skin. All growing warts, moles, and nevi (so-called

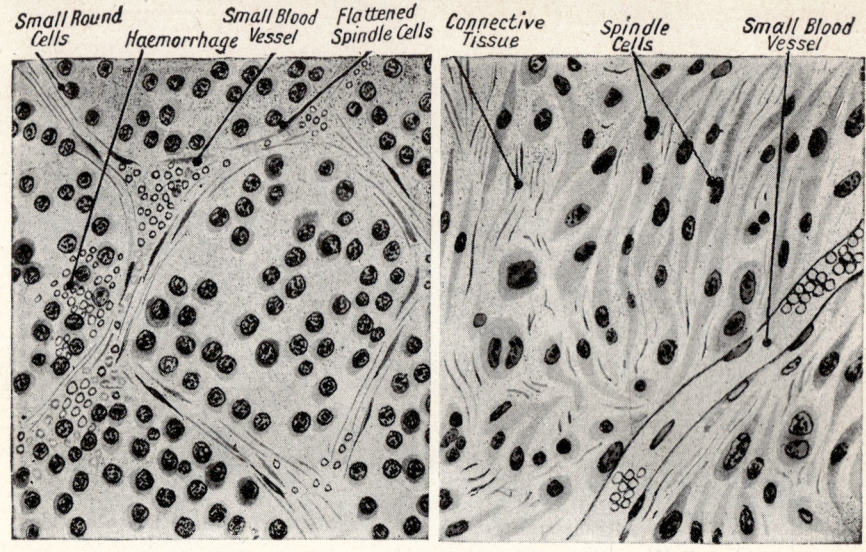

ROUND-CELLED AND SPINDLE-CELLED VARIETIES OF SARCOMA

Consisting of rounded cells, with large nuclei, the round-celled sarcoma (left) may make its appearance in practically any tissue of the body and at any age, sometimes occurring even before birth. The cells in the second type of tumor (right) may be stumpy, like oat grains, or elongated and narrow. Wherever it begins in the body a sarcoma spreads by metastasis to other parts.

birthmarks) should be regarded with suspicion and reported to a doctor if increasing considerably in size. In the breast a lump is often the first indication of a cancer. Many lumps in the breast are not cancers, but in women over forty they often tend to become cancerous. In the breasts of fat women a lump may form and remain unnoticed for months (being painless), but may betray its presence by a dimpling of the skin. Dimpling of the skin of the breast in a woman over forty may indicate an underlying malignancy which has already invaded the skin. In younger women lumps in the breast are not usually due to cancer, but it is a safe rule to advise removal of a lump in the female breast at any age.

A more diffuse and less well-defined lumpiness and hardness of the breast, accompanied by aching pain, especially at the monthly periods, should be carefully watched by the doctor.

Deeper cancers (*e.g.* abdominal) do not appear as a lump until the growth is of a considerable size. Usually other symptoms call attention to the tumor. Pain is often absent until the growth has attained considerable size and is causing pressure or obstruction by reason of its bulk.

It should be universally known that pain is neither a necessary nor an early symptom of cancer.

Discharge is met with only in those cancers which soon reach a surface. It is of the utmost importance in cancers of the uterus (cervical portion) and rectum. The discharge may be either bloodstained, watery, or mucoid. Any woman who has an irregular discharge of blood from the vagina between the periods or after they have ceased needs a medical examination. Similarly, any person who has a discharge of blood or mucus from the rectum should be medically examined.

GENERAL CONSTITUTIONAL DISEASES

Interference with the function of an organ may be the earliest symptom of a deeply situated cancer. Gastric or intestinal cancer nearly always leads to pains which are too readily attributed to indigestion. Cancer of the pancreas may stop the entrance of bile into the intestine and cause severe jaundice.

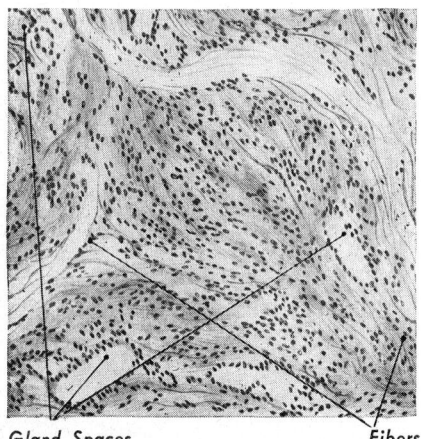

FIBROADENOMA: A GLAND TUMOR
In this microscopic section of a breast tumor, while there are spaces resembling those of the normal gland, there is also a large amount of fibrous tissue. This constitutes a fibroadenoma; the gland spaces do not function as glands.

Cancer in the gullet causes difficulty in swallowing; in the larynx a husky voice.

In the case of some deep-seated visceral cancers the first symptom noticed may be a gradual loss of strength and weight. In most instances, however, the onset of wasting and weakness denotes the final stages. Any change of bowel habit in the adult, especially the male, is significant and should be investigated.

There is no set period for the course of cancer. Some cancers of the breast are so slow in formation that they may continue for ten or fifteen years without causing death or even any serious inconvenience; rodent ulcer of the face may slowly extend for twenty years or more. On the other hand, some sarcomata kill quickly by secondary deposits, and many internal cancers are fairly rapid in their growth. After the diagnosis of an internal cancer, and in the absence of treatment, the duration of life is between six months and three years. Treatment of various kinds modifies this period considerably.

Diagnosis. With regard to the diagnosis of cancer, although in very many cases it is possible to say at once that cancer is present, yet there are numerous instances in which certainty is only obtained when the microscope demonstrates cancerous changes.

In the case of deep-seated cancers special methods of examination are neces-

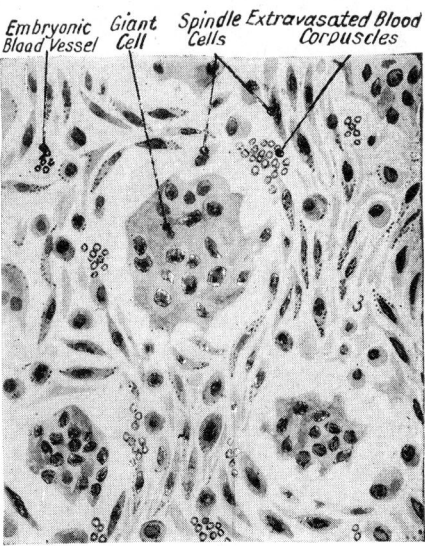

MYELOID VARIETY OF SARCOMA
This type of growth owes its name to the large giant cells it contains, some being shown here. It is so little malignant that it is doubtful if it should be classed as a sarcoma.

sary, and need specially trained physicians and surgeons to use them. The esophagus, the bladder, the rectum and the larynx can be examined by an electric light passed or reflected along a tube; and the intestines and abdominal viscera can be examined by X-rays or inspected by exploratory opening of the abdomen. If there is any doubt about any accessible tumor it can be cut out and examined under the microscope.

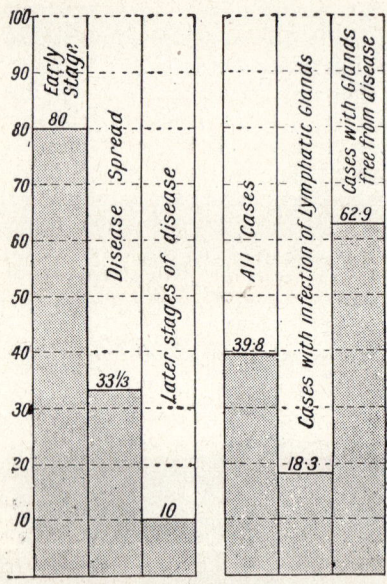

VALUE OF EARLY OPERATION
These two sets of statistics show clearly the value of early operation, the shaded areas indicating percentages of success.

There is no evidence to show that cancer is infectious or contagious. Nurses and doctors who are in frequent contact with cancer patients do not develop cancer in any greater proportion than other people. There is therefore no likelihood and certainly no proof that cancer is infectious. Although there is not proof that cancer is hereditary, the predisposition to cancer is certainly greater in some families than others, and this predisposition is possibly transmissible.

Prevention and Treatment. In considering the treatment of cancer it will be well first to consider what means we have for preventing it. The only causative factor upon which most authorities agree is that of irritation, so every means possible should be taken to prevent chronic irritation in the various parts of the body.

Any warts that are located in positions in which they may be frequently knocked or injured should be removed. Irritation of the cheek and tongue should be prevented by seeing that any jagged or septic teeth or tooth plates that cause pressure sores should be dealt with. Constipation should be treated, for the large bowel may be irritated by hard masses of feces, and the results of constipation may by their effect on the tissues very possibly predispose to cancer elsewhere in the body. Finally, diet and habits must be persistently directed towards a high standard of health. It should be

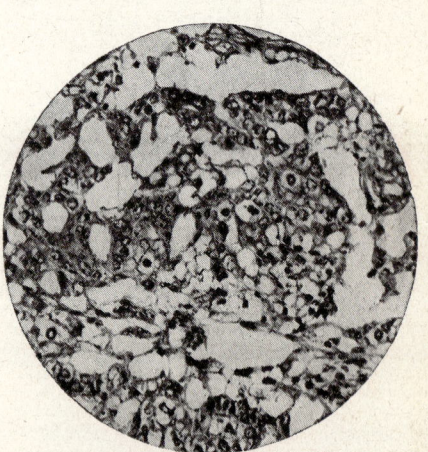

CARCINOMA OF THE BREAST
The cells of carcinoma in a particular epithelial tissue bear some resemblance to those of the tissue itself, but present differences in size, shape, and otherwise. Here masses of cancer cells are seen in the breast.

emphasized that the most important preventive measure is the periodic health examination.

If we cannot prevent the development of cancer, the next most important thing is to diagnose the condition early so that treatment may have the best chance of success. Early medical advice must be sought if any suspicious symptoms arise.

GENERAL CONSTITUTIONAL DISEASES

The American Society for the Control of Cancer is carrying on an educational campaign in an effort to teach the patient to see a physician in time so that a cure may be obtained.

It cannot be insisted upon too strongly that the patient who broods in secret over a tumor and purposely avoids obtaining medical advice is simply throwing away the chances of relief that operation provides, for the disease constantly spreads until it reaches a stage when all hope of cure is lost even after the most extensive operation. The folly of delay will be seen from the following extract from the English Ministry of Health's Report on Cancer of the Breast: "It was found that of patients subjected to early operation, *i.e.* before the disease had extended beyond the breast itself, 94 per cent were alive and well at the end of three years, 91 per cent at the end of five years, and 87 per cent at the end of ten years."

When the diagnosis of cancer is definitely confirmed, what measures are of avail?

Surgical operation still holds out the best prospect of cure for cases of early cancer. The results are very favorable for early growths of the lip, breast, uterus, intestines, and on the limbs and skin. In the case of the stomach and rectum the results are also good. The more cancer is advanced the greater the risk of the operation.

Radiation. The most conspicuous advance in the treatment of cancer in late years has been in the use of radium and X-rays. According to Professor Woodburn Morison, radium and X-ray treatments have the same physical basis, and in many cases the methods should be combined. Of one thing we may be certain. We have profited by our past experience, and if radiology is unstable and more or less in a transition period at present, this is because so many ad-

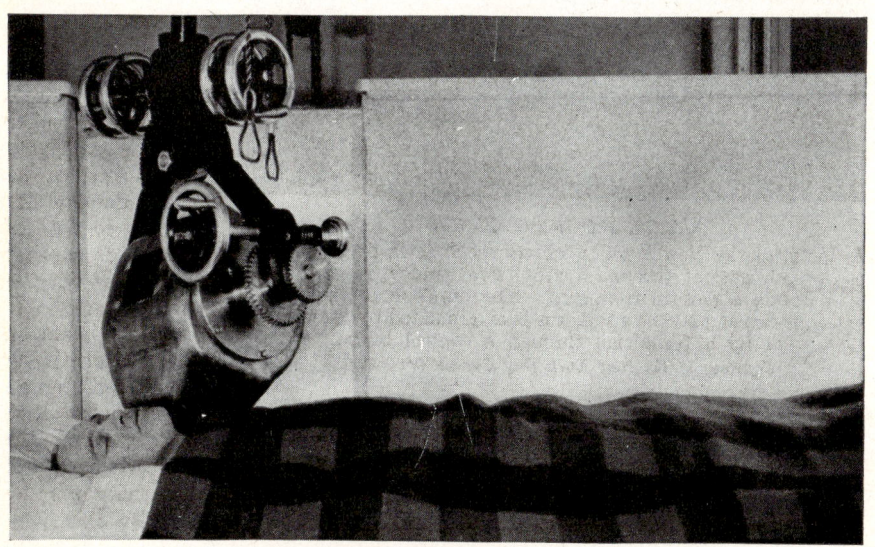

RADIUM TREATMENT FOR CANCER

At the State Institute for the Study of Malignant Diseases in Buffalo, New York, treatment is given by means of a radium pack, the apparatus shown above. Radium for such intense doses (this is equivalent to a million-volt X-ray tube) must be kept inside a lead-lined container. Heavy and bulky as this seems, an X-ray tube giving comparable radiation is so big as to fill several ordinary-sized rooms.

Courtesy of the New York City Cancer Committee

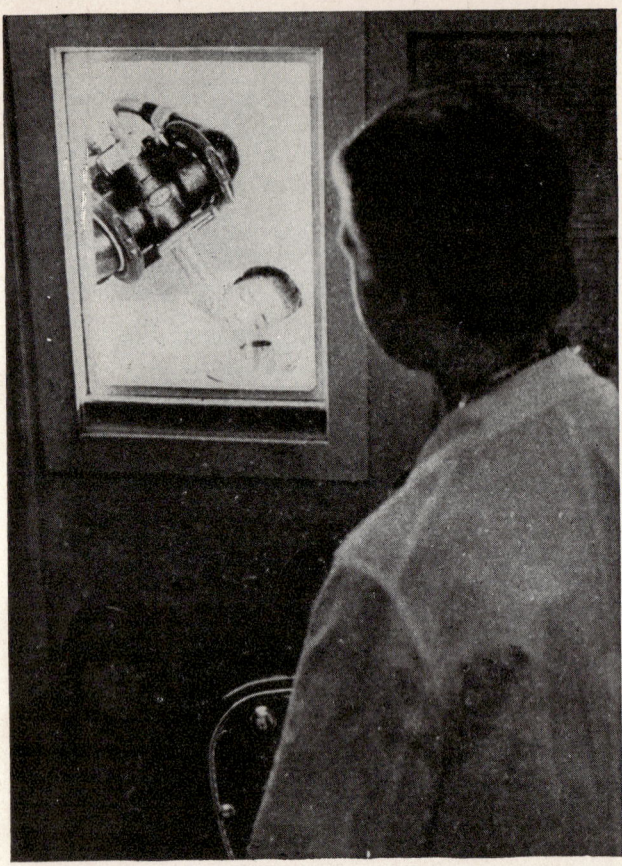

RADIUM TREATMENT CONTROL

A doctor at the New York Infirmary for Women and Children observes a patient through a protective window in a wall of lead during a radium treatment. The duration of the application is timed, and the apparatus is manipulated by the doctor or by a technician through a control board.

Courtesy of the New York City Cancer Committee

been established an international unit of X-ray dosage, referred to among experts as *"r."*

Various methods of giving radiological treatment have been devised. Within the last fifteen years, so many improvements in machinery have been effected that what is known as the massive dose can be prescribed, *i.e.*, the maximum amount of concentrated rays which can be tolerated by the tissues in a given period, without any damage being caused. But owing to the difficulties associated with intolerance in some patients, it was found more satisfactory to give the split dose, a series of smaller doses the aggregate of which equalled the massive dose. Other methods consist of dosage depending upon skin testing — the fractional dose; of systems based on keeping the tissues "saturated" by an initial big dose and subsequent loss-replacement doses; of regulating the amount of rays so that certain cells of a known degree of sensitivity are destroyed (Coutard's method). Skin damage, when it occurs is temporary and with newer techniques is being rapidly eliminated.

It should be realized that the aim of radiologists is to produce apparatus that will give the highest voltages and the shortest wave lengths. Numerous ex-

justments have had to be made in order to bring the therapeutic methods into conformity with the findings of clinical observers.

It is possible to say that nowadays the dosage of X-rays or of radium are more appropriately estimated with regard to the particular condition under treatment. The old-fashioned methods of using the pastille (an almost crude trial-and-error system) have given way to modern instruments, and there has

GENERAL CONSTITUTIONAL DISEASES

periments are continuously carried out both in the United States and in Great Britain and in 1940 it is too early to estimate the results; but the facts are that an X-ray beam may be generated which is in co-ordination with the gamma ray of radium.

With regard to radium, the various methods of application include seeds, needles, and plaques. Modern opinion is that the best way to get any appreciable result is to put the radium container on the surface so that the rays will spread out in all directions. The term "bomb" has been applied to such containers. The dosage is accurately measured so that only the required amount is given.

It is still clearly a policy of blind optimism to hold that cancer is being conquered even with all the above advances in therapy. There is agreement among experts as to the benefits of X-rays and radium in many types of cancer. Radiation is the only measure available for patients who are poor operative risks, *e.g.* cases of advanced malignancy or where medical contraindications to surgery exist. Radium masks can be fitted over growths on the lips, cheek, and other parts of the face, and are very effective.

Probably the best area for radiation in cancer is the cervix of the uterus, and very good results are being shown. Early cases respond very well to the treatment. Both X-rays and radium should be used.

Radiation combined with surgery often succeeds in amplifying the work

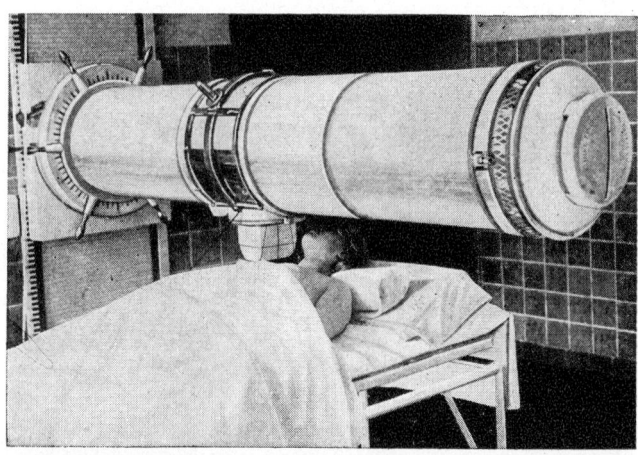

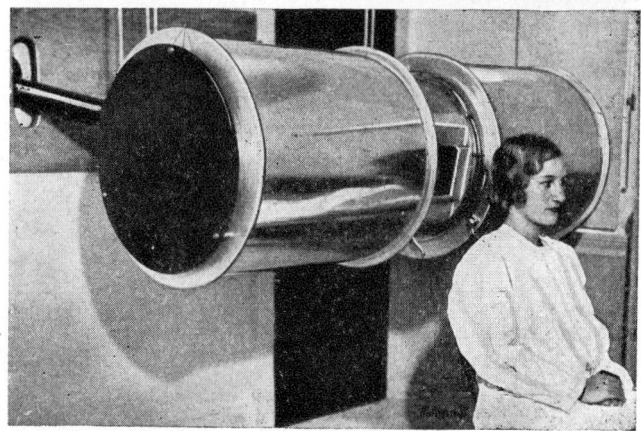

MODERN APPARATUS FOR TREATMENT BY X-RAYS
As in the case of radium, the application of X-rays in cancer is largely restricted to cases which cannot be operated upon and to following up cases which have undergone operation. Above: an elaborate German apparatus which is completely protected and can be placed in any desired position for treatment. Below: a special deep therapy tube in use at the Temple University Hospital, Philadelphia.

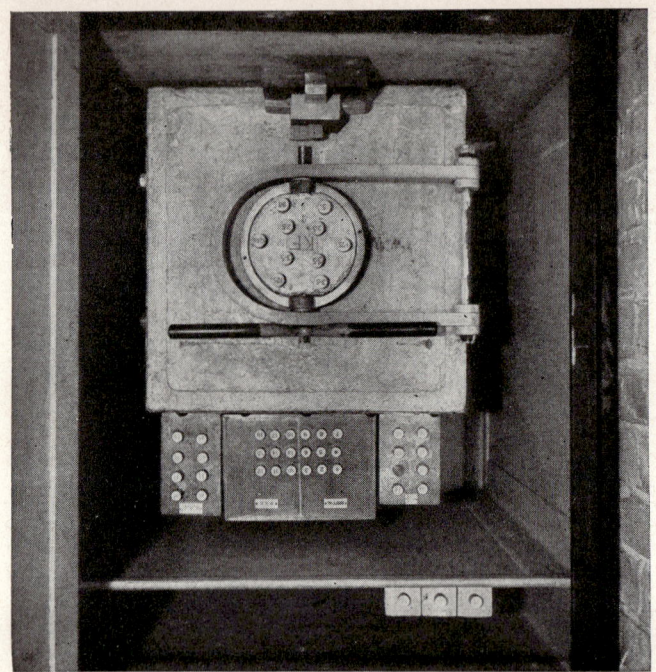

nant cells, but others may multiply, and after a time the tumor may be as bad as ever. From the point of view of prolonging life and dulling pain, deep X-ray therapy is justifiable. In all cases of application, however, it must be remembered that we are dealing with a very powerful and unknown agent, and it would appear, therefore, that the resistance of the individual is the dominating factor in the success of the dosage, and, so far, very

STORAGE OF RADIUM

The radium salts which are used in radium therapy are extremely potent sources of radiation, and the rays which are emitted are so powerful as to be dangerous, especially since they have high penetrating power. Therefore radium is stored when not in use in safes thickly lined with lead. These are typical. The one at right is in Bellevue Hospital, New York.

Courtesy of the New York City Cancer Committee; Joel photo

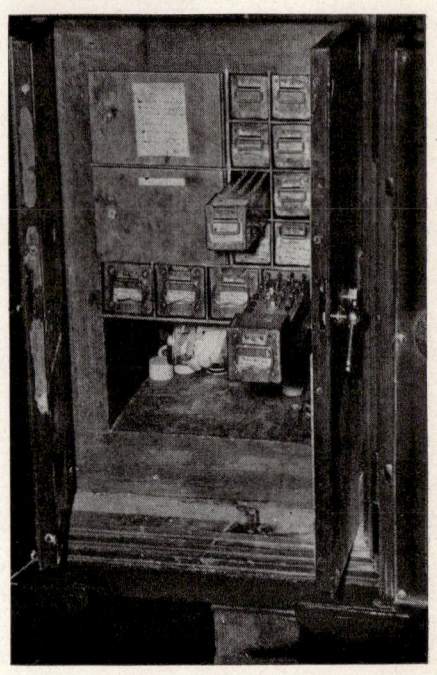

of the operator, and although surgery remains as the oldest therapeutic weapon against cancer it is becoming more and more frequently supplemented by combination with X-ray or with radium or with both. Postoperative radiation is quite commonly recommended for patients under treatment for cancer of the breast.

It must be remembered, though, that where there is a deeply placed cancerous growth, the inaccessibility of the growth to X-ray or radium presents a difficult problem; the effect of treatment is to destroy some of the malig-

little definite knowledge is available to us as regards the assessment of this resistance.

Coley's Method. Treatment by Coley's fluid has obtained many good results in the hands of the originator of the method. Coley based his treatment upon the fact that some cases of sarcoma got well after an accidental attack of erysipelas or other streptococcal infection. The fluid which he used was a sterilized culture of the Streptococcus pyogenes and Micrococcus prodigiosus in bouillon.

Treatment starts as small doses of one or two minims and is continued with increasing dosage until a definite reaction is obtained. The reaction consists of fever and malaise. Though the fluid is so toxic, Coley worked up to a dosage of as much as sixty minims on occasion. Doses can be given daily or every second day until a reaction has occurred, and treatment should be continued so long as it is considered that there is any chance of a beneficial effect.

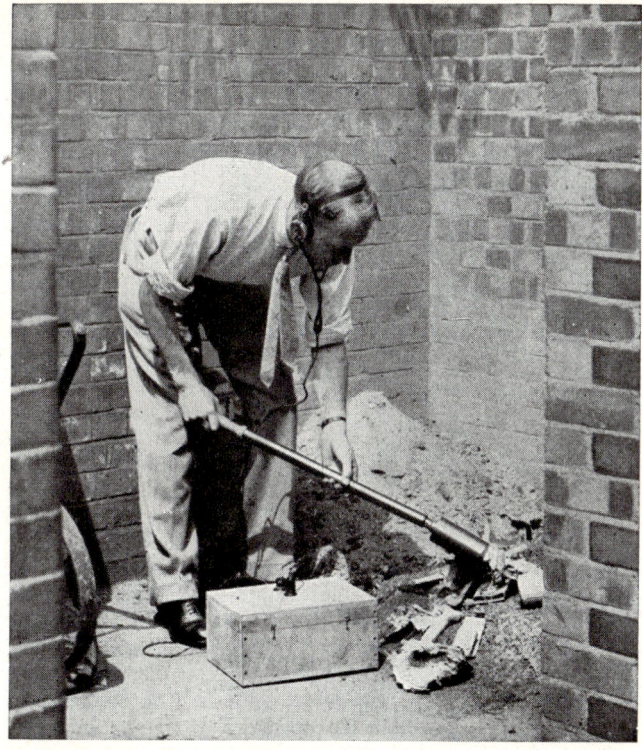

LOCATING LOST RADIUM

So great would be the calamity of losing even the smallest quantity of radium that the most sensitive kinds of apparatus have been invented for locating it. When near the radium this apparatus gives out a warning clucking sound to the searcher wearing earphones.
Photopress

RHEUMATISM

The term rheumatism is often loosely used to cover a great variety of conditions associated with pain in the skeletal and supporting structures of the body, but conveys no exact meaning in a pathological sense.

Changes in joints and fibrous structures which cause the pains are of various kinds, and there are probably many kinds of causative agent. It would probably be better to abolish the term altogether. In popular usage the tendency is to label all painful conditions affecting the framework of the body as "rheumatic" and therefore of no great importance. Doctors, too, in the past have been too ready to classify a host of disorders under this heading, whereas now these are proving to **be of very** varying natures.

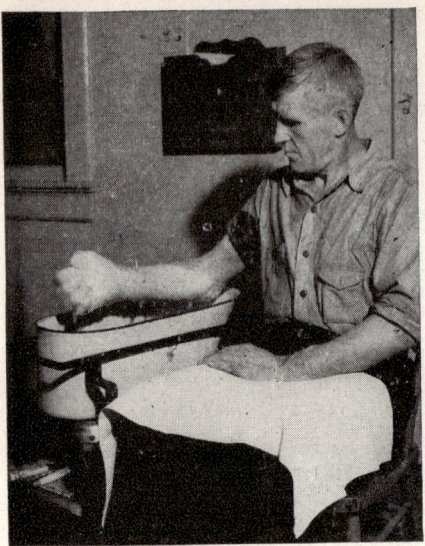

PARAFFIN BATH

This treatment has been found extremely beneficial in all conditions of the extremities for which the application of heat is indicated, such as arthritis, contractures following laceration, fractures, strains, sprains, etc. The paraffin is heated to temperatures ranging from 120° to 135° F. and applied over joints and other affected parts of the extremities. The advantages of paraffin over water baths are that paraffin can be used with safety and relative comfort at higher temperatures than water and that it does not wrinkle or roughen the skin. This picture was taken at The Curative Workshop in Milwaukee.

Courtesy of The Curative Workshop

Disease of the joints leading to severe disability and associated with inflammatory destruction of the joint and its surrounding structures occurs in many pathological conditions. We may describe these conditions as five in number, of which the first is arthritis due to injury.

The second of the five conditions is specific infection by the bacteria of known diseases, such as those causing gonorrhea, syphilis, and tuberculosis; by the pneumococcus, septic, typhoid, and other organisms responsible for general infection of the body, and in these cases attacking the joints and fibrous structures. Acute rheumatic fever comes into this category, although the specific agent is not yet definitely known.

Gout and other metabolic disturbances constitute the third of the five conditions.

The fourth condition is disease of the nervous system, as in locomotor ataxia.

The fifth condition may be any of several deficiencies in the diet, as in rickets and scurvy.

The commonest type of so-called rheumatic disease of the joints and fibrous structures, however, is that large group of cases included under the terms rheumatoid arthritis, osteoarthritis, and arthritis deformans. These are dealt with under their special headings, but here it may be said that these again fall into several groups according to their causation and the nature of the pathological changes present. Many of the cases are undoubtedly due to infections of various kinds, some of them known, others as yet unknown. They may therefore be classed as arthritis due to nonspecific infection. Other types are beginning to be recognized as due to metabolic disorder accompanied by the

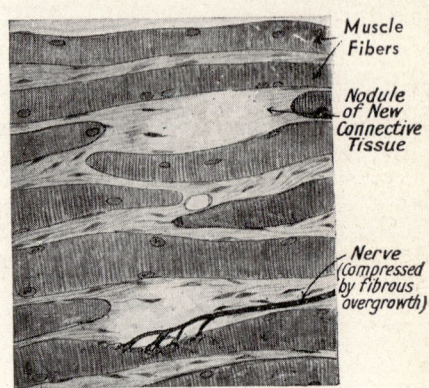

INFLAMMATORY NODULES IN MUSCLE

The above illustration shows how, in muscular rheumatism, overgrowth of connective tissue takes place at various places on the sheaths or in the fibrous intersections between muscle tissues proper and presses on nerves, causing pain.

GENERAL CONSTITUTIONAL DISEASES 1271

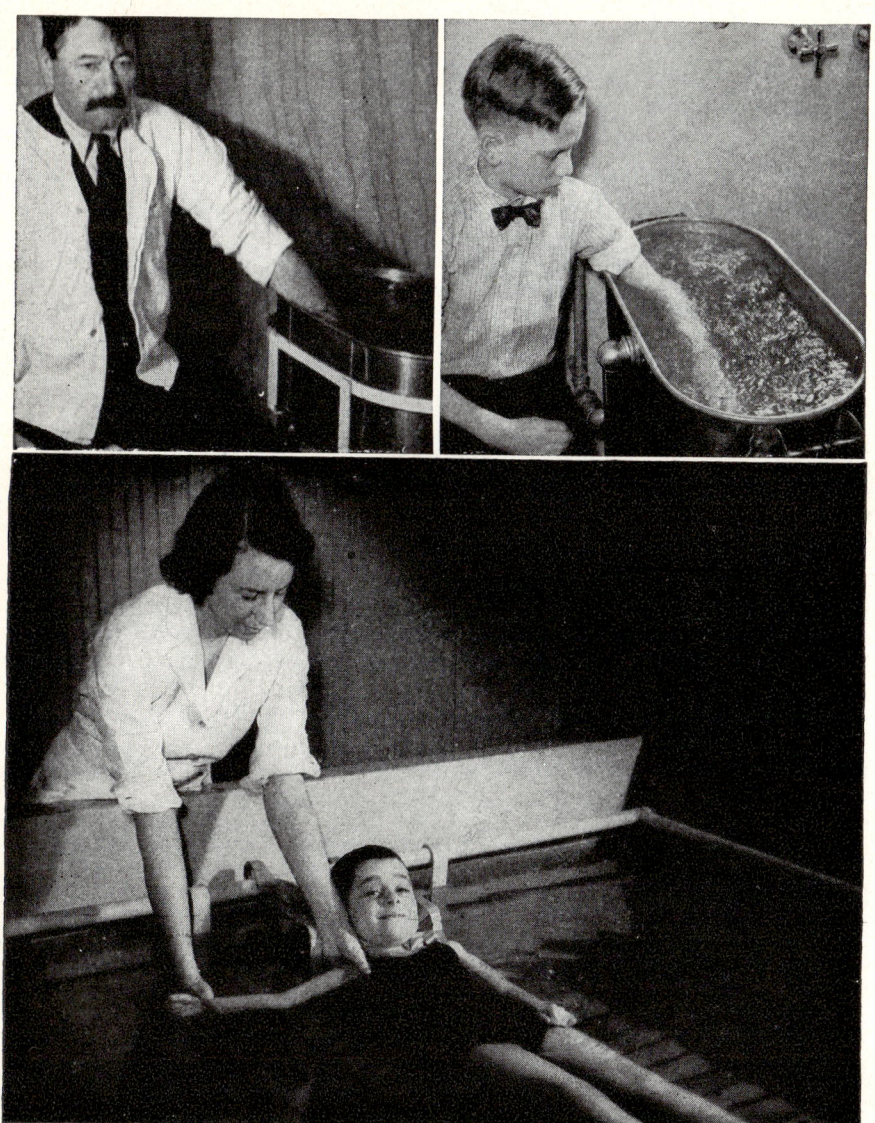

HYDROTHERAPY

The mechanical action of water is used to advantage in hastening recovery from injuries, from arthritis, and from many other ailments. Above are shown small underwater massage tubs in use. In these, strong currents of water are directed against the part of the body needing attention, and the effect is one of massage. The water's velocity and temperature can be varied by the operator according to the doctor's prescription. The boy is a patient in The Curative Workshop of Milwaukee, the sailor in a marine hospital in New York City where he is being treated for an arm injury. The child below, recovered from infantile paralysis, is receiving assisted exercise in a bath of warm water at the Milwaukee institution.

Courtesy of The Curative Workshop; © *Harris & Ewing*

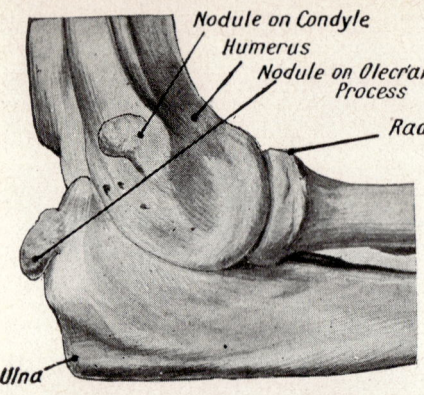

RHEUMATIC NODES ON ELBOW

In true rheumatism an overgrowth of fibrous tissue may occur in many situations, forming little nodules. Here two of these are shown, attached to bones at the elbow joint. In children, nodules are commonly found in the skin.

production in the body of poisonous substances which directly attack the joints and fibrous structures and may destroy them. In other cases both factors may be at work, and the infection may act indirectly by affecting the metabolic processes. The foregoing types are dealt with in the section on Diseases of the Locomotor System in a later volume.

The term "rheumatism" is, however, applied to many conditions in which the joints are not affected. The affection is one of fibrous structures alone. These include the fasciae, the sheaths and supporting fibers of the muscles and nerves, the tendons and ligaments. These cases are best considered under the general name of fibrositis. This group includes a very large proportion of the disorders prevalent principally in industrial communities and spoken of as "chronic rheumatism."

Other so-called rheumatic manifestations in the course of rheumatic fever include skin conditions such as erythema and the "rheumatic nodule," chorea, inflammation of the tonsils, and other less clearly defined troubles. In all cases the underlying cause is that which has led or will lead to the painful joint or to fibrositis, and is believed to be of the nature of a specific infection. In some cases these manifestations, or at any rate some of them, may have origin in metabolic disturbances.

The so-called rheumatic affections constitute the most frequent cause of bodily pain and disability. They have been found, to account for as much as 14 per cent of total sickness and disability. This represents enormous waste of time, loss of work, expense to the community, and suffering. With further research into the causative factors this suffering and waste of human energy could well be prevented. Meanwhile, much can be done both by the individual and by the community to prevent the ravages of this disabling disease along the lines of dental clinics, medical supervision of school children, and health

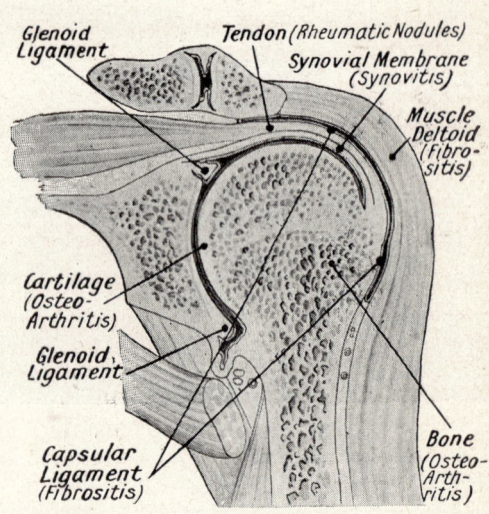

SITES OF RHEUMATIC DISEASE

Bones forming a joint are covered with cartilage. Where they come into contact, the joint cavity is lined with synovial membrane, and outside this are ligaments and tendons; various affections of these are named.

education of the people. The treatment clinics set up by hospitals in most large cities are a great step in the right direction, if treatment is sought at a sufficiently early stage of the trouble.

Chronic Rheumatism. Chronic rheumatism is liable to affect any part of the body, but a few varieties have acquired distinct names. Thus, stiff neck, the form of chronic rheumatism most frequently met with in young people, affects the muscles of the right or left side only, so that the head is held stiffly in a fixed position on one side.

In lumbago, one of the most painful and notable of the chronic rheumatic affections, the seat of the fibrous patches is in the muscles of the loin and back, on one or both sides. In pleurodynia the site of the rheumatism is the chest wall, the pain being generally confined to one side of the body. These special forms are dealt with later.

Individuals of both sexes and of all ages are liable to chronic rheumatism, but the complaint is most frequently met with in the middle and later part of life.

The true cause in the great majority of cases is some focal infection in the body. This focus is most commonly to be found in the teeth, tonsils, or bowel. Pyorrhea, chronic tonsilitis or hidden infection in the tonsils, constipation with some chronic infection of the bowel as a consequence —one or more of these conditions can generally be discovered and must be effectively dealt with if the liability to attacks of rheumatism on slight provocation is to be dispelled. Less commonly septic foci in other parts of the body, the ear, uterus, etc., are responsible. Heredity is doubtless an important factor in most types of so-called rheumatic disorder, though its exact influence is little understood.

The condition which may induce an attack in the presence of some source of infection is actual exposure to wet, cold, or keen winds, which is extremely likely to set up an attack. So common is this happening that the word rheumatic inevitably calls to mind the idea

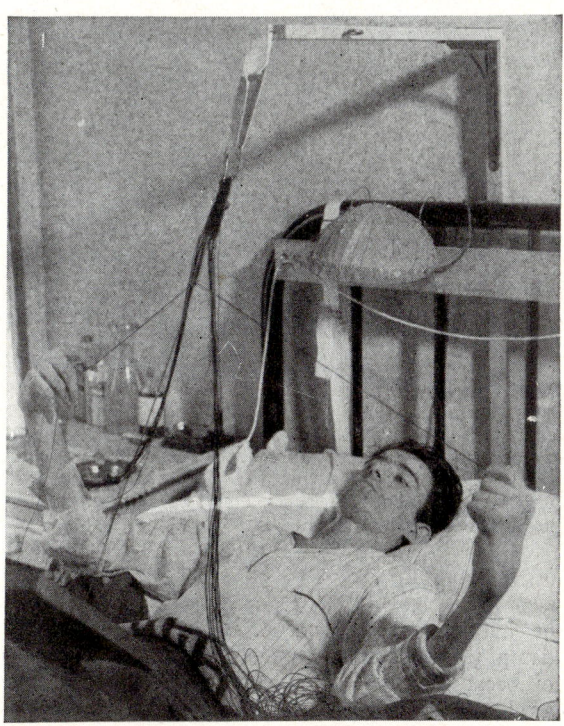

TREATMENT OF RHEUMATISM
Maintaining the mobility and usefulness of affected limbs and joints is one problem in the care of arthritis patients. Exercises under careful medical direction are used for this purpose, and occupational therapy is one promising procedure toward this end. This young man, bedridden by arthritis, is tying knots to make a belt, which helps to increase the strength and motion of fingers, wrists, and arms. The treatment is guided by a therapist from the Curative Workshop in Milwaukee, Wisconsin, as prescribed by the patient's physician.
Courtesy of The Curative Workshop

1274 THE CONCISE ENCYCLOPEDIA OF HEALTH

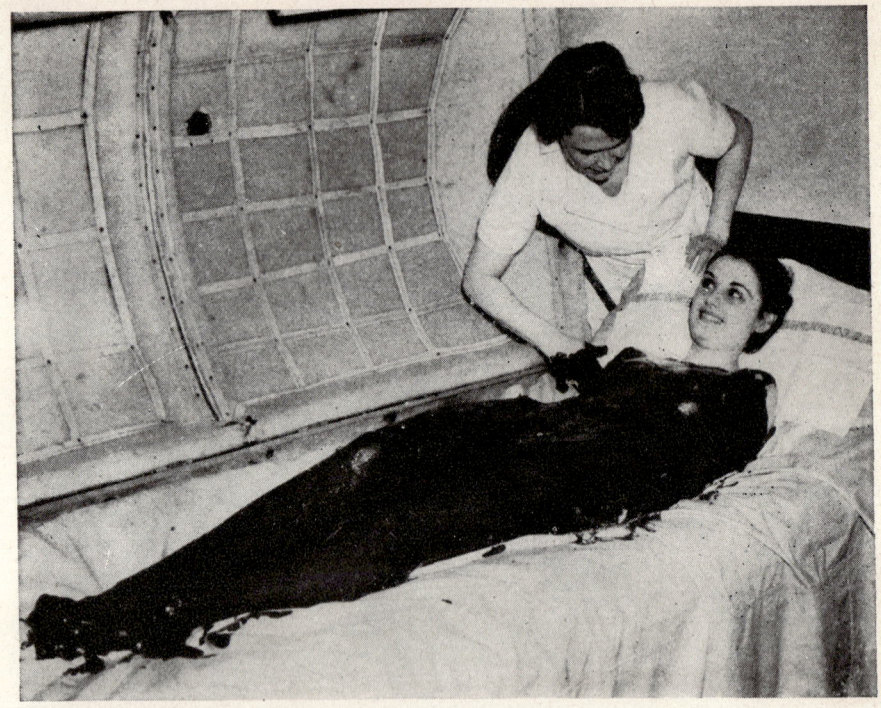

MUD BATH FOR ARTHRITIS AND SKIN DISEASES

Mud baths have been known for a long time to afford relief to sufferers from some types of arthritis and many skin diseases, though it is not certain whether the chief contribution is from the physical or chemical properties of the mud. One famous and effective mud, *fango,* is taken from the bottom of a lake in an extinct volcanic crater near Naples, in Italy. Quantities of this mud are dried and exported. This picture was taken at Sharon Springs, New York, where such imported mud is mixed with a local mineral water and used to treat patients at the resort. A physician should be consulted before any such treatment is undertaken.

© *International News Photos*

of chilly dampness. Lying or sitting on damp ground, resting on a stone seat, or being in a draft are very liable to awaken a chronic rheumatic condition. In some people heat has a similar effect.

Sudden changes of temperature and of barometric pressure may determine an attack, and sudden or prolonged muscular strain is a common exciting cause in those predisposed. There appear to be some cases in which dietetic errors and disorders of metabolism play an important part even in the absence of any condition of focal infection. Overuse of a muscle or group of muscles may also lead to a fibrositis in the tendons and ligaments. Tennis elbow is a common example. Finally, care must be taken to arrive at an exact diagnosis of the cause of localized pain resembling that of fibrositis, lest in reality it be due to some underlying disease in the deeper and more vital structures.

General Treatment. With regard to the treatment of chronic rheumatism the essential thing is to seek out and eradicate any source of chronic infection. This being done, the sufferer should then be able to lead a normal life with only the ordinary precautions to secure good health. At the same time it is well to attend to such matters as suitable clothing to make sure of warmth and protection without undue overclothing, which latter will certainly increase the liability to attacks; the avoidance of overexertion and fatigue, and removal from a damp, cold locality to a dry, warm one. It is also necessary to abstain from severe sudden or awkward muscular efforts. Diet must be attended to. Any tendency to acidosis must be checked by the free use of green vegetables, juicy fruits, and dairy produce, and by limitation of carbohydrate and meat foods. If there is a tendency to constipation the diet must include ample roughage. Vitamin deficiency in food may well lead to rheumatism owing to the consequent lack of resistance to infection and the poor quality of bone substance.

No reliance must be placed on drugs. No known medicine, injection, or liniment, no fanciful diet or much-advertised patent medicine, has any curative influence on chronic rheumatism.

It is necessary to emphasize this warning against trusting in proprietary medicines claiming to cure arthritis, because very large sums of money are still wasted on them. When salicylates and

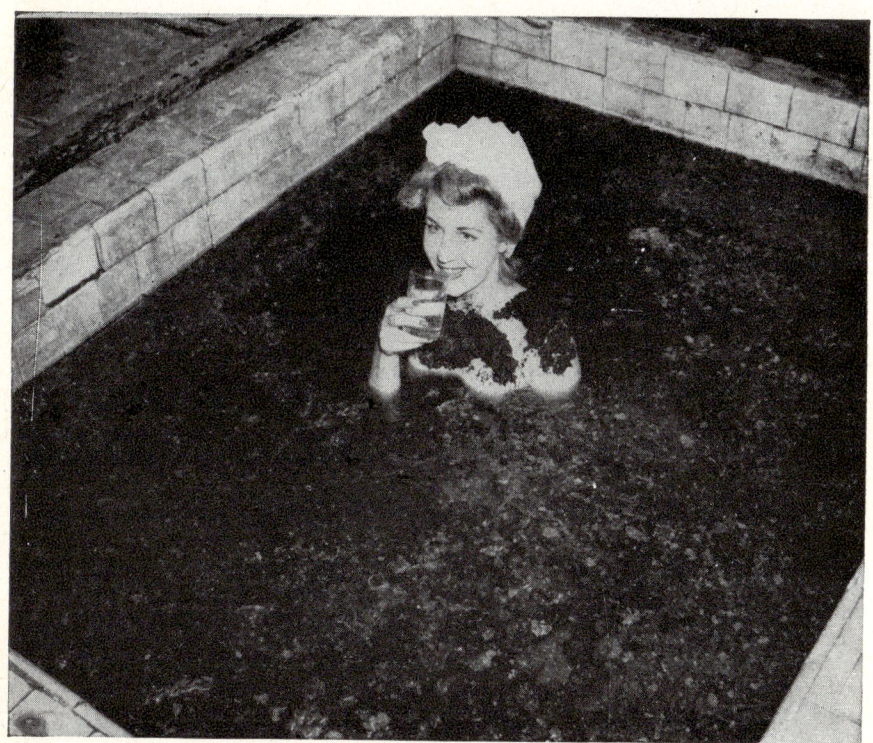

SPA TREATMENT FOR ARTHRITIS IN CALIFORNIA

Paso Robles Hot Springs, in San Luis Obispo County, California, offers treatment for neuritis, arthritis, and some other conditions by means of mud baths, massage, and the drinking of the waters. Operated as a resort since 1889, the region and its properties had some earlier reputation among white men and among the Indians before white colonists came. A patient is shown in a bath of peat mud mixed with the local lithia water. Such treatment should be taken only under a doctor's direction, like any other medical treatment.

© *International News Photo*

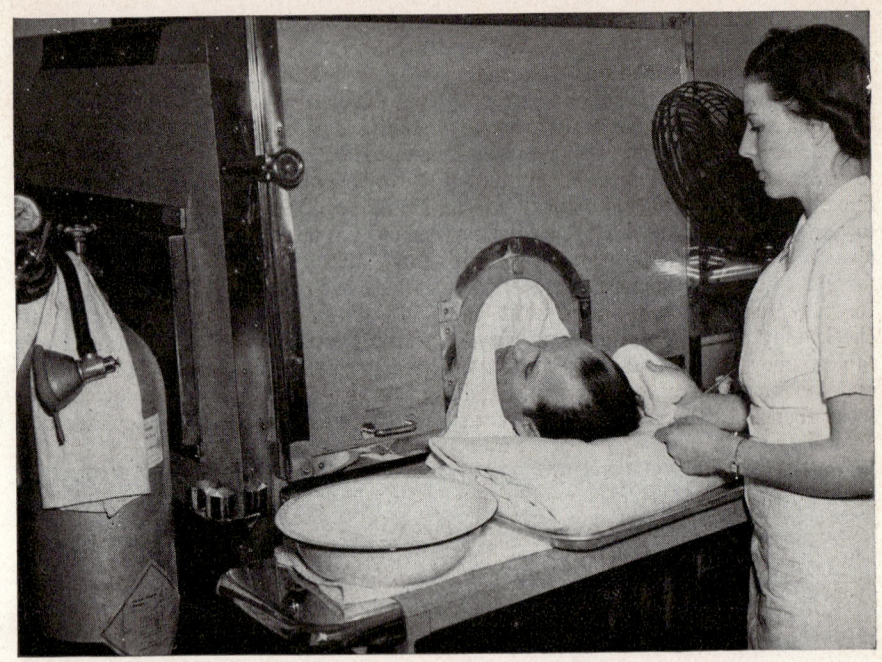

ARTHRITIS TREATED BY HEAT

The fever therapy which has been so successful in helping patients suffering from a variety of other diseases has also had strikingly successful results in rheumatic arthritis, one reviewer reporting cures in 30 per cent of the cases (Dr. Clarence A. Neymann of Northwestern University Medical School). Here a patient is enclosed in a cabinet where the heat may be raised as high as 106.7° F. for periods running as long as twelve hours. The constant attendance of a nurse is required for safety, and the head is cooled by fanning and by sponging.

© *Ewing Galloway*

similar drugs are used they should always be administered by a physician.

Good results in the treatment of chronic rheumatism in addition to more radical treatment are obtained from massage, baths, and counterirritants. Certain health resorts make a point of providing all the conditions requisite for the treatment of this disorder in its various forms. Residence at a mineral-water spa has many advantages. The hotter waters are specially helpful, and they may be assisted by douches and manipulation. Hot bathing immediately before the massage renders it more effective and less painful, and massage under a steam of hot water is very valuable. So also is the whirlpool bath, in which the water is in violent circulation around the immersed patient. In early and mild cases a Turkish bath, with manipulation of the affected muscles, may give great relief. Hot-air baths, hot sandbags, or any other method of applying dry heat are very useful forms of counterirritation. Diathermy (see page 583) is probably the most effective method of applying heat locally and deeply. Ultraviolet radiation is recommended by some, but has, as yet, to prove its general efficacy. Infra-red treatment is much more successful.

Lastly, some reference must be made to vaccine treatment in cases of long-standing infection which do not respond to removal of the original source. The value of this treatment is variable but is often very satisfactory. Much depends

GENERAL CONSTITUTIONAL DISEASES 1277

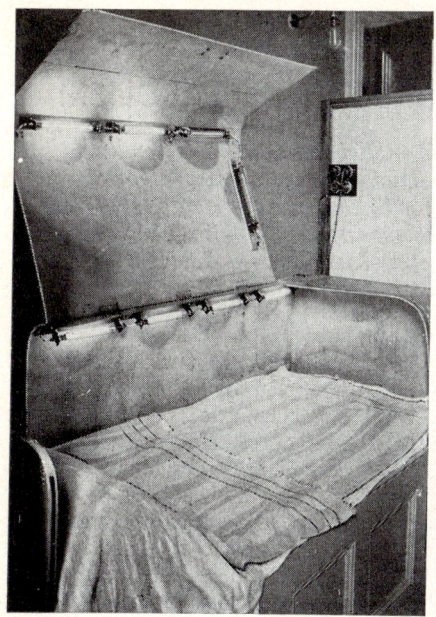
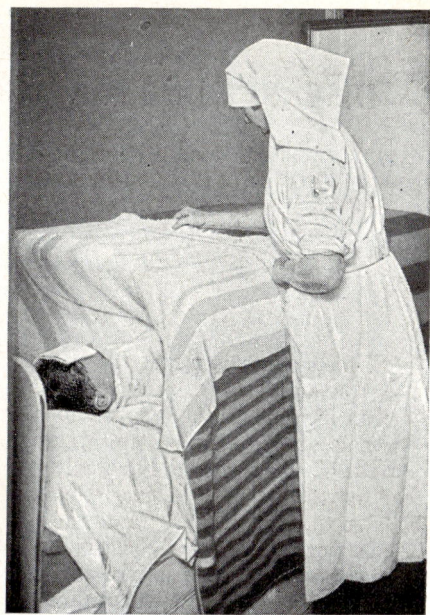

DEALING WITH CHRONIC RHEUMATISM BY BAKING TREATMENT
Raising the body temperature and free sweating contribute to the cure of complaints of a chronic rheumatic nature by improving metabolism and getting rid of deleterious waste matters. The apparatus shown here may successfully accomplish these purposes. Left: the apparatus opened up; electric bulbs contribute to the heating, but there are also steam vents beneath the couch. Right: in operation: cold cloths are put on the patient's head.

on the character of the infective agent, the powers of response left in the patient after a long fight against the infection, and other factors some of which are of an unknown character. Recently attempts to treat the condition have been based on the isolation of certain chemical substances from the urine, the result of disordered metabolism. Research work along these lines may prove of considerable assistance in dealing with this and the chronic joint manifestations of rheumatism.

With regard to the local and particular manifestations of rheumatism, these are dealt with in the section on Diseases of the Locomotor System. It is considered that some time will elapse before it may be possible to group all these "rheumatic" complaints under one name, and for various reasons it is advisable that the old-established classification should be continued. At the same time, care has been taken to incorporate information about the most recent discoveries wherever these apply.

CHAPTER 94

DISEASES DUE TO DISORDERED METABOLISM

Diabetes Mellitus—Symptoms—Diet Treatment—Insulin Treatment—Diabetic Coma—Diets for Diabetics—Home Cooking for Diabetics—Tests for Sugar—Gout—Acute Gout — Chronic Gout — Complications of Gout — Preventive Measures — Obesity — Diabetes Insipidus — Acidosis — Alkalosis.

BY metabolism is meant the total of the various processes by which food is transformed in the body into the inorganic chemicals which are absorbed into the blood stream and lymphatic system for the purpose of nourishing the body so that it can carry on its work.

The work of the body chemicals is divided into two sets of activities. These are anabolism, or the building up of the body tissues, and catabolism, the breaking down of them. The health of the body depends upon the well-balanced use of the body chemicals. The processes both of anabolism and catabolism are chemical changes, and chemical changes liberate or require energy, depending on their character. This energy is commonly in the form of heat.

In order to measure the efficiency or otherwise of the bodily metabolism heat has therefore been used as a "yardstick." The unit of heat is the calorie, which, as explained in Chapter 34, is the amount of heat required to raise the temperature of a kilogram of water one degree centigrade. To secure a uniform standard of measurement the difference in bulk between one individual and another must be allowed for, so it is usual to state the rate of heat production (that is, the metabolic rate) in terms of so many calories per square meter of the body surface per hour—the body surface being measured upon calculations from tables based upon body weight and height. These calculations are used to discover how many calories per hour the body of any individual is producing in order to compare it with the rates of heat protection by other bodies. The basal metabolic rate is defined as the least rate of chemical activity which will maintain the absolutely essential functions of the body sufficiently to keep an individual alive. This basal metabolic rate is determined by measurements taken after a subject has had complete rest for a period of twelve to fifteen hours after ingestion of food.

All sorts of considerations vary the metabolic rate, such as rest or exertion, calm or emotional stress, heat or cold, so it is impossible to determine any constant figure for a given person, but it is possible to determine an average rate in normal circumstances, and this is what is considered the basal rate of metabolism. The rate in males is from forty-five or forty-six calories per square meter per hour in the late teens to thirty-five in old age. Females have a slightly lower rate. A normal basal metabolic rate having been determined, it will be found that this rate is greatly altered in states of ill-health, and thus it has a valuable diagnostic significance. Roughly, the process consists in attempting to measure the amount of oxygen absorbed by the lungs in a measured time. It is known that the thyroid gland plays a very important part in the basal metabolism of the body, and others of the ductless glands, such as the pituitary, may also have their role. Certain diseases are called diseases of metabolism, notably diabetes, gout, and obesity.

DISEASES DUE TO DISORDERED METABOLISM

DIABETES MELLITUS

We shall deal first with this condition, called simply diabetes as a rule. It must be distinguished from diabetes insipidus, which is discussed later in the present chapter.

Diabetes is a disease which most people know by name, but about which, until comparatively recently, even the best informed had to confess to knowing very little. Even now the knowledge that has been acquired leaves a great deal still to be discoverd. The name diabetes, derived from the Greek, means "a flowing through," and it is so called because one of its most marked symptoms is the loss of sugar from the body, which "flows through" the kidneys and appears in the urine. It is called diabetes mellitus (from the Greek *mellita*, a bee) to distinguish it from diabetes insipidus (see page 1296), in which no sugar is present.

In ordinary conditions of health no sugar is present in the urine, and if it is found there we look upon it as abnormal. But not every case in which we find sugar in the urine can be called diabetes, for it is met with in many other diseases temporarily, but without the other important symptoms which, all put together, make diabetes. The temporary presence of sugar in the urine is called glycosuria, which means "sweet urine," and is not a serious condition. It may occur as the result of some dietetic error, as after a meal containing large quantities of sugar or starch.

If, however, the sugar is present in the urine day after day, the symptom becomes a matter of serious import.

The pancreas is a gland which produces an internal secretion in addition to that secreted by a duct, and is situated in close proximity to the stomach on the right side of the upper abdomen. Its internal secretion is formed in the parts of it that are known as the islands of Langerhans, and it is now recognized that most cases of diabetes are due to deficiency of this secretion, for when the secretion, isolated from pancreatic extracts obtained from oxen, is administered to diabetic patients, it causes a rapid reduction of the sugar in the urine and the blood. The substance which produces this remarkable effect is called insulin from *insula* (Latin, island). Why the islands of Langerhans sometimes fail to produce their normal secretion, or produce it in insufficient quantity, is not known.

The result of the failure of the internal secretion of the islands of Langerhans is

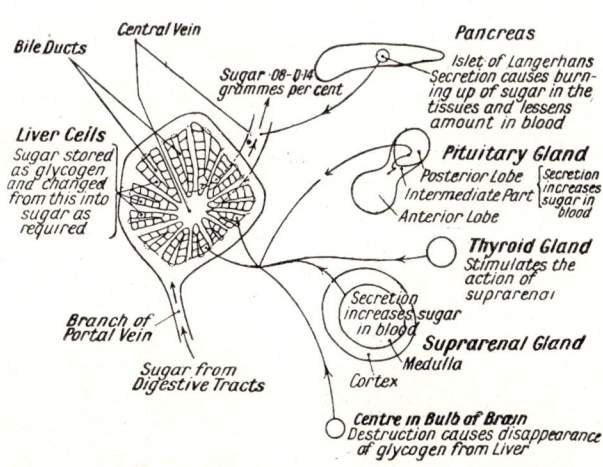

CONTROL OF THE BLOOD SUGAR BY ENDOCRINES

The quantity of sugar in the blood is controlled by the action of the secretion of various glands, which may stimulate the liver cells to pass sugar into the blood or, on the other hand, may increase the burning of the sugar in the tissues.

From The New People's Physician

that the carbohydrate metabolism of the body is gravely upset as well as the metabolism of fats and proteins, with the result that sugar and acetones are found in abnormal quantities in the urine.

Diabetes occurs much more frequently among men than women, and is a disease of middle age. It certainly sometimes occurs in young persons, and is then acknowledged to be far more serious. There appears to be an hereditary tendency. Diabetes is sometimes associated with brain trouble, such as a tumor or other disease, or an injury. It may be produced in those hereditarily predisposed by certain errors of diet, such as excessive use of starchy or sugary food with resulting obesity. Many cases occur, however, in which no definite predisposing cause can be discovered. Recent work indicates that a disordered relationship between the pituitary gland and pancreas may be the underlying factor.

Symptoms. Diabetes may come on suddenly and acutely. In this case there is great thirst and extreme weakness, and the patient may slip rapidly into a coma and, if untreated, die without the trouble having been diagnosed, though in these days many people are acquainted with the danger of diabetic coma and are able to recognize the possibility of such a state. In the majority of cases, however, the symptoms come on gradually, and may long go unnoticed. The first thing which usually attracts attention is the large amount of urine that is passed. With this there is an excessive thirst, which cannot be satisfied even by enormous quantities of fluid. The appetite becomes voracious, and yet, in spite of the amount of food eaten, the body grows rapidly thinner and the strength fails daily. The urine has a characteristic odor, like that of apples or new-mown grass, and if a drop of it falls on the carpet or elsewhere, it leaves a white spot on drying. If the urine is examined, its specific gravity is found to be raised to 1030, or even to 1070, according to the amount of sugar present. The quantity passed may be as much as fifteen quarts, and sometimes even more, during a period of twenty four hours. The urine of a diabetic is characteristically of a pale greenish color.

While the kidneys act with excessive freedom, the skin hardly acts at all; it becomes dry and harsh, and is very liable to eruptions and boils. The bowels are very constipated and the movements hard and dry. The mouth and tongue are parched and sticky, and the breath gives off a peculiar sweet odor (acetone breath).

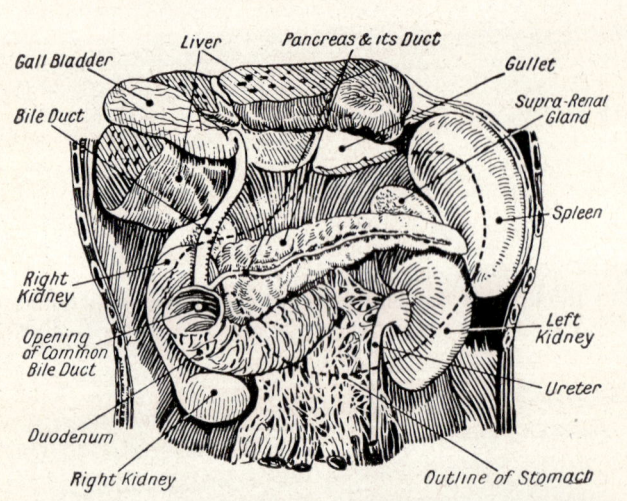

PANCREAS: AN ORGAN IMPORTANT TO METABOLISM

The pancreas lies in the loop of the small intestine forming the duodenum. In addition to the secretion of its duct, which plays a part in digestion, the pancreas supplies to the blood an internal secretion which is essential to life.

DISEASES DUE TO DISORDERED METABOLISM

Nervous symptoms such as neuralgia, numbness, and tingling are frequently mentioned. When these latter symptoms occur, it shows that the nerves have become inflamed, the condition being known as peripheral neuritis. Severe sciatica and shingles may sometimes occur. These ailments are seldom related directly to the diabetes but are usually due to an arthritis or neuritis of independent origin. Fully one-tenth of the cases of diabetes are symptomless.

On the other hand, patients may show mental symptoms, and may become depressed and sometimes melancholic. Cataract of the eye may set in accompanied by sudden blindness. Formerly it was rare for diabetic women to have children, but now 50 per cent of the pregnancies of diabetic mothers terminate successfully. There has been no known instance of a diabetic mother bearing a diabetic infant. Only one child in 8000 contracts the disease before the age of fifteen.

The disease is easy to diagnose, and the outlook is changed considerably as a result of discoveries and methods of treatment. On the whole, the outlook is much more favorable in old than in young patients (see chart, page 1282). The prognosis depends to a great extent on the common sense and intelligence of the patient. If he co-operates he can expect a long and interesting life.

Fevers of any kind or infections, like a sore throat, may severely complicate the disease, and finally diabetic coma as a rule manifests that the disease is gaining ground, and, if untreated, heralds the early approach of death. The majority of cases terminate with complications, such as septicemia as a result of a local infection or gangrene, pneumonia, or tuberculosis. Diabetic coma is much more frequently a cause of death in elderly patients than it is in children.

Though the expectancy for different ages is much less for the diabetic than for the general population the life expectancy of diabetics has been increased markedly by modern treatment.

ISLANDS OF LANGERHANS
Groups of cells within the pancreas, called islands of Langerhans, pour their secretion into the blood and this effects the burning of sugar in the body. Disease of these islands causes diabetes.

Diet Treatment. Until very recently the methods of treatment in general use involved undernutrition and prolonged fasting, but today less rigorous methods are employed, and diets are allowed which are more liberal in fat, and which therefore provide more food, and therefore energy.

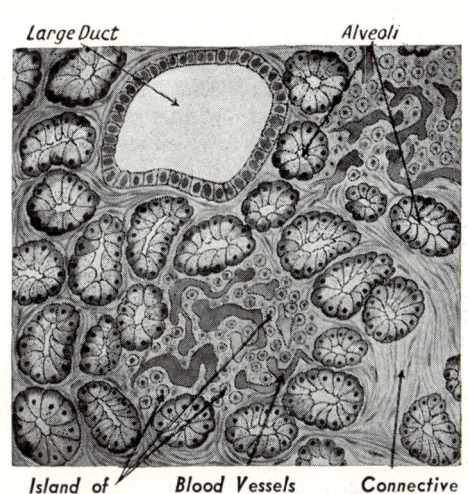

Fats will not burn in the tissues unless a certain amount of sugar is burned with them. If fat fails to burn completely, acid bodies are produced and coma may result. Hence there is a limit to the amount of fat that can be used by the diabetic or that may be included in a diet mixture which is low in carbohydrates, and therefore the content of fat diets must be planned exactly to fit the condition of the patient. Furthermore, in the beginning of the treatment the urine must be examined frequently, and the patient must be carefully watched for evidence of acidosis.

If the patient be unable to go into a hospital, he is advised to place himself under the care of a doctor.

After the urine has been made sugar-free, the sugar tolerance is determined. The actual procedure may vary with different patients. The general rule is to increase the diet a little at a time, raising the daily intake of sugar-forming food until the limit is reached, beyond which any further addition of food causes an excretion of sugar. This is the point of tolerance, and when arrived at the diet can be precisely planned.

A food mixture is then prescribed which will provide enough albuminous (protein) food for tissue building, and enough heat energy from fat and carbohydrates to carry out the patient's bodily wants.

Insulin Treatment. Insulin is a watery solution of sugar ferment from the pancreatic glands of slaughterhouse animals. When injected into the body it makes it possible for a definite amount of sugar to be used, and thus assists the diseased pancreas. Furthermore, insulin makes larger diets possible and helps the patient to regain his former weight and strength.

DEATH RATES PER 100,000

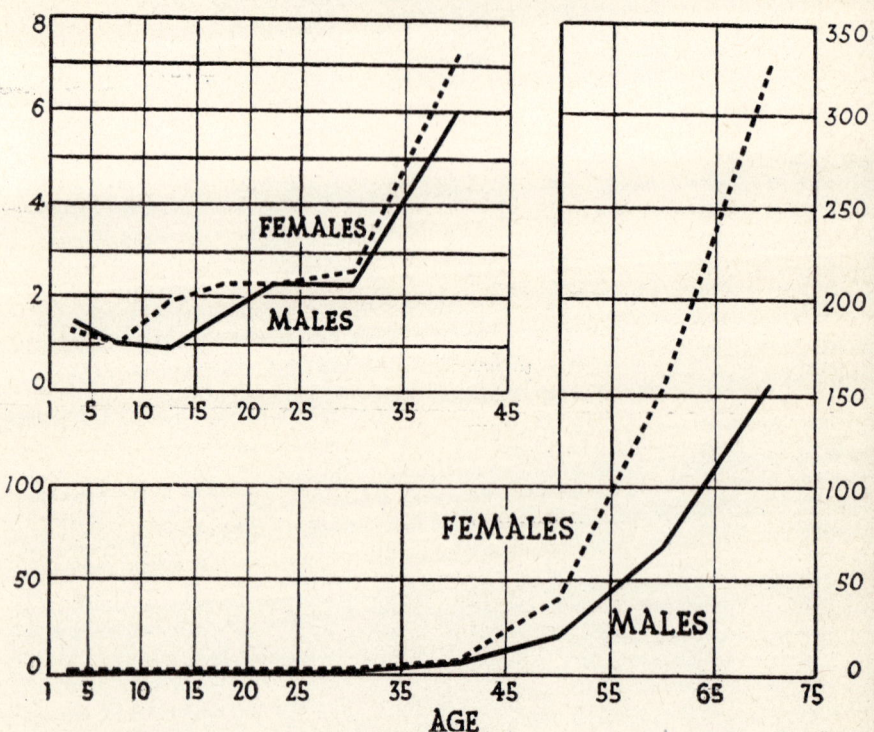

WHERE DIABETES KILLS

This chart prepared by the Metropolitan Life Insurance Company shows that diabetes mortality in the late nineteen-thirties was markedly concentrated in middle-aged and older women. The Company's report remarks that this tendency is becoming accentuated. Though diabetes deaths at ages under twenty-five are few in number, many more girls in the teens die of diabetes than boys in the same age group.

DEATH RATES PER 100,000

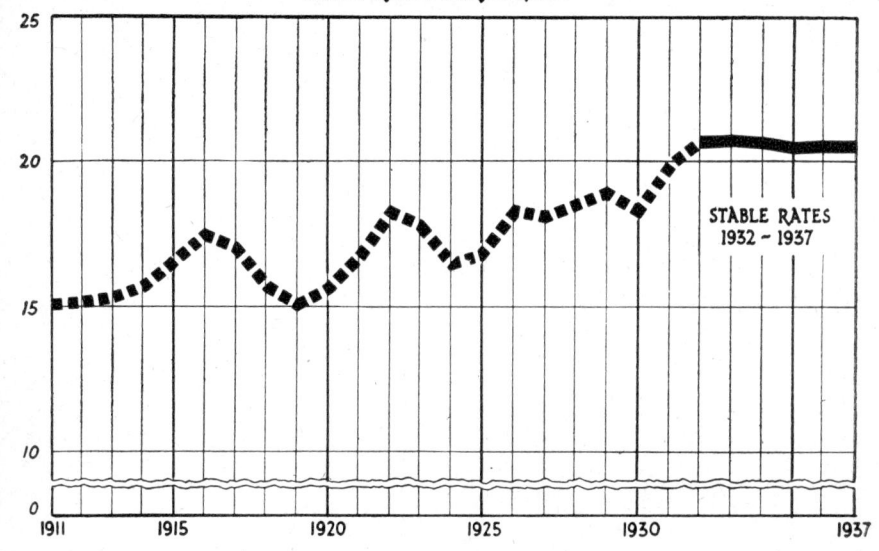

HOLDING OUR OWN AGAINST DIABETES

Only among old people have diabetes deaths been increasing since 1932; at the younger ages the death rates have continued to show great improvement. This graph, prepared by the Metropolitan Life Insurance Company, illustrates this hopeful development. There is a continuing increase in what statisticians call crude mortality from diabetes, but this reflects merely the growing proportion of old people in the population of the world. Diabetes has not been increasing recently if allowance is made for shifts in the age and sex make-up of the population; the adjusted death rates, as shown above, were unchanged from 1932 to 1937.

The daily dose is a matter which must be determined separately for each patient. The amount of food for which this dose will provide is also a matter that must be carefully determined. This requires careful planning by the physician and intelligent co-operation on the part of the patient. The dose of insulin is expressed in terms of units, one unit being enough to ferment about two grams of sugar. The daily dose will vary from ten to forty units. This is a small volume of fluid, not more than two cubic centimeters, (thirty-three minims), and it is injected beneath the skin of the upper arm or the thigh with a syringe and needle.

The course of treatment with insulin begins just as does the dietary procedure previously described. It is necessary for the patient to rest in bed. The tolerance is determined, and a diet is mapped out which will support the patient without insulin. This is important, inasmuch as if the supply of insulin should be interrupted he can then go back to the low diet and take to his bed. Next, a food mixture is planned which the patient will be able to tolerate with the help of not more than from thirty to forty units of insulin. This higher diet and the daily administration of insulin are then started.

The patient is permitted to be up and about, and he rapidly gains strength and bodily weight. The best time to give insulin is in the morning before breakfast. If for any reason insulin has to be discontinued, the high diet must be discontinued. The patient must return to the fasting diet, and must rest in bed. It is an absolute necessity that this diet and rest be continued until insulin be resumed.

Insulin is dangerous unless properly used. It must be balanced with food, otherwise it will cause the necessary sugar in the blood to disappear. Whenever blood sugar falls below a certain level, alarming symptoms may occur. There may be drowsiness, muscular weakness, hunger, and fear. The muscles may tremble, and sweat usually breaks out all over the body. Recovery from this condition may be spontaneous, but in many cases it requires an antidote. Fortunately there is a very simple antidote in sugar taken in any form. The juice of a small orange is usually sufficient. Should mild reactions occur on two or three days in succession then the insulin must be reduced or the diet adjusted.

The introduction of protamine insulin has decreased the number of daily injections needed. This mode of treatment is still in its early stages and very careful medical supervision is essential.

The majority of patients under forty-five are severe diabetics and require insulin. Past this age dietary care often suffices. This is also true for the obese diabetic.

Diabetic Coma. This complication is due to the collection in the blood of the products of the incomplete metabolism of fat—acetone and fatty acids. As a result the excretion of carbon dioxide gas from the lungs is insufficient to counteract the acidosis which develops, and when this reaches a certain severity the condition of coma sets in.

It occurs in very acute cases, in untreated cases, and as the result of some intercurrent acute infection. Treatment of coma is by prompt and large doses of insulin and sufficient liquids to bring back the depleted fluid supply in the patient's system to normal.

The patient must be kept warm and treated as for shock. Usually thirty to fifty units of insulin may be safely given at once without waiting for a blood examination. Two ounces of sugar should be given with the insulin, if necessary by a nasal tube. An ounce of castor oil should be given, and water in as large amounts as possible—if necessary by the rectum, or, better still, intravenously if the patient cannot be roused to drink. Subsequent treatment is by carefully adjusted doses of insulin.

The following facts must be clearly grasped before the subject of diabetes can be thoroughly understood: (1) Starches are absorbed by the alimentary canal in the form of sugar. (2) The sugar is turned into glycogen in the liver. (3) The glycogen is reconverted by the liver into sugar. (4) Blood acts purely as a means of transport and communication, and the kidneys act as safety valves when the blood sugar rises too

SELF-INJECTIONS OF INSULIN
At the University of Michigan, Ann Arbor, children under treatment for diabetes are successfully taught to measure out their own dietary as prescribed, and also to make injections of insulin. Thus they need pay only occasional visits to the hospital.

high. (5) The muscles utilize sugar to produce energy. (6) As blood sugar is consumed "by muscular exertion" the liver supplies more. (7) In the absence of pancreatic ferment the muscles refuse to make use of the sugar carried to them by the blood, and the safety valves in the kidneys remove this excess and produce sugar in the urine.

Of the complications, coma has already been mentioned. Pruritis (itching) and eczema are often present in neglected cases and are best treated by controlling the disease and applying a cooling lotion of boric acid. Arteriosclerosis, both of the peripheral vessels and of the heart, is a severe and important complication. Poor blood supply to the extremity results in frequent infection and in some instances gangrene. Cataract and anemia may also be mentioned as complications. There is a surprisingly high incidence of tuberculosis among diabetics.

Patients suffering from diabetes should be clothed in such a manner as to protect them from the effects of cold weather, as the malnutrition caused by the disease exposes the patient in an exceptional degree to the risk of catching cold. A moderate amount of outdoor exercise, graduated according to the severity of the disease, is beneficial. A systematic use of the muscles aids digestion and contributes to the general well-being. The large muscles when given work tend to reduce the sugar content of the blood and thus encourage the tolerance of starchy food. Rigid foot care in diabetics is essential if infection is to be avoided. The feet should be washed daily with soap and water and dried thoroughly. The nails should be kept clean and cut straight across after bathing. The patient should not attempt to cut corns or calluses. Lanolin may be used to keep the skin soft.

Diets for Diabetics. There are numerous systems of diets for diabetics—Allen's, Lawrence's, etc. Broadly speaking, foods are given in the forms of vegetables and fruits because the carbohydrates in them are dilute. Therefore these foods are very useful in planning diabetic menus. On the other hand, foods like bread, rice, sugar, and potatoes are less suitable, because of their richness in carbohydrates.

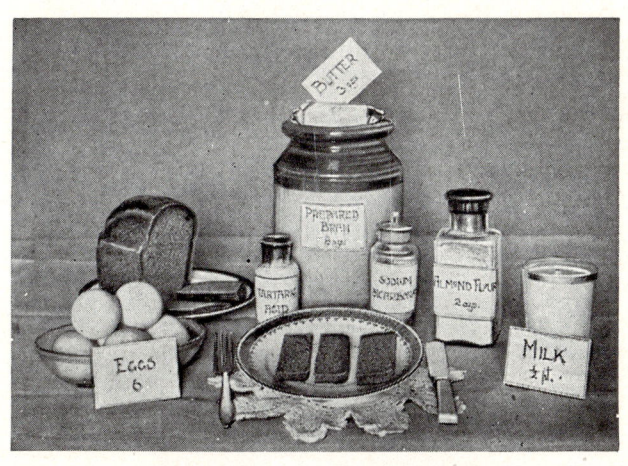

DIABETIC BREAD AND ITS INGREDIENTS

Small squares of bran bread, fried in butter, are quite palatable. The photograph also shows the ingredients, and a detailed recipe for making the bread is given in the text.

As regards fats, pure fat foods are lard and oil; butter is almost pure fat. The meats nearly all contain a certain proportion of fat, and, whereas in the process of digestion carbohydrates are completely changed in the body to sugar, only about one-tenth of the fat content in food is changed in the body to sugar.

The dietary for a diabetic patient should be selected from fresh meat, game, poultry, fish, tongue, ham, bacon, meat juices, and extracts; soups made

BASIC DAILY DIABETIC DIET AS COMPUTED BY THE
METROPOLITAN LIFE INSURANCE COMPANY

Food	Portion or unit	Number of portions	Weight of each portion, grams	Weight of food elements in each portion, grams			Total weight of food elements in each food, grams		
				Carbohydrates	Proteins	Fats	Carbohydrates	Proteins	Fats
Bread......	slice	3	30	18	3	—	54	9	—
Oatmeal....	large serving	1	30 (dry)	20	5	2	20	5	2
Orange.....	each	3	150	15	—	—	45	—	—
Vegetables, 3%-5%...	serving	4	150	5	2½	—	20	10	—
Milk.......	¼ pint	1	120	6	4	4	6	4	4
Cream, 20%	¼ pint	1	120	4	4	24	4	4	24
Egg.......	each	1	—	—	6	6	—	6	6
Meat.......	serving	2	60	—	16	10	—	32	20
Butter......	chip	3	10	—	—	8	—	—	25
Grand total weight of food elements, grams...................							150	70	80
Calories per gram, approximate.............................							4	4	9
Calories of each food element, approximate.................							600	280	720
Total calories, daily diet, approximate.....................							1600		

without flour; eggs, butter, cream, cream cheese, ordinary cheese; salad, watercress, green vegetables, such as cabbage, Brussels sprouts, lettuce, spinach, broccoli, French beans, endive, cucumber; pickles, almonds, cobnuts, walnuts; almond biscuits, coconut biscuits, protein bread; hock, Moselle, claret, brandy, whisky if the patient feels a need of alcohol and the doctor permits it; tea, coffee (sweetened with saccharin, if any sweetening is desired); and possibly a little milk.

The fact that ordinary white bread contains between 50 and 60 per cent of carbohydrates gives rise to the chief difficulty in arranging a dietary for diabetics. Ordinary bread, when allowed, is usually well toasted before being eaten by a diabetic patient, the sole advantage being that he will probably eat less toast than he would eat of the same bread untoasted.

Bread prepared from ordinary flour from which the starch has been washed away has long been used as a substitute for ordinary bread; this is called gluten bread, and is a most unsuccessful substitute—it is dry, chippy, and tasteless; it is very expensive, and it usually contains more than half as much starch as ordinary bread. Almond bread contains about one-fifth the amount of starch that is present in ordinary white bread, and is therefore serviceable; but the most starch-free substitute for wheat bread is that made with protein flour (prepared from milk), which contains less than 3 per cent of carbohydrates.

The following substances should not be allowed when a strict dietary is prescribed:

Wheat bread, white soups, shellfish of all kinds; all farinaceous foods; potatoes; sweet fruits, such as cherries, apples, pears, dates, figs, and all dried fruits; cocoa, milk, sweet wines, and malt liquors.

Home Cooking for Diabetics. The diet to be followed by a patient suffering from this disease has been detailed above. In particular carbohydrates must be forbidden or restricted to such amounts as the patient can assimilate—a matter for experiment with each individual. Hence almond flour, bran, casein, gluten and ground nuts are used to make bread, biscuits, and puddings, etc., and the sugars are replaced by glycerine, saccharin, or dulcin.

To test for the presence of starch in food, add a few drops of a solution of iodine in potassium iodide. If the material turns a deep blue or black a definite proportion of starch is present.

Bread and biscuits, etc., prepared from these diabetic flours have been placed on the market under many trade names. It should, however, be noted that all reliable diabetic foods are expensive, and in many cases, therefore, it will be necessary to select from the ordinary foods those which are suitable for use (see tables, page 1286 and below, and also the recipes in this chapter).

For soups no root vegetables should be employed, and no starchy thickening materials added. If a thick soup is required, egg yolk or almond flour may be used for thickening.

Gluten flour may be used for sauces, cream and egg yolk being used partly or wholly to replace these when desired.

Ordinary cakes and cookies contain flour and sugar, and cannot be allowed; but a large number of cakes may be prepared from almond flour, bran flour, coconut flour, and so on, using the permissible sweetening agents already mentioned.

Eggs, fish, cheese, custards, meat, game, and poultry may all be cooked by the ordinary methods, provided any gravies and sauces served are free from starch, root vegetables, and flour. Most fruits and puddings are forbidden, but unripe gooseberries and a few other unripe fruits may be cooked in water sweetened with saccharin and served with junket, cream, or diabetic custard (see page 1175). Rhubarb and tomatoes, and vegetables such as cauliflower, may be given.

The following recipes for bread substitutes suitable for diabetic patients will also be useful:

Bran Bread. Beat three ounces of butter to a cream in a basin, beat thoroughly into it two ounces of almond flour, and then add six eggs, one at a time. Partly mix in eight ounces of prepared bran, add a cup of milk, a teaspoonful of tartaric acid and two teaspoonfuls of sodium bicarbonate. Finally, thoroughly mix the whole together, pour into a buttered tin, and bake in a moderate oven for an hour.

Gluten Bread. Make a dough as for ordinary bread, using a pound of gluten flour, four ounces of prepared bran, an ounce of ground almonds, two eggs, an ounce of yeast, and a pinch of salt, and leave to rise, a process which will require from three-quarters of an hour to an hour. Then bake as usual. The ground almonds and eggs may be omitted, but are an improvement. This bread, cut into small slices and toasted or fried, is very palatable.

Gluten and Almond Bread. Mix together four ounces of gluten flour and two ounces of almond flour, and rub in one ounce of butter; then add a half teaspoonful of baking powder and one well-beaten egg. Mix with a scant cupful of water, allow to stand for three or four minutes, and then add another scant half cupful of water. Mix and bake for twenty minutes to half an hour in a hot oven.

Two other recipes for the diabetic are as follows:

Gluten Omelette. Break three fresh eggs into a basin and add a tablespoon-

PORTIONS OF ORDINARY FOODS CONTAINING APPROXIMATELY TEN GRAMS OF CARBOHYDRATES, AS COMPUTED BY THE METROPOLITAN LIFE INSURANCE COMPANY

Food	Household measure	Weight, grams
Orange	1, small	100
Banana	½	50
Oatmeal, cooked	½ saucer	120
Oatmeal, dry	—	15
Vegetables, 5%	2 large saucers	300
Vegetables, 10%	1 large saucer	150
Bread	½ slice	15
Potato	1, size of egg	—

ful of cream. To this add a half ounce of butter in small pieces, a dessertspoonful of gluten, salt and pepper to taste, a teaspoonful of chopped thyme and parsley, and, if desired, a little finely minced ham. Well mix all these together and pour into a frying pan in which another half ounce of butter has been melted; stir carefully until the eggs begin to set, then shape and serve.

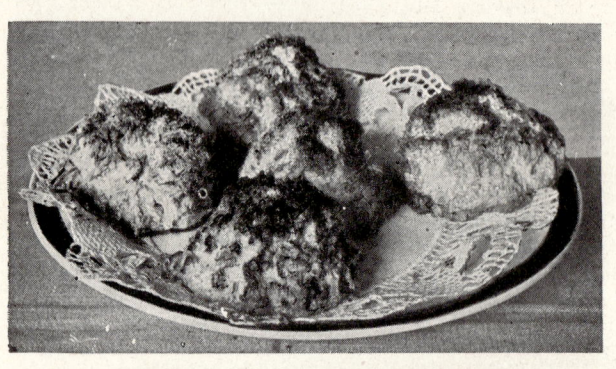

GLUTEN BREAD FOR DIABETIC PATIENTS
These little rolls are made with gluten flour, prepared bran, and almonds according to the recipe given on page 1287, but instead of being baked in one loaf, the dough is divided roughly into small portions before being put into the oven.

Gluten Pancakes. Break an egg into an ounce and a half of gluten flour, beat well, add a pinch of salt, and then gradually pour in a half cup of milk, stirring continually. With this as a batter, fry very thin pancakes in the usual manner, using butter, and serve the pancakes rolled up, after sprinkling with lemon juice and a very small quantity of saccharin powder.

Tests for Sugar. The first test for sugar is with the urinometer, a little instrument used to measure the specific gravity. It consists of three parts. The lowest part forms a small globular glass chamber containing some mercury. This part is connected by a narrow neck with a cylindrical air-containing chamber which is in turn surmounted by a hollow glass stem sealed at the top. The stem contains a scale marked in equal divisions, usually from 1000 to 1050.

If the urinometer is placed in a tall vessel containing urine, it will float upright but partially submerged, so that the upper level of the fluid is at some point on the scale. This reading is the specific gravity. The instrument is usually graduated to give the specific gravity of a fluid at 59° F., which is about the ordinary room temperature.

If the specific gravity is found to be high the presence of sugar must be suspected. To prove its presence a special preparation, Fehling's solution, is used. As this keeps badly it is usually sold in two bottles, one containing a solution of copper and the other a solution of potash. Equal quantities of these solutions are mixed together in a test tube, when they make a beautiful dark blue liquid, which is boiled. To this hot liquid add the suspected urine a few drops at a time, and boil again. If sugar is present in the urine a red or orange cloud forms in the solution.

This shows the presence of sugar, but not its amount. If sugar is found or suspected in the urine, a doctor should be seen at once. If by reason of distance, etc., this cannot be done, the next task is to find the amount, which is really the important matter in watching a case of diabetes.

The urinometer is again used for this, together with two glasses long enough to receive it, and a cake of yeast, which can be purchased at any grocery store. Dry yeast may be easier to use, but moist yeast will serve. The two glasses should be nearly filled with some of the urine, and the specific gravity of both taken; we will assume this to be 1040. Now put a pinch of yeast into one, and keep the other as a standard, for comparison; cover them both up, and put

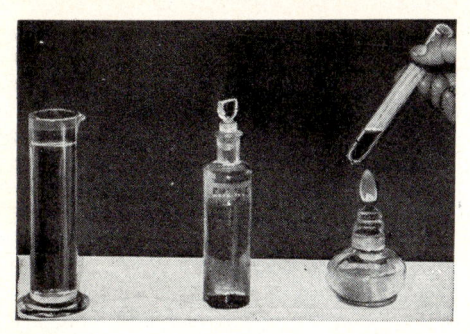

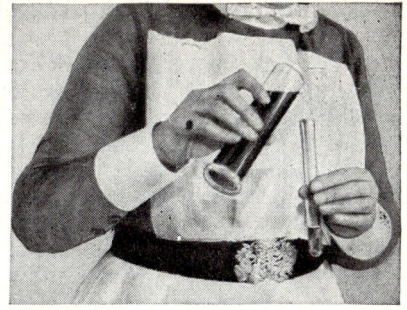

TESTING A SAMPLE OF URINE FOR SUGAR

Left: a small quantity of Fehling's or a similar solution is put into a test tube and brought to the boil. If any alteration takes place in the color on boiling some fresh testing solution must be obtained. Right: a few drops of the sample of urine are then added to the test solution, which is again boiled; if there is no change more urine is added and again boiled; the appearance of a brick-red color means that sugar is present in the urine.

them to stand for twenty-four hours in a warm place—the mantelpiece or a shelf in the kitchen will do. At the end of this time take the specific gravity of both specimens again, and you will find that the specimen in which you put the yeast has a much lower specific gravity than the standard one: the specific gravity will be perhaps 1010. This is because the sugar, which caused the high specific gravity, has been changed by the yeast, and in its place have been formed alcohol (which is lighter than water) and carbon-dioxide, which has escaped into the air. Every degree of specific gravity that has been lost represents a grain of sugar in the ounce of urine. As in this sample experiment the specific gravity fell thirty degrees, the urine contained thirty grains of sugar in every ounce. By multiplying this by the number of ounces of urine passed in the twenty-four hours it is easy to find the amount of sugar that is being lost daily, and also the improvement, or the reverse, as the result of treatment.

Should the diabetic who is testing his urine at home notice sugar, it is urged that he notify his physician who can if necessary carry out exact blood and urine sugar determinations by precise laboratory methods.

GOUT

Gout is perhaps the best example known to medicine of a diathesis, *i.e.* an inborn tendency to disease coloring all the reactions of the body to the influences by which it is affected through life. The individual member of a gouty family may himself be the subject of acute gouty troubles in his joints as age advances; on the other hand, he may escape the classical symptoms altogether and yet find that he is the victim of minor degrees of ill-health affecting in turn one or all of his physiological systems.

The best-known theory of the nature of gout ascribes its occurrence to a disturbance of the chemistry of uric acid in the body. This hypothesis has many incontrovertible arguments in its favor, but it fails altogether to explain why such a disturbance should arise. The connection between gout and uric acid was first brought into prominence when it was found that in the blood of the gouty individual there was an excess of uric acid.

It has since been demonstrated that uric acid exists in the body in the form of various salts with sodium, potassium and magnesium; these salts differ in their solubility in the blood and tissue juices, and they easily change their form and composition.

It is supposed by the supporters of the uric acid hypothesis that such changes, sudden and only partly understood, are the cause of acute gouty symptoms; it is rightly pointed out that a gouty paroxysm is associated with the excretion of urine rich in salts of uric acid and of a highly acid nature; it is also known that the familiar deposits in the neighborhood of the joints in gouty persons are largely composed of relatively insoluble salts of uric acid, and that these undergo physical changes corresponding to the onset and course of an acute attack of gout.

A more modern view is to regard gout as an indication of a change in the physical condition of uric acid and its salts in the body; it is suggested that in health and between the periods of acute gout these substances are in a colloid state, and that under the influence of some abnormal factor they suddenly change their state from that of a colloid to that of a crystalloid, which owing to its relative insolubility is deposited in the tissues and sets up the

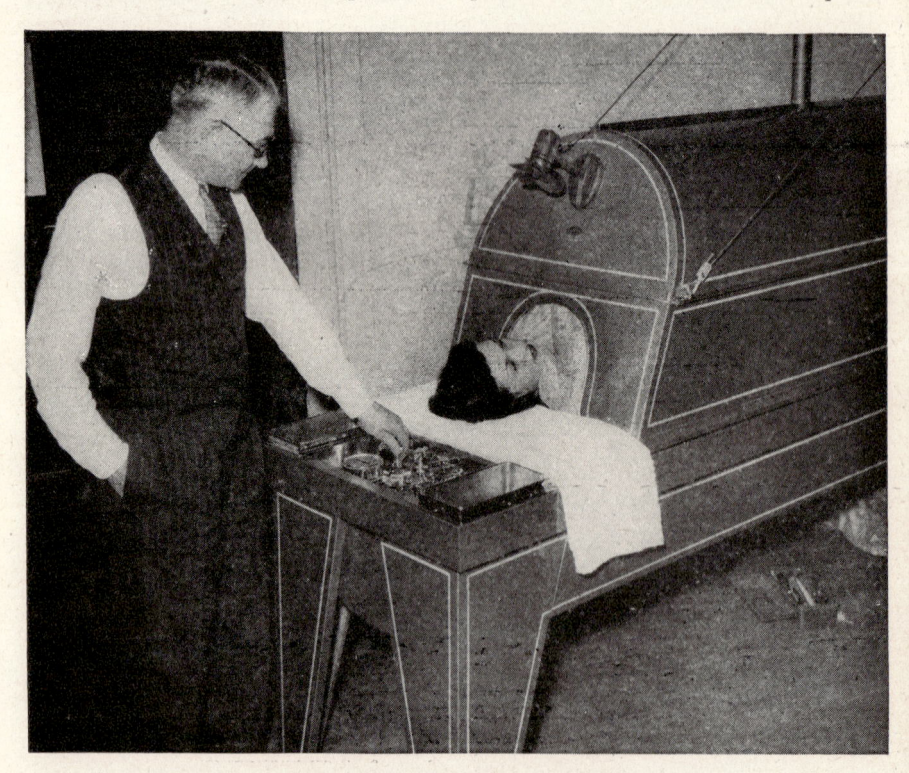

HIGH HEAT FOR "FEVER THERAPY"

The advances in knowledge relating to the effectiveness of heightened body heat in combating various diseases have stimulated the design of technical devices for the safe administration of this therapeutic measure. As might have been expected, one problem was to reduce the likelihood of burns. The device shown was demonstrated before the Academy of Physical Medicine in the Willard Hotel, Washington, D. C., and is designed to avoid burns by the use of atomized water for heating the patient's body.

© *Harris & Ewing*

acute symptoms. This suggestion has much to recommend it, but it leaves unexplained the reason for this change in the uric acid.

Many possible explanations have been advanced, but the true cause is still undetermined. It has been suggested, for instance, that gout is an instance of protein sensitization on a par with nettle rash, and induced by the taking of minute quantities of nitrogenous substances that are poisonous to the individual concerned; the well-established relationship between gout asthma and certain forms of skin rash lends a good deal of support to this view. Absorption of poisons from the bowel has been held to offer a solution of the problem, and here again a good deal of support is forthcoming in the well-known influence of constipation and digestive disturbances in precipitating an attack of gout. Poisons such as lead and certain forms of alcoholic drinks are liable to cause gout.

Retention in the body of certain normal products of its activity which in the healthy individual are excreted by the skin has also been blamed for gout; there is much to recommend this view also, for under the influence of warmth and free sweating great relief of gouty changes can be produced.

The gouty individual presents certain fairly constant characteristics that distinguish him from his more fortunate brethren. He comes from a gouty family; among his near ancestors are those who have had gout in its classical form or have suffered obviously from allied disorders; he himself has very likely suffered in infancy from obstinate eczema or attacks of asthma; he is usually "full-blooded," of an active nature and alert mentality; he is prone to indigestion and his blood pressure is usually above the normal for his age; he has a special tendency to early degeneration of blood vessels and kidneys, and is liable to mild diabetes.

Acute Gout. The first attack of acute gout is usually a surprise; it is very liable to arise in the small hours of the morning, waking the patient with a severe pain in some joint, most often in the great toe; the painful part is red, swollen, acutely tender to the touch and intensely painful on movement or jarring. There may at the same time be considerable constitutional disturbance, with fever, headache, and sometimes vomiting. It is unusual for more than one joint to be affected at first. Under treatment and in the course of a few days the pain, swelling, and redness diminish, and the joint may apparently return completely to a normal state. There is often an interval of months or years before a fresh outburst occurs, and all the original symptoms are repeated; the intervals between attacks grow shorter with each recurrence, and gradually the joint acquires the signs and deformities of chronic gout. Before this happens other joints have become involved, and acute attacks in these may alternate or coincide with paroxysms in the part first affected.

Classical gout, as above described, is much less common nowadays than was the case even a few years ago; possibly the greater observance of simple rules of health, especially in restriction of intake and promotion of excretion, affords an explanation.

Treatment. Treatment of acute gout consists in measures to promote local warmth and sweating; the sweat secreted by the skin over such an inflamed joint is intensely acid, far more so than that of other parts of the body at the same time, and this observation affords a reason for the promotion of skin activity. The joint should be warmly wrapped up, enveloped in hot, moist coverings, or exposed to an atmosphere of warm steam to promote sweating; it should be supported in the position of greatest comfort and protected from jarring and movement. The patient should be purged, starved for forty-eight hours, and encouraged to drink large quantities of water, preferably containing alkalis, such as the citrates and carbonates of potassium; when food is again allowed him it must be given in small quantities, and meat and meat extracts must be excluded for a time.

Many drugs have been advocated; their numbers are constantly being added to, but reliance is best placed on three old-fashioned remedies; colchicum, or meadow saffron; potassium iodide; and guaiacum, a tree resin. Of these colchicum is of greatest value while the gouty attack is at its height; the others are more useful when it is subsiding, though they may sometimes be used with advantage to assist the action of the indispensable colchicum. More recently drug therapy has included atophan and the salicylates. There are very successful reports of the latter when used in combination with bicarbonates.

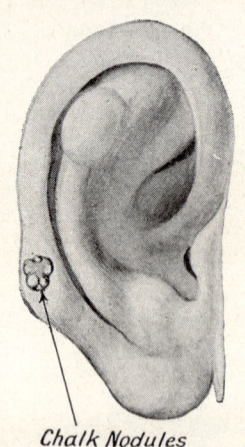

During the attack of acute inflammation what has been called metastatic gout may occur; this is a serious complication taking the form of a severe disturbance of the brain, causing delirium or unconsciousness, or affecting the alimentary tract, producing severe diarrhea or vomiting, with dangerous collapse.

Chronic Gout. Chronic gout is usually the sequel to several attacks of acute inflammation of the joints, but it may come on more insidiously in persons who have never suffered from such intense symptoms.

Chronic gout is associated with the deposition of chalky material in the neighborhood of the joints or tendons, and in time leads to marked deformity and loss of power. These deposits are composed of almost insoluble salts of uric acid; they accumulate gradually and may grow to very considerable size; their most common situations are the external ear, the large toe joints, and the backs of the hands, but they may be met with in any situation where tendons and ligaments are to be found.

These deposits are known as tophi, and when they are found they constitute an absolutely certain indication of gout.

When a joint bearing tophi in its neighborhood becomes inflamed, these deposits soften; as the attack subsides they again become hard and stony; sometimes they grow to such a size that the skin overlying them becomes stretched and ulcerates, exposing them. When this happens they exude a semisolid material whose chalky consistency accounts for the name chalkstones often applied to them.

Complications of Gout. No hard and fast distinction can be drawn between the symptoms of anomalous or irregular gout, about to be described, and those which might perhaps be regarded as complications of gout.

Chalk Nodules ulcerating through skin

AURAL TOPHI
The ear is a very common site of gouty deposits; these form little nodules known as tophi.

Skin ailments are very common in gouty subjects; they usually take either of two forms: they are an obstinate eczema, or an intense itching pruritus resembling nettle rash. The former condition often appears first in infancy, and may be very resistant to local treatment and recur again and again throughout life; the latter itching condition is more common after adult years have been reached.

Both of the conditions are apt to follow a mild dietary indiscretion, usually the taking of some animal or fish food for which the affected individual displays a peculiar intolerance. (See also Allergy, page 101.)

Dyspepsia is an almost constant manifestation of gout, it generally takes the form of an excessive acidity of the stomach juices, causing burning pain a short time after meals, tenderness on pressure over the stomach, a sense of fullness after taking food, and a tendency to flatulence. Less commonly the gouty patient is apt to suffer from periodical attacks of diarrhea with the passage of definitely acid feces.

Changes in the heart and vessels are very common complications of gout. The rise of blood pressure, which is so apt to occur, leads to hardening and degenerative changes in the walls of the smaller arteries and to an impairment of the nutrition and power of the heart, allowing some degree of dilatation to take place, with consequent weakening of the reserve force and the occurrence of palpitation and breathlessness on moderate exertion.

Closely connected with these changes are degenerative processes in the kidneys. It is possible that the altered chemical activities of the body that are responsible for gout throw an extra strain upon the excretory mechanism of the kidney cells and thereby induce early degeneration of these organs. Signs and symptoms of chronic nephritis appear to be among the normal consequences of gout, for whatever reason.

Preventive Measures. Treatment of the gouty state is necessary as soon as it is recognized, irrespective of whether acute symptoms have or have not appeared, for the condition is insidious in its onset, widespread in its effects and steady in its progress.

Treatments based on general measures, of perhaps small influence individually, can in combination accomplish much. They must include the enforcement of regular bowel action, adequate exercise, restraint of emotional indulgence, the habit of efficient sweating and sufficient sleep.

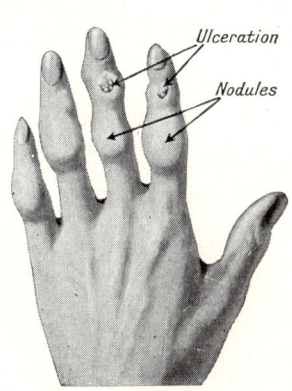

CHALKSTONES IN FINGERS
Chalkstones, tophi, or gouty deposits consist of urate of sodium; they may ulcerate through the skin.

Diet is important, but its value in the prevention and treatment of gout must not be overemphasized. Every case differs in some particulars from others, and due allowance for idiosyncrasy must be made, but certain well-established rules may be suggested. The gouty individual, as a general rule, drinks too little water and eats too much food.

Foods whose effects must be carefully watched in a case are all meats, eggs, starchy puddings, and sugar; most gouty people are well advised to cut their intake of these foods down to a minimum. All gouty persons must avoid glandular meat, such as liver, kidneys, and sweetbreads.

Potatoes are, perhaps, rather undeservedly under a cloud; many gouty subjects can eat them without ill effects. Tomatoes and cucumber, rhubarb, bananas, and strawberries are usually unsuitable for gout sufferers.

Alcohol is bad for gout; port is poison to the gouty, but light wines, such as hock and Moselle, are sometimes permissible. Dry wines and sparkling cider are harmful to most patients, but dry still cider may be taken by most without harm.

Medicinal treatment is of great value. Colchicum is useful, though its effects are not so rapid as in acute gout. As mentioned before, atophan or large doses of salicylates and bicarbonates may be effective.

Guaiacum resin is a valuable drug, as it aids in the removal of uric acid from the body. It can be obtained in capsules containing five grains each, and two of these should be taken two or three times a day.

For local treatment, in order to remove stiffness and pain, iodine may be painted on or the part rubbed with camphor liniment. Blisters are sometimes useful, or long-continued warm compresses; the application of great heat, by some method of electrical treatment or artificial sunlight, or by hot-air, vapor, or water baths is very useful and comforting. These treatments can be obtained at almost any spa and in therapeutic establishments in almost any large town.

Treatment of gout by brine baths is recommended, although it is open to question whether the salt content of the waters used has any real effect. What is helpful is the stimulating effect upon the sweat glands, the effect of temperature changes and physical applications to stiffened and painful parts, and the general tonic influence of a change in a pleasant and invigorating spa.

OBESITY

Obesity is the name given to the condition in which the body develops an excessive amount of fat. There are many races of the world in which a condition of fatness which we would consider abnormal is normal, or at least habitual. Among these are the Dutch and most Germanic races, Jews, and some native races of Africa and India. There is also a considerable element of heredity, and one is inclined to label people as belonging to either fat or thin families. The condition of obesity may arise at any age, but childhood and middle age are the most usual times for it to make its appearance, and women are more liable to it than men. This is easily understood when it is considered that one of the functions of fat is to store up nourishment, and woman's metabolism up to a certain age is designed in many respects to support another life besides her own. This condition of obesity is not necessarily a sign of disease, and may indeed be a proof of health, for fat deposited in the body denotes an active condition of the digestive organs. But it must be looked upon as a disease if it exists to such an extent as to interfere with the health, usefulness, and comfort of the individual; and if it will not yield to the ordinary dietetic measures of treatment. The common form of obesity due to simple overeating and physical inertia is dealt with in a later chapter. In the present section it is assumed that ordinary measures have failed and that the condition is due to some error of metabolism.

Most of the cases of obesity which are not the result of overfeeding appear to be due to some factor which is controlled by one or other of the ductless glands. Of these, the chief is the thyroid gland, and its effect on the fat consumption of the body is well known. When the thyroid is not functioning up to standard, that is, when the condition known as hypothyroidism is present, the basal metabolic rate is low and there is a tendency to gain weight. The typical case is myxedema, where the correcting of the error in the functioning of the thyroid gland, by administration of thyroid extract, results in an immediate loss of weight. In the opposite case of hyperthyroidism or over-functioning of the gland, there is a rapid loss of weight, as in exophthalmic goiter.

The next ductless gland in point of importance with regard to obesity appears to be the pituitary gland. When the pituitary is abnormal from birth the child may become a giant; when the gland is damaged later in life by some such occurrence as a tumor, characteristic changes take place in the metabolism, and the individual becomes fat abnormally, and in some cases where the fat is deposited on the breasts and hips the appearance of a male becomes feminine. The sex glands probably play a part in the production of obesity, since it is at the time that their function changes, as during a pregnancy or at the change of life, that many women tend to lay on fat. It is well known that the removal of the male sex glands produces obesity, as in the classical example of eunuchs. It is known also that the suprarenal bodies are concerned to a certain extent in the production of obesity.

Another type of obesity may be regarded as constitutional and is not well understood. Persons with this type become and remain obese with a diet which is far below that required for their physiological maintenance. There is no evidence of disease in any of the organs. All that can be said about this class of case is that there is some disturbance of the normal processes of energy exchange, and that this causes accumulation of fat.

Treatment. In those cases of obesity due to some disorder of one or more of the ductless glands, treatment by dieting has no effect, and the basal condition must be dealt with. Thyroid or other glandular extracts may be taken in some cases under the supervision of a doctor, but it must not be forgotten that such drugs are dangerous if wrongly used, and in any case careful watch must be kept for the onset of such symptoms as palpitation, sweating, tremor, faintness, etc., indicating that the glandular extract should be stopped or that the dosage should be decreased.

Formerly 2,4 dinitrophenol was widely used because of its potent weight-reducing qualities. Many fatalities were reported from its indiscriminate use (especially in proprietary preparations) so that at present it has practically disappeared from the therapeutic armamentarium.

In all forms of obesity a second line of treatment may be directed to increasing the metabolism of the body. Exercise in the form of walking, physical exercises carried out in the bedroom, swimming, golf, and gymnastics are all suitable, and should be carried on with great regularity, but carefully avoiding overexertion at first.

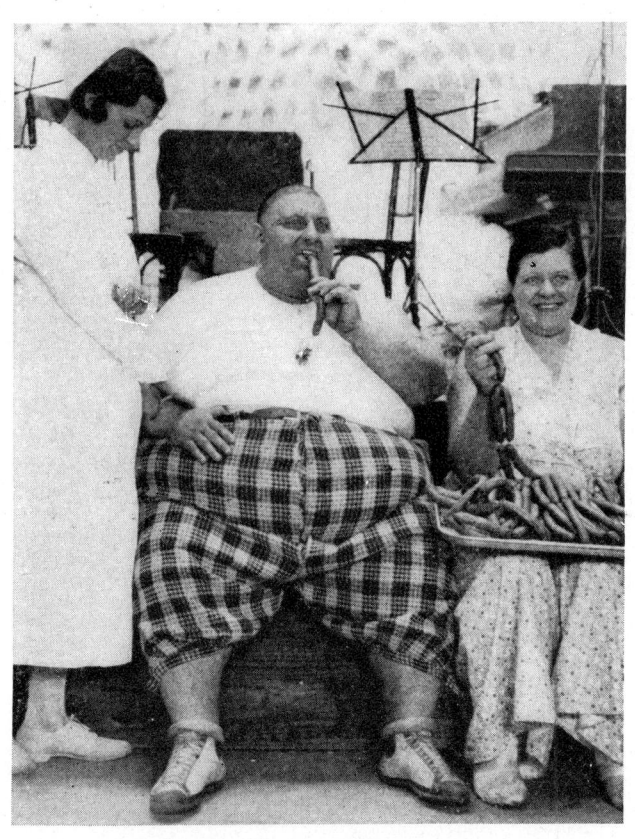

EXTREME OBESITY

This Philadelphia man weighed 950 pounds when this photo was taken. Although the food in the picture might truly intimate that he had eaten himself into this tremendous bulk, the usual cause of such extreme deviations is likely to be an abnormality in the functioning of some of the endocrine glands. © *International News Photos*

DIABETES INSIPIDUS

This is a chronic malady characterized by the passage of large quantities of normal urine of low specific gravity. It must still be classified with the diseases of disordered metabolism. Diabetes insipidus must be distinguished from diabetes mellitus, and from such complaints as Bright's disease and hysteria, which are also characterized by the passage of large quantities of urine. The disease is generally due to some interference with the secretion of the pituitary gland, or with the hypothalamus, but very little is definitely known. The interference may be due to injury or to a growth or to syphilis. In a number of these cases an affection of the eyes known as hemianopsia may occur. Various changes have been found in the nervous system, as, for example, tumors of the brain, and meningitis, or inflammation of the membranes.

The disease usually progresses in a gradual manner, but may come on rapidly, as, for example, after fright or injury. Its most prominent feature is the passage of a large amount of urine, with an increased thirst. The amount of urine passed may range from ten to twenty quarts in twenty-four hours; the specific gravity is low — 1001 to 1005; the color is very pale, but abnormal ingredients are seldom met with. Traces of sugar have occurred.

While there is an excessive amount of thirst, the appetite is usually good and sometimes excessive. The mouth is usually dry, and, moreover, these patients can tolerate a tremendous amount of alcohol. The skin is harsh and perspiration is slight. The patients, as a rule, rapidly lose weight and strength, but in some cases good health may be maintained for a very long period. The disease has been known to persist for fifty years, and finally cures may take place spontaneously.

Diabetes insipidus can be distinguished from diabetes mellitus by the absence of sugar in the urine, with a low specific gravity, and from Bright's disease (see Chapter 120, page 1686) by the presence of albumin and casts in the urine.

Treatment. It is important that the patient should lead a tranquil and carefree life. Injections of extract of the posterior lobe of the pituitary gland offer the most hope for the alleviation of symptoms but do not cure the disease. Some cases improve on large doses of thyroid gland. Syphilis must be looked for and treated. A liberal and varied diet should be allowed, and though no limitation should be placed on the amount of liquid drunk by the patient, tea, coffee, and alcohol should be avoided as far as possible. In some cases gradual reduction of protein and salt is useful. Finally nitroglycerine and large doses of antipyrine have been known to give results, but these in particular should only be used under medical observation, perhaps of specialists.

ACIDOSIS

Acidosis consists in the accumulation in the blood and body tissues of certain acids along with which a substance called acetone is found. Acetone is excreted in the urine and in the breath, imparting to these what may be described as a sweet, fruity odor. The acids in question are believed to be derived from a faulty metabolism of fat in the body in consequence of a scarcity in the tissues of glucose or grape sugar. This is excreted from the body in the urine of the diabetic in large quantities, and to prevent this the supply of starchy food in the diabetic diet must be severely restricted.

Often such a restriction as is necessary to prevent the patient from passing sugar results in a high degree of acidosis and a consequent danger of coma. This constitutes one, and perhaps the chief, difficulty in treating diabetes.

Acidosis occurs in other forms of tissue starvation. It is the cause, for instance, of what is known as delayed chloroform poisoning. A patient who has had chloroform for an operation comes out of the anesthetic all right, but, later suffers from incessant vomiting, becomes drowsy, and may lapse into unconsciousness and die. Acidosis is treated by attempting to restore the electrolyte equilibrium. This is best done by the administration of large amounts of normal saline solution. In diabetic acidosis, insulin and glucose are needed in addition.

A similar but much less severe or serious condition is of somewhat common occurrence in children, especially those of nervous, excitable, and wayward disposition. These children have considerable difficulty in digesting fat, and from time to time, unless carefully fed, a mild condition of acidosis is set up. The principal symptoms are those of the so-called "bilious attack"—pallor, vomiting, dark rings beneath the eyes, a coated tongue, drowsiness and fretfulness. There may be a rise of temperature. The breath and the urine have a pronounced disagreeable, sweetish odor which once perceived is quite unmistakable and immediately recognized.

It should be treated by confinement to bed, warmth, and quiet. While vomiting continues, drinks of sweetened water and fruit juices should be given freely, but no other food. If the water is vomited, then try giving some slowly by rectum through a funnel and small rubber tube. Glucose in doses of two or three teaspoonfuls to half a pint of water should be given by the mouth or the bowel, and half-teaspoonful doses of bicarbonate of soda every two or three hours may be also given. As the vomiting subsides, rusks, barley sugar, and cornstarch puddings made with water can be given, but milk and all fatty foods are forbidden until the attack has completely subsided. From one-half to one grain of alcohol at night followed by one-half to a whole seidlitz powder in the early morning is useful.

To avoid the attacks fatty foods, especially fried foods, should be limited, and extra sugar such as barley sugar or glucose given at meal times. Orange juice and other fruit juices should be given daily in good quantity.

Many grown-up people suffer from a chronic mild condition of acidosis quite apart from any tendency to diabetes. The body in health should have a considerable reserve of alkaline salts to ensure the proper alkalinity of the blood and tissues. This reserve may become depleted by a long continued diarrhea with the subsequent loss of alkaline salts in the feces and the lowering of the body's alkaline reserve.

Foods such as meat, sugar, bread, and fats tend to produce "acidity" in the body—others, such as the juice of fruits and green vegetables, increase alkalinity. The latter applies also to acid fruit juice, such as that of the lemon and grapefruit, the action being similar to that of dilute mineral acids.

ALKALOSIS

While acidosis may be said to be the result of decreased reserve of alkali in the body, with consequent upsetting of the normal balance between acid and base, there may be also the opposite condition, namely, alkalosis, in which there is either a loss of acid leaving normal unfixed alkali, or increase in the amount of basic alkali itself.

Sodium bicarbonate is the chief buffer of the blood against acidosis, and it is closely allied with the supply of carbon-dioxide gas. In alkalosis, therefore, any increase in the number of respirations per minute may be looked for as a primary cause. But so far as alkalosis is observed in the sickroom, the symptoms of irritability, with headache, lack of appetite, nausea, vomiting, loss of sensation, and very marked dryness of the mouth, mean that the natural supply of alkali has increased. In conditions accompanied by persistent vomiting, hydrochloric acid is lost through the gastric juices and a state of alkalosis results. Excessive ventilation of the lungs and ingestion of large quantities of alkalies *e.g.* too much sodium bicarbonate, are less common causative factors. Severe alkalosis generally results in tetany.

Treatment. Treatment here, as in acidosis, aims at restoring the electrolyte equilibrium of the body. Wherever possible the cause of the alkalosis should be eliminated. The administration of normal salt solution by a doctor or under his direction is the most reliable aid to recovery.

CHAPTER 95

DEFICIENCY DISEASES

Beriberi and Rickets—Prevention by Vitamins—Scurvy—Infantile Scurvy—Prevention of Scurvy.

BY this term is meant diseases which are due to the partial or complete absence from the diet of some element which is necessary to bodily metabolism, and more particularly to absence of vitamins. The best-known examples of deficiency diseases are rickets, due to deficiency of vitamin D; beri-beri, due to deficiency of vitamin B_1; scurvy, due to deficiency of vitamin C; and pellagra, believed to be due to deficiency of a vitamin provisionally known as vitamin G or vitamin B_2, (see Chapter 157).

The secret of scurvy was discovered long ago, before the name vitamin had been heard of. In those days it was noticed that scurvy broke out on sailing ships which had been away from land for considerable periods of time, and which carried no fresh meat or vegetables. It tended to disappear or become cured when fresh supplies were obtained. Experience showed that ships which carried lemon juice — called "lime juice" but actually obtained from lemons—were free from scurvy if the crew members were given a small quantity of the juice, each day.

Beriberi and Rickets. In the year 1897, Eijkman pointed out that beriberi, a disease characterized by neuritis and digestive disorder, could be prevented and cured by the use of hand-milled rice. Prisoners fed on "red rice" did not contract the disease, while those fed on white rice were very prone to develop it. The disease, in turn, could be cured by giving the whole rice. The germ of the cereal therefore contains some food factor in the absence of which the disease develops. This, however, is

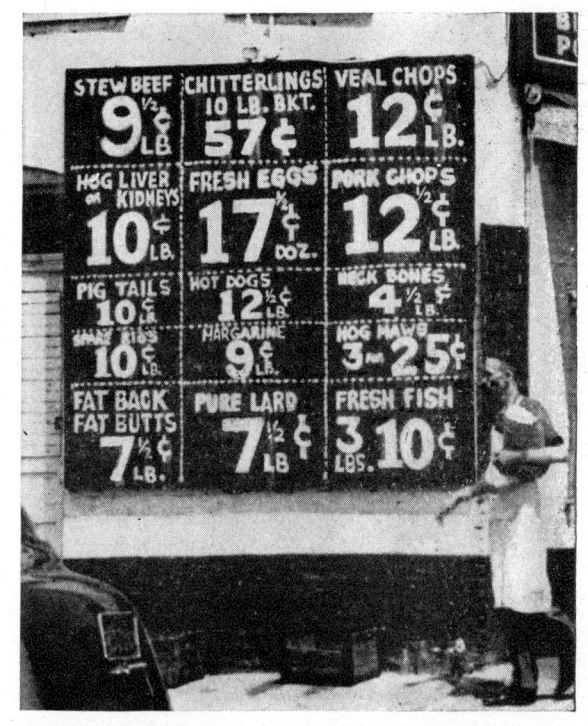

DEFICIENCY DISEASES WILL BE FOUND NEAR THIS SIGN
A grocery-store sign in Washington, D. C., in a low-income section. Some of these foods are almost wholly lacking in vitamins, and none are rich enough to supply normal bodily needs—unless the eggs chance to be fresh, as alleged. *Courtesy of The Washington Post*

(1299)

Lobulated Swellings

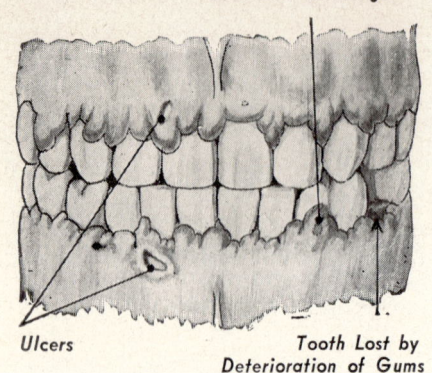

Ulcers — *Tooth Lost by Deterioration of Gums*

HOW SCURVY AFFECTS THE GUMS
In scurvy the gums are swollen and softened, fleshy masses occurring irregularly on the margins; often there is ulceration, and consequent on these changes teeth may drop out.

not the same factor as that which prevents the onset of scurvy, because no amount of fruit juice will take the place of the germ of cereals as a cure for beriberi.

The symptoms and treatment of rickets are dealt with in Chapter 196, while beriberi and pellagra are described among the tropical diseases in Chapter 157. Here we will consider the remaining deficiency disease, namely scurvy.

The work on beriberi led to the discovery of the nature of rickets—another deficiency disease. This study is one of the romances of modern medicine, thanks in large measure to the work of a group of English doctors, among whom Harriette Chick was prominent. It was found that rickets was due to diet poor in those vitamins present in animal fats. It was also found that even with the poor diet the disease would be prevented and cured by exposure of the children to good sunlight. The inference seemed to be that strong sunlight is equivalent, in its effect on the body, to the administration of animal-fat vitamins.

This idea has since been amply confirmed. It explains most of the past doubts and difficulties existing about rickets. That disease is prevalent in slums, because there food is inadequate as to quantity and furthermore is usually deficient in animal fat, while the smoky atmosphere deprives the inhabitants of the actinic or ultraviolet rays of the sun. They may, even when they get fats in their food, have those which lack vitamins—sowbelly, fatback, and salt pork, to cite a few examples, offer very little vitamin protection if they offer any. Thus slum children obtain too little fat and too little sunlight, and so suffer from a double deficiency. If they are supplied with the fat-soluble vitamins, or taken into the country and sufficiently exposed to sunlight, their disease disappears.

Animal fat, therefore, contains some quality in the absence of which rickets develops, and this quality is related in some way to the power of the sun. In countries where sunlight is plentiful the inhabitants avoid animal oils and do their cooking with olive and other vegetable oils; but in the Arctic regions, blubber and oil are staple articles of diet.

Prevention by Vitamins. To this food principle, contained in animal oil, the name vitamin D has been given. Vitamin B is the food principle contained in the germs of cereals. Vitamin C is the food principle contained in lemon juice and fruit juices generally. Any deficiency disease is simply prevented by securing the necessary vitamin-containing substances in the diet.

Exception for rickets, well-marked deficiency diseases are seldom now seen but they occur very frequently in a modified form. Defective growth, lowered resistance to infection, disorders of digestion, and nerve weakness can all be traced to a dietary lacking in one or other vitamin.

It has been repeatedly shown that most of the common diseases of civilized people can be produced in animals by a dietary lacking in these essential substances. Many people who believe that they are enjoying an entirely satis-

DEFICIENCY DISEASES

factory diet are actually suffering in slight degree from one or another of the deficiency diseases.

A diet consisting principally of meat and potatoes, white bread and white flour, margarine and sugar, is still much too common among people whose means could permit them a better diet; for such a diet is decidedly lacking in vitamin substances and needs supplementing with whole cereals, dairy produce, green vegetables, and fruit, both raw and cooked. The spectacularly bad diets—restricted to "hog and hominy," "grease and grits," salt pork and corn meal, spaghetti and salt fish—are frequently the accompaniment of poverty and of lack of information, and are less common in this country than in the recent past.

Children fed on patent foods, tinned milk, and other similar preparations are apt to lack vitamins, and so to develop rickets or other deficiency troubles.

SCURVY

As already noted, the particular vitamin concerned in this disease is that known as water-soluble vitamin C. It is discussed in greater detail elsewhere in this work and under the paragraph on treatment, so that it will here suffice to point out that it is present in largest amounts in fresh raw fruit and vegetables. As these could not be obtained and preserved during the long voyages of the sailing ships of olden days, the inevitable appearance of this disease is explained.

In adults mild conditions are indicated by anemia, lack of energy, failure of appetite, and a tendency to lose weight.

The onset is insidious, with progressive weakness, languor, and loss of weight gradually becoming evident. The patient may then begin to complain of bleeding from the gums, which are seen to be dark purple in color, swollen, spongy and sometimes even deformed by fungous excrescences. These local changes are often accompanied by loosening of the teeth, some of which may fall out. The breath is extremely foul and nauseating, and the tongue is likely to become swollen and red.

Hemorrhages form the outstanding feature of the whole picture. Bleeding from the nose is frequent, and blood may also be present in the sputum, vomit, urine, and bowels. Most commonly, however, the hemorrhage is most obvious in, and may be confined to, the skin. The skin itself becomes rough and dry, while tiny pin-point hemorrhages (petechiae) appear in the neighborhood of the hair follicles on the legs. These rapidly spread to the arms and trunk and often increase in size themselves. In severe cases the effusion strips the periosteum from the bones to form

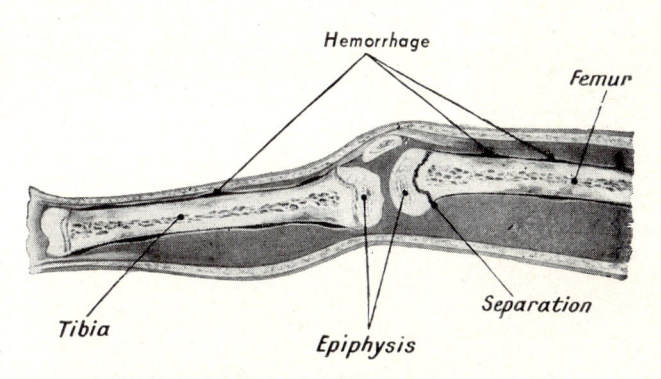

HOW THE BONES MAY BE AFFECTED IN SCURVY

In infantile scurvy hemorrhage beneath the periosteum of the long bones is a common event and is associated with considerable pain and tenderness. Separation of an epiphysis, as shown here at the lower end of the femur, is another possibility of infantile scurvy.

nodes which may extend to the surface and form foul ulcers.

In scurvy-sclerosis the whole of the subcutaneous tissues and muscles become so infiltrated with blood as to form a hard, solid-feeling mass. This is not common, but when it does appear it most usually affects the legs. More often, however, these are swollen around the ankles from the presence of edema. These severe injuries to the blood and blood vessels naturally involve the heart as well, and in this palpitation, irregularity, and feebleness of action are prominent. The appetite becomes more and more impaired as the soreness of the gums increases. Constipation also appears.

The early mental depression, headaches, and languor are gradually succeeded by delirium and convulsions as the patient gets worse. The bleeding may occur into the thin tissues covering the brain and spinal cord (meninges) and can also involve the eyes, so that blindness may result. As the disease advances, necrosis of the bones may occur, but effusion of blood into the joints is more common.

Despite the severity of the picture, the outlook is excellent so long as the causative conditions are brought to an end, and so long as the disease is not too advanced when first the patient submits himself for treatment. In the early stages it has to be very carefully distinguished from all the affections, such as the purpuras, which can cause similar hemorrhages into the skin.

Infantile Scurvy. While the above description applies to scurvy in adults, there is a very similar entity known as Barlow's disease, or infantile scurvy.

Onset occurs between the fourth and the fifteenth month of age in infants who are being artificially fed. These extreme periods are well maintained, as the supply of vitamin in the newly born child lasts some time, while the feeding on devitaminized milk or other defective food alone is very seldom carried on after the age of one year by even the most ignorant of mothers. During this period the processes of growth and development naturally modify the site and types of the hemorrhages, for these are still the outstanding feature of the disease. They now occur chiefly between the periosteum and the bone. Therefore an indefinite and rather obscure swelling can be felt deeply beneath the muscles of the limb. Similar extravasations occur at the ends of the bones, where the epiphyses are joined on, and these latter may become displaced thereby.

These changes give rise to extreme pain on movement, so that the child lies quietly with the legs drawn up. A change of position is never voluntarily carried out, and when this is effected by the nurse there is immediate and continuous crying. Indeed, the child often starts to whimper on seeing anyone approach it. The changes are nearly always in the lower limbs and but rarely elsewhere. The legs therefore become somewhat larger in bulk and later lie everted and motionless in a state of pseudoparalysis. The wrists, forearms, and shoulder blades may be affected, while the sternum or breastbone and the adjacent ribs may sink backwards bodily. Occasional thickenings appear over the skull and bones of the face.

Sometimes the bleeding occurs behind the eye so that this is forced forward and the surrounding lids are blackened. The conjunctiva may be infiltrated with blood. Anemia and weakness become marked, and at this stage a few small subcutaneous hemorrhages may appear, but they are far from common. Blood may be present in the urine and feces. The characteristic changes in the gums are never seen unless the child has teeth or is just on the point of cutting them. Even then only a little local purple puffiness is seen, but a large node of blood may in some cases appear on the hard palate. Very mild cases may show only pallor, loss of appetite, fretfulness, and failure to gain in weight.

Prevention of Scurvy. The prevention of this dietetic disorder lies, of course, in the consumption of a sufficiency of such foods as contain a supply of vitamin C, the antiscorbutic substance. In this respect the juicy fruits —orange, lemon, grapefruit, and raw tomato—are by far the most valuable. One ounce of the juice of these fruits in the case of adults and a quarter of an ounce for infants is sufficient, when taken daily, to protect against the disease, however deficient the rest of the diet in this substance. Other fruits are less valuable. Thus two apples or two bananas are necessary. Berries and grapes have little anticorbutic value. Raw vegetable leaves, as in salads, are very valuable sources. Of other vegetables, turnips are good in this respect, carrots and potatoes of moderate value. The cooking of vegetables impairs their vitamin value, but quick cooking by boiling is less harmful than slow cooking.

The addition of soda in order to retain the color of vegetables is very destructive of vitamin C.

Fruits and vegetables canned by modern methods do not lose appreciably in vitamin value. Lime juice is of uncertain value, some varieties being better than others, but never as good as lemon juice. Milk, even when unheated, is comparatively poor in vitamin C. An infant needs at least a pint daily and an adult about two quarts if milk alone is to be depended on to protect against scurvy. Heating it makes it still less dependable and so does the addition of citrate of soda. Infants, therefore, should be given orange or lemon or tomato juice when artificially fed. Germinating seeds are very rich in this vitamin. Meats, on the other hand, contain very little.

The treatment of the established disease lies in giving the fruit juices above mentioned in generous amounts. In marked cases it may be advisable to give concentrated preparations of the vitamin in the form of cevitamic acid. Other treatment is designed to be symptomatic and palliative.

CHAPTER 96

DISORDERS OF THE ENDOCRINE SYSTEM

Disorders of the Thyroid Gland—Goiter—Cause of the Condition — Treatment of Goiter — Exophthalmic Goiter — Cretinism — Myxedema — Disorders of the Suprarenal Glands—Addison's Disease—Other Diseases Affecting the Adrenal Cortex—Disorders of the Thymus Gland—Status Lymphaticus — Disorders of the Parathyroid Glands — Tetany—Excess of Parathyroid Action—Disorders of the Pituitary Gland—Acromegaly—Gigantism—Cushing's Disease—Infantilism—Thyroid Infantilism—Renel Infantilism—Pancreatic Infantilism—Frölich Infantilism—Sexual Infantilism — Rejuvenation — Transplantation of Testicles—Vasectomy and Vasoligature—Medication.

THE endocrine glands preside over the anatomical structure of the individual, and as certain mental and moral characteristics are now believed to be associated with certain types of physical conformation, these glands must be regarded as determinants of the general make-up of any given person. An outstanding example is furnished by the pituitary. Overactivity of this gland, especially of the anterior part of it, during the growing period causes an overgrowth of the bony skeleton, giving rise in extreme cases to gigantism.

The endocrine glands preside over growth, development, and nutrition of the body, including the brain and nervous system. They seem also to determine to a great extent the character and personality of the individual. The suprarenals, from their very intimate connection with the sympathetic nervous system, preside over the bony and muscular tissues, the large vital organs, and the purely animal functions of digestion, assimilation, excretion and reproduction; while the central nervous system, brain, and spinal cord preside over the higher functions and are dependent upon such endocrine glands as the thyroid and pituitary for their efficiency.

The substances secreted by the endocrine glands are called hormones. The influence on the endocrine system exercised by means of these hormones is of paramount importance. It presides over development and nutrition; it determines stature and temperament; it affects sex both as regards secondary sex characteristics and reproductive capacity; it furnishes our main defenses not

ACTION OF MAIN ENDOCRINE GLANDS

From the glands, which are distinguished by crosslines and are named, lines go out to various destinations, indicating the effects of the internal secretion of the gland in question. Although these effects are shown separated, it must be understood that they are not actually so.

only against microbes introduced from without, but also against poisons and toxins which are created within the body by the functioning of the ordinary process of metabolism.

Defects in the endocrine system are known to be responsible for disorders and abnormalities which used formerly to present insoluble problems. Such defects are, for example, the cause of gigantism, of dwarfism, of obesity, of feminism in men and mannishness in women. It is now thought that many cases of abnormal sexual behavior are due to disturbances of the endocrine system.

The disturbance of the hormonic equilibrium is the cause of severe nervous and physical troubles of the climacteric in women, and it is the gradual exhaustion of the endocrine system which accounts for many of the signs and symptoms of old age. Failure and disorder on the part of the endocrine glands are probably in many cases secondary to other conditions. These consist of focal centers of infection giving rise to blood infection which will influence these glands in common with other parts of the body. It is a vicious circle, since the effect on the gland further damages the body.

DISORDERS OF THE THYROID GLAND

Goiter. A goiter is the name given to an enlargement of the thyroid body, or gland. Goiters are of three main kinds —simple, exophthalmic, and malignant.

The thyroid, which is one of the ductless glands, lies in front of the windpipe in the lower part of the neck. It is a small, fleshy body weighing about an ounce, though this is subject to great variation even in health. It is closely applied to the larynx and trachea and moves with them.

Goiter is far commoner in women than in men, for the thyroid plays a greater part in the female organism than in the male. In fact, slight enlargement of the gland is almost a normal occurrence in young women at the monthly periods. Such a temporary swelling of the thyroid need not cause any anxiety, for it is, of course, not a goiter.

The condition called goiter, however, often arises in girls soon after menstruation is established and frequently persists throughout life. The swelling is quite painless, but is important for other reasons. From its close relation to the windpipe it may give rise to interference

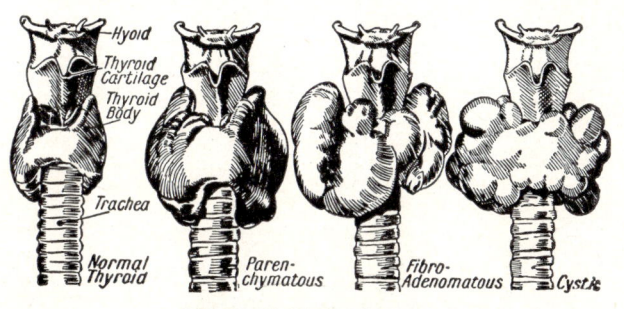

GOITER OF VARIOUS KINDS

The thyroid gland, the normal relative size of which is indicated on the left, may undergo general enlargement (parenchymatous), from fibrous and abnormal gland tissue (fibroadenomatous) or develop large fluid-containing spaces (cystic).

with breathing; it is often a gross disfigurement, and a simple goiter may cause symptoms akin to those of mild exophthalmic goiter.

As regards the difficulty in breathing, a goiter may reach a large size without inconvenience. Occasionally, however, a part of the tumor has grown down behind the breast bone and is thus prevented from enlarging forward; and it can only enlarge backwards by pressing the windpipe against the spine. In other cases the early onset of difficulty in breathing marks the onset of malignant disease in the goiter. In yet other cases the cause of breathing difficulty remains somewhat of a mystery. For the same reasons difficulty in swallowing may arise, inasmuch as the esophagus lies directly behind the windpipe.

The enlargement of the thyroid giving rise to goiter may be a general increase in the bulk of the gland with very little alteration discoverable in its structure; and it is possible such an increase in size is the response of the gland to some call for more thyroid tissue on the part of the body generally. Such cases are undoubtedly the most amenable to treatment. In other forms of enlargement, however, small tumors may arise in the gland, and the goiter is then seen and felt to consist of rounded projections varying from the size of a pea to that of an orange. Such tumors are called adenomata of the thyroid, and may be solid masses of cells closely resembling developing thyroid tissue, or cysts containing fluid. General increase in the size of the thyroid nearly always affects the whole gland; adenomata are more often localized to one part of it.

Cause of the Condition. That goiter is due to insufficient iodine in the food and water is now generally accepted. The disease is prone to attack the inhabitants of mountainous limestone regions, and thus it is very common in the Swiss and Himalayan valleys, and the valleys of other mountain ranges of less note. In America, goiter is most common in the Great Lakes regions and the northern Pacific Coast.

It has been shown that the cause is closely connected with the question of water supply, and the incidence of the disease has been proved to diminish when the inhabitants of a given district have added sodium iodide to the municipal water supply. An alternative prophylactic measure is the administration of sodium iodide either as tablets or in the form of iodized table salt. Where the natural water supply is deficient in iodine the common practice is to add iodine to the water twice a year for a period of two weeks.

Treatment of Goiter. Three lines of treatment are possible, namely, the administration of medicine, local applications to the thyroid, and surgical treatment.

When the tumor is due to uniform enlargement of the gland medicines offer a good prospect of cure, but they will require the supervision of the medical attendant. Iodine in some form is usually given, either alone or in addition to thyroid substance obtained usually from the sheep. The latter is obtainable in the form of tablets or as a liquid extract.

Thyroid extract is a dangerous drug, and sufferers are earnestly advised never to take it unless under the advice of a qualified doctor. They should also adhere strictly to the amount prescribed, for overdosage is liable to lead to thyroidism, a condition dealt with in Chapter 145.

When the goiter consists mainly of adenomata or cysts, treatment other than surgical is not often of much service. It is certain that the goiter as a whole will often diminish in size as a result of nonsurgical treatment, but often the individual tumors of which it is composed remain, to become prominent again when treatment ceases.

As regards local treatment, exposure to X-rays and to sunlight has given variable results, and should be regarded as invariably a shot in the dark. Sunlight treatment (see Chapter 42), in which the rays of the sun or sunlight lamp are directed upon the swelling, may be useful if the goiter has first been submitted to a good rubbing with an ointment containing iodine. X-ray treatment should not be continued unless improvement is immediate and obvious.

In any case, if difficulty in breathing is a prominent symptom it is wiser not to postpone operation unless nonsurgical treatment affords rapid relief, for the anesthetic dangers are increased by postponement, and the patient becomes less fitted to undergo the operation. When this is decided upon, the surgeon always leaves a portion of the gland untouched, as the removal of the whole results in myxedema. After an operation by a skilled surgeon the scar that remains is almost invisible, and the relief from the operation makes it a most gratifying procedure.

Whatever form of treatment is adopted, the general health of the patient must receive due attention, aside from pressure symptoms. The existence of a goiter may give rise to psychic disturbances which must be recognized and treated as such by the physician.

Hygiene and diet should be carefully adjusted. The importance of regularly evacuating the bowels cannot be overestimated. A diet rich in vitamin substance is indicated, with a minimum of animal flesh. A change of air, especially a visit to the seaside, is often of benefit, from the fact that sea air contains a proportion of iodine.

Malignant disease of the thyroid gland may take the form either of sarcoma or carcinoma (see Chapter 93), and for a long time may not extend beyond the capsule of the organ, but sooner or later it invades the neighboring parts; in the blood or lymph stream portions of the tumor may be carried to distant organs. Removal by operation is here the only treatment likely to yield to permanent results. Thyroid tissue is very sensitive to irradiation and this method is used postoperatively to prevent recurrences. It may be the only mode of therapy for advanced cases.

Exophthalmic Goiter. Also known as Graves', Basedow's, or Parry's disease,

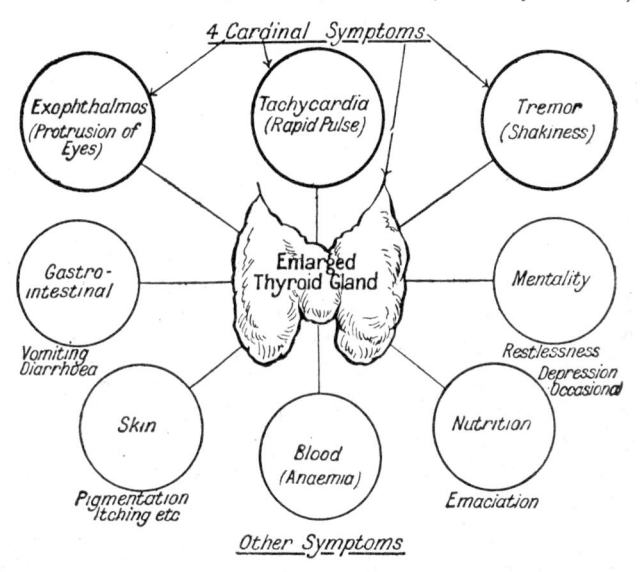

EXOPHTHALMIC GOITER: SCHEME OF SYMPTOMS

Enlargement of the thyroid gland, protusion of the eyeballs, a rapid pulse, and tremulousness are the cardinal symptoms of this disease, but other signs shown in this diagram are also met with. An excess of thyroid secretion only partially explains the disease.

exophthalmic goiter is a morbid condition due to abnormal functioning of the thyroid gland. The gland has not ceased to perform its work, but is producing an excess of thyroid secretion as a result of the increase in the number of functioning glandular units.

An advanced case of exophthalmic goiter presents a very characteristic appearance. The patient's eyes seem to be bulging out of his head. The eyeball is thrust forward; the white of the eye, uncovered by the lids, gleams in a most alarming fashion. The patient's whole face is dominated by this condition of "exophthalmos" or protrusion of the eyeballs. (Hyperthyroidism may, however, exist with very little or no exophthalmos.)

Nor is this expression of fear confined only to the face. The whole attitude of the body is one of anxiety. Thus there is always a fine tremor of the muscles. The rate of the heart is enormously quickened and the patient's skin is usually covered with perspiration. Intense nervousness is the rule, so that life becomes a heavy burden. Moreover, the flushed skin gives its owner a sensation of warmth even in cold weather.

In addition to these symptoms, swelling of the neck is usually found, in front, just above the top of the breast bone. This swelling may not be very large; indeed, it never approaches the size of an ordinary goiter. But it is almost invariably present and is usually quite obvious. This swelling is the enlarged thyroid gland. Other prominent symptoms are palpitation, undue rapidity of the pulse rate, loss of flesh as a result of the increased metabolism, and alternating nervous excitement and depression.

The actual nature of the disorder is not fully understood. the underlying factor which brings about the increase in thyroid activity is as yet unknown. One school adheres to the belief that a certain constitutional type predisposes to the disease. Psychic disturbances are known to play an important role. Some observers hold that the thyroid disturbance is secondary to influences arising elsewhere in the body. It is know that overstimulation of the sympathetic nervous system will produce all the symptoms of Graves' disease in an animal, and it has been suggested that the disease in man is primarily due to some cause acting as an irritant to this part of the nervous system. It is known that adrenalin, the secretion of the suprarenal glands, will act as a stimulant to the sympathetic nervous system and perhaps an abnormal secretion of this hormone is responsible for some of the symptoms.

Exophthalmic goiter may arise suddenly. There are many cases on record in which, immediately after a severe fright or shock, the symptoms showed themselves fully developed. In other cases the onset is more gradual. Infections also seem to play a part in causing the disease, prompt recovery occurring after subsidence of the infection.

Sometimes, again, the disease goes away as mysteriously and suddenly as it arose. And there may be relapses of as severe a nature as the original attack. Some of the patients never recover. Some of them become very seriously ill and die; some live to old age—even extreme old age—with their trouble fully active. About half the cases with proper treatment recover to a very considerable extent.

Mild forms of the disease show all the symptoms except the bulging of the eyes or the trembling. Indeed, a quick pulse and a slight swelling of the throat may be the only signs present. It must be remembered, however, that the thyroid gland swells slightly at certain times in the normal course of living. Thus it always tends to become a little larger during menstruation. During pregnancy it is usually swollen, and also during convalecence from some illnesses. As already stated, these enlargements are normal and need cause no anxiety.

Methods of Treatment. Operation seems still to be the most successful method of treatment, although some cases may derive little or no benefit from it. Since cases of the disease vary so greatly in the course they run, it is difficult to assess the value of various treatments adopted. Surgical treatment of the thyroid gland, either by tying off some of its blood vessels or removing part of the gland, has shown a very considerable success in the hands of surgeons who have specialized in this operation.

Short of this, the application of X-rays or radium has sometimes succeeded. Medical or palliative treatment consists of prolonged rest, treatment of any intestinal infection, and the use of small daily doses of iodine. The diet must be very carefully regulated and be very liberal in respect of energy-producing foods, namely, fats and carbohydrates.

A quiet life free from excitement of any kind and careful all-around living are of the utmost importance.

Cretinism. A cretin is a child who suffers from congenital absence or deficiency of the secretion of the thyroid gland. The disease occurs either endemically, *i.e.* in certain definite localities constantly, or sporadically, in any locality. It is common in the villages in the mountain valleys of Switzerland, France, and Germany, localities in which goiter is common. The parents of many of these endemic cretins suffer from goiter.

Up to the age of six or nine months nothing unusual about the child is noticed. Thereafter it will be observed that the child has ceased to grow, is dull, and takes little interest in his surroundings. The tongue is unusually large and tends to protrude. Later the skin is observed to be dry, the hair scanty, the face broad with flattened nose, and the eyelids puffy. No attempt at walking may be made, or, if the child learns to do so, he moves in a slow, waddling fashion. The eruption of the teeth is irregular and late, and they decay rapidly. Speech is late and defective, or absent. When the child is made to stand the abdomen is seen to be prominent with protruding umbilicus, and the back is much hollowed. Large pads of fat may develop above the collarbones. The hands are stumpy and spadelike, and the finger ends square.

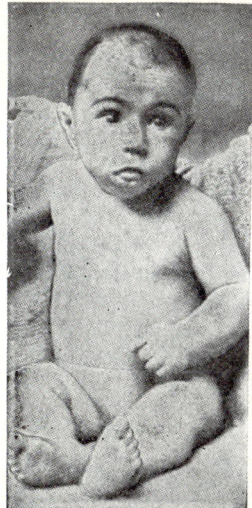

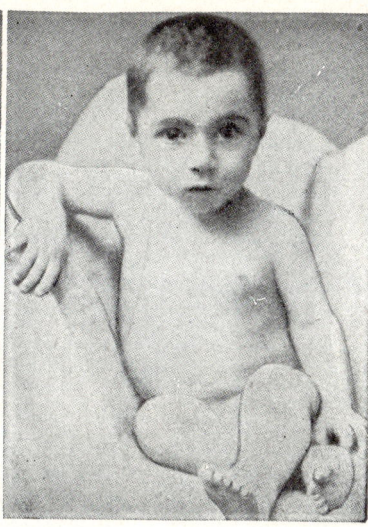

CRETINISM: A TRIUMPH OF MODERN GLAND TREATMENT
A child may be physically and mentally defective because of absence or deficiency of secretion from the thyroid gland in the neck (left). Right: the same case after regular doses of thyroid-gland extract. Below: reversion due to parents' mistake in discontinuing treatment. Further regular treatment would restore the child again to normal.
From "The Journal of Heredity," Baltimore

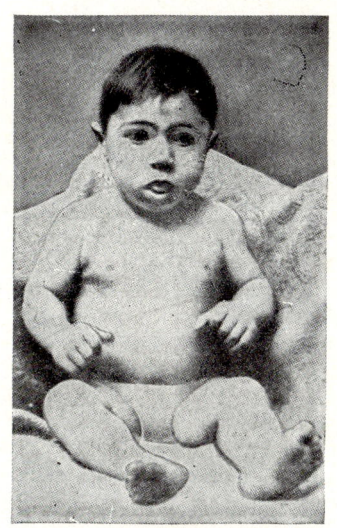

Unless treated, cretins remain stunted physically and are feeble-minded. Treatment consists in the continuous administration of thyroid gland or an extract made from it. If this is done early and no remission allowed in the taking of the thyroid gland extract, the child will immediately begin to develop, both mentally and physically, and will ultimately reach almost normal standard.

It is one of the triumphs of modern medical science that so many infants, formerly condemned to a life of idiocy, may now be compensated by the administration of regular doses of the dried thyroid gland and thus become normal human beings.

Myxedema. This is a condition having many manifestations, which is due to a deficiency of the internal secretion of the thyroid gland. It may occur as the result of illness in childhood, in which case development, both mental and physical, is considerably impaired, or, as is more usual, it may become manifest in later middle life. Like goiter, it is more often seen in women than in men, and is very common in mild degrees at the time of the menopause. The name was given to the condition by way of describing an appearance of edema or swelling of the body from infiltration of the tissues with a gelatinous mucuslike material.

Slight degrees of myxedema are very common, and are often missed owing to the slow progress of the changes to which they give rise; but when myxedema is well developed the appearance is unmistakable. Coarsening of features, growth in bulk, increasing slowness of speech, thought, and movement, together with a marked intolerance of cold, combine to form a group of symptoms that is produced by no other cause than thyroid deficiency. The face becomes bloated, with puffy swelling of the eyelids simulating the edema of Bright's disease; there is roughening of the skin and a change in complexion to a muddy, sallow tint except for a pink flush over the bones of the upper jaw. There is loss of hair from the scalp and eyebrows, especially from their outer parts, and a coarsening and lack of growth in the hair that remains.

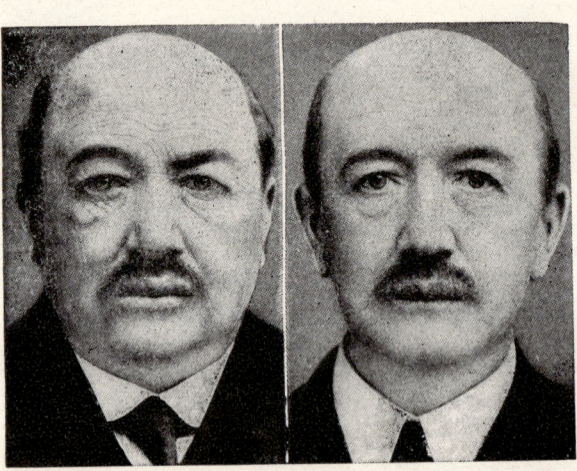

MYXEDEMA: THYROID DEFICIENCY
Left, the devitalizing effect of insufficient thyroid gland secretion, with the coarsened myxedematous features, is well seen. Right, the same adult after thyroid treatment.
Courtesy of The Editor of "The Practitioner"

There is a marked tendency for deposits of fat to form in certain situations, especially above the collarbones, in the abdominal wall, and in the breasts. The hands become spadelike owing to thickening of the fleshy parts of the fingers, and the whole conformation of the body tends towards a massive shapelessness. The action of the heart becomes feeble and slow, there is a persistent fall of blood pressure and a sluggishness of the functions of the stomach, the bowel, and the kidneys.

Causes of such a marked failure of thyroid activity include the effects of severe infective illnesses and abnormal growths and degenerations of the thyroid gland, but in many cases no definite cause can be assigned, and the condition must be regarded as a premature exhaustion of the gland.

Treatment by Gland Extract. The improvement that follows the administration of thyroid-gland preparations to such a case is startling. Under the influence of doses of dried thyroid gland of animals all the signs and symptoms may disappear and the unfortunate victim be restored to the appearance and reality of health.

So powerful are the effects of this remedy in these cases that there is some danger of thyroid-gland substances being given to excess. Their action must be closely watched, and when once definite improvement has set in it is often wise to reduce the dose and the frequency of its administration. Harmful effects that must be looked for are rapid heart action, with or without symptoms of distress, diarrhea, nervousness, flushing, breathlessness, and loss of sleep. But cessation of the treatment is followed in almost every case by a return of the symptoms.

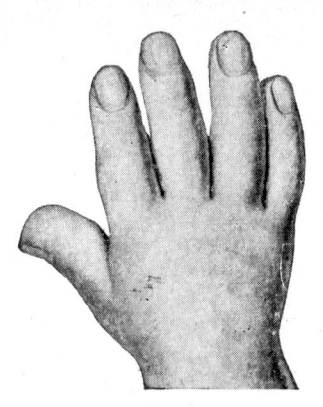

HAND IN MYXEDEMA
A broad, short, spadelike hand is characteristic of myxedema and occurs along with other changes, coarsening of the skin, etc., and with mental dullness.

At first the dosage is small, namely, two grains of the dried extract of the thyroid gland of sheep. If no symptoms of intolerance appear with such a dose it may profitably be increased gradually till the patient is taking ten grains a day, but such a heavy dosage should never be administered unless the patient is under skilled supervision. It is advisable to determine by experiment the smallest dose that will keep the myxedematous symptoms in abeyance and from that time forward to restrict the amount to this minimum.

DISORDERS OF THE SUPRARENAL GLANDS

Addison's Disease. Named after its discoverer, Thomas Addison (1793-1860), this is an example of the very grave illness which arises when the vital juices supplied to the body by certain small glands are not forthcoming, owing to deficient size, activity, or disease in those glands.

At the upper end of each kidney there is a small, flattened body of a yellowish color. These bodies are sometimes called the adrenal glands, but they are more exactly described as the suprarenal glands or the suprarenal capsules because of their shape and position. They pour the vital juice or essence which is formed in their substance into the blood as it flows through them, and this essence stimulates to activity the muscles of the heart and of the arteries, and thus helps to maintain the normal pressure of the blood in the arteries and to keep the muscles in tone.

This powerful drug, called adrenalin, is prepared from the suprarenal capsules of sheep, and its action on the muscles of the blood vessels is made use of in the control of hemorrhage.

If the suprarenal capsules are removed, death ensues from paralysis of the muscles which control the breathing apparatus; if they become diseased and so fail to supply their necessary secretions, a very grave train of symptoms sets in.

Failure of the adrenal cortex results in a general state of weakness; the heart's action is feeble and sufferers are easily tired. They complain of pain in the back and of indigestion, nausea, and vomiting. A curious pigmentation of the skin sets in, and this may be the first symptom noted; it varies from a light yellow to a deep brown color, and is always deeper on the exposed parts of the body and in those places where there is normally some excess of pigmentation. At first it may be noted on the face and hands only, giving them a bronzelike appearance. In the later stages patients may become very anemic and suffer from severe headaches, delirium, and convulsions. The disease occurs twice as frequently in men as in women, but is, however, distinctly rare.

The disease which affects and destroys the suprarenal glands is in the great majority of cases tuberculosis. The germs of tuberculosis find their way into the capsules and there produce destruction and degeneration, with consequent arrest of hormone producing power. In many sufferers from the disease other organs of the body are found to be affected by tuberculosis also.

There is, as yet, no known cure for Addison's disease. It is, however, possible to keep most patients in a reasonably good state of health through certain dietary measures. A high-calory diet, containing liberal amounts of salt and low in potassium, is now generally accepted. Adrenal cortical extract is most valuable, and often life-saving, in times of crises. In the more favorable stages of the disease it may or may not be of benefit.

Sufferers must be protected from all injurious influences. They should avoid strains and excesses of any nature.

Other Diseases Affecting the Adrenal Cortex. Of late there has been a great deal of fresh information obtained from research into the functions of the cortex of the suprarenal gland. The cortical portion may be overgrown or be the site of a tumor. In these cases signs of false hermaphroditism may be seen, but a common evidence is an interesting and almost unbelievable condition of premature adolescence called progeria. This is generally associated with congenital deficiency of the cortical matter, and the victim may be thin and wizened like an old woman, although her age may be only eight years.

In other conditions children are in possession of all the usual secondary sexual characteristics by the age of six or seven; the child may be excessively precocious. A similar condition arises in certain diseases of the pituitary body. Indeed, as will be observed later, many of the functions of the suprarenal gland and of the pituitary gland are closely allied.

In women, tumors of the cortex of the suprarenal gland lead to the development of male characteristics, such as the growth of a beard, the deepening of the voice, and increased muscular power. The mental attitude may change considerably, so that the former timid female may become the aggressive male. Recent reports in newspapers show that such cases are on the increase. Several women have succeeded in proving that they have actually turned into males. In many of these states, degeneration comes on at the menopause, with marked weakness and obesity. In some cases there have been successful operations which put an end to the threatening virilism and hirsutism as well as the changes in the sexual apparatus, and effected a resumption to the normal female state.

DISORDERS OF THE THYMUS GLAND

Status Lymphaticus. This condition, which is also known as lymphatism and as the status thymicolymphaticus, may fortunately be numbered among the rare diseases. It is most commonly present in infants, but is not unknown in young adolescents. The subjects are usually plump and flabby, with a pasty complexion and possibly some anemia. These appearances, however, are never sufficiently marked to prevent the child being regarded as in good health.

Death is often dramatically sudden, and this fact has called particular attention to the disease, for it is found in those victims who succumb readily to such trifling causes as the prick of a hypodermic needle. They take anes-

DISORDERS OF THE ENDOCRINE SYSTEM

thetics very badly, and so form a large percentage of those patients who die during operations. Occasionally there are preceding symptoms of heart failure and asthma. It is thus seen that the first possible knowledge of the existence of the affection is only too often gained too late. Some of the sudden deaths that occur during swimming, or in the course of convalescence from fevers, etc., are probably due to disorder of the thymus gland.

On examination the most important feature is found in the thymus. This structure is large at birth and lies just beneath the breastbone or sternum. Normally it shrinks and atrophies as the child develops, but in these cases it persists and may measure as much as four inches in length. This gland can then be felt during life in some patients, for it may just bulge up into the notch at the base of the neck. It can also then be detected by percussion and by means of the X-rays.

Three hypotheses have been offered to explain the sudden death. Pressure on the windpipe and the vagus nerve might occur, involvement of the latter causing the syncope. The idea of sudden and extensive clotting of the blood in the vessels is now generally discredited. It is possible that death is the terminal event of a chronic and unknown poisoning, a theory which is somewhat supported by the widespread enlargement of the lymphatic tissues, the condition which is alluded to in the two scientific names already mentioned—status lymphaticus and status thymicolymphaticus.

Fortunately, this is a disease out of which the child will generally grow, and many cases of successful treatment of status lymphaticus have been reported. General tonics, such as iron and arsenic, are given, and endeavors are made to cause an atrophy of the thymus by exposing that area to the action of the X-rays. It has been observed that the spleen enlarges if the thymus is removed or becomes atrophied, and in status lymphaticus this organ is found enlarged as well as the thymus.

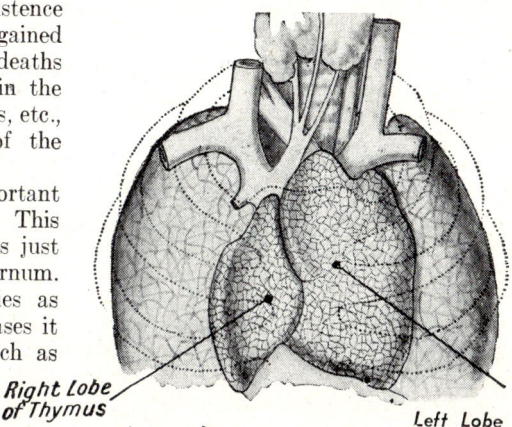

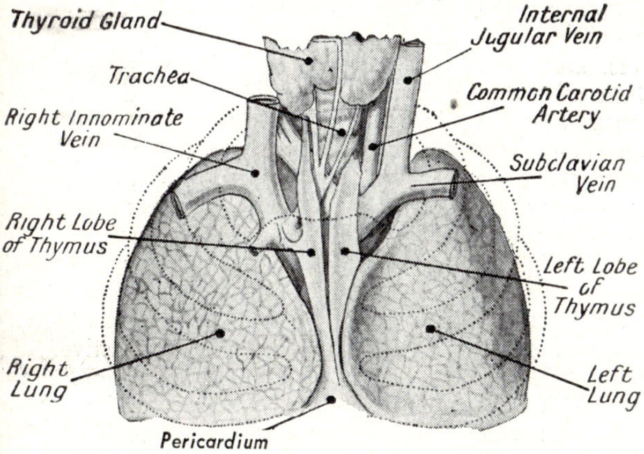

THYMUS GLAND: SITUATION, SIZE AND STRUCTURE
Above, right, the thymus gland of a child; it is a relatively large organ extending down into the chest behind the breastbone or sternum. At or before puberty it begins to atrophy and in the adult (lower illustration) it has almost disappeared.

DISORDERS OF THE PARATHYROID GLANDS

During the past ten years, great advances have been made in the understanding of the work of the parathyroid glands (see page 1304), which lie often unobserved in the substance surrounding the thyroid gland. Small though they may be, they are proved to be of inestimable value in the metabolism of phosphorus and calcium, two of the basic minerals of the body. When there is excessive output of the hormone of the parathyroids (parathormone) the calcium of the bones is absorbed, and the bones are thus left brittle and studded with minute pores.

Tetany. Lowering of the blood calcium leads to a well-known disease of children called tetany. In this condition, which is characterized by muscular spasms, the result usually of some atrophy or disease of the parathyroid glands, the metabolism of calcium is abnormal. Tetany may be allied to one of the infectious diseases and may thus be found in epidemic form. Sometimes tetany is found in mothers who have had several pregnancies with very short intervals between. Vomiting, diminution in acid with accompanying alkalosis, and general wasting of bottle-fed babies, usually form the preliminary picture of the disease. False croup may be one of the first symptoms.

When the case is fully established we find a typical posture of the child, who lied in bed with the forearms turned inwards in a spasm across the chest, while the hands are formed into a cone by the stiffening and approximation of the fingers. The legs are held in the extended position, but the toes are flexed on the soles of the feet, while the arches are raised. Sometimes there are spasms of the face, like those of lockjaw, but not quite so alarming. Depending upon the seriousness of the case, the spasms of the limbs may be maintained for several days, but they may be very transient—a few hours and they are past. Pulse and temperature may be raised. Sometimes a spasm may be set up by even very slight tapping upon the muscles.

Children usually recover when the digestive disturbances are rectified and when a carefully balanced diet is given. In the attacks it is sometimes necessary to give calcium chloride by intravenous methods, but the necessary elements may be given in foods such as milk, and especially foods which contain a good amount of vitamin D.

Indeed a substance has been isolated, called calciferol, which is for all practical purposes concentrated vitamin D. The latter has been proved to act not by stimulating the parathyroids, but rather by increasing the absorption of calcium. Apart from the concentrated vitamin D preparations, the best way to supply the natural form of vitamin D (irradiated ergosterol) is to give the child the foods which contain it. Milk is one of these.

Many authorities continue to advocate the giving of parathormone, although it is established that this acts merely by withdrawing bone calcium and using it as an emergency supply for the blood. Injections of parathormone are therefore given usually in very acute conditions, and they are then effective.

Excess of Parathyroid Action. A set of parathyroid glands working above normal limits may cause, as stated above, excess of blood calcium, rarefied bone tissue (osteitis fibrosa, or Recklinghausen's disease), and great cysts of bones with multiple fractures. Females are more susceptible than males. Large amounts of urine are secreted and there is excessive thirst. Ultimately the softening of the bones leads to widespread deformities, with pain. In these cases, the affected parathyroid glands should be removed, or at least the overgrown portions of them. Extra calcium, such as calcium lactate, is freely given, also parathormone, while vitamin D is also helpful to counteract the condition.

DISORDERS OF THE PITUITARY GLAND

In order to appreciate fully the various diseases which are based on abnormalities of the pituitary gland, some accurate estimate must be made of the importance of this small body which lies on the Turkish saddle of the sphenoid bone, about the size of a bean and almost smothered by the great mass of the cerebrum above. In that minute gland there are actually centered the powers of reproduction, of the fundamental instincts of sleep, hunger, and thirst, of development, of nerve control, and of the emotions. The pituitary gland is, in fact, the chief member of the endocrine system.

Of the three lobes, the anterior contains two different kinds of cells — eosinophil and basophil. It is unnecessary to go fully into the complex physiological chemistry of these cells, and it will suffice if we remark that when the eosinophil cells are excessive, the overproduction of hormone causes a disease, acromegaly, described below. When the hormone is too active in infants, they become giants in a very short time (see illustration on this page); on the other hand, the disease progeria, already mentioned in connection with suprarenal disease, is associated with eosinophil hormone deficiency.

The basophil cells control the development of the sexual characteristics, and puberty can be explained by the careful adjustment of the eosinophil and basophil cells just as the acids and alkalis of the tissues are measured one against the other. Up to the age of fourteen it is presumed that the eosinophil cells have the mastery; after that the basophil cells take command. By knowing these simple points, we can readily understand and make allowances for many of the abnormalities of precocity and backwardness of both physical and mental quality.

The rhythm of sexual activities is apparently controlled by two hormones, now known as prolan A and prolan B. It is known also that certain neutral cells found in the anterior lobe have some connection with obesity. Other hormones present affect the thyroid, the suprarenals, the pancreas, and the parathyroids.

From the posterior lobe there is produced a secretion which contains at least two great hormones. One is called

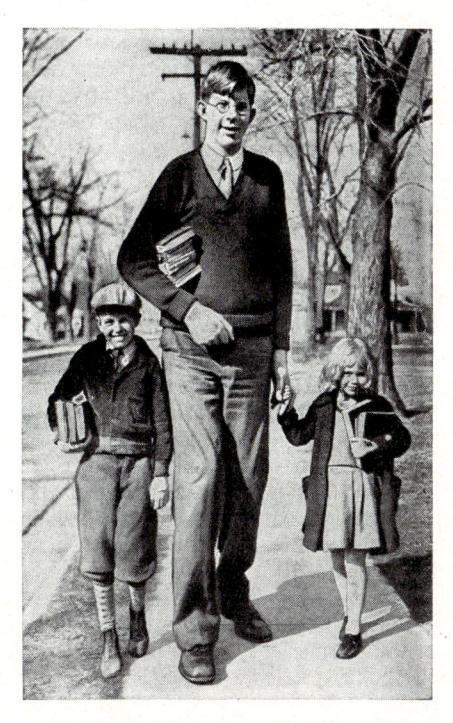

GIGANTISM: A YOUTHFUL EXAMPLE

Robert Wadlow of Alton, Illinois, was perhaps the tallest man of authenticated record. Born February 2, 1918, he was eight feet eight and one-quarter inches tall and weighed 491 pounds on his twenty-first birthday, in 1939, according to a magazine article published at that time. He was about an inch taller at the time of his death, July 15, 1940. This picture was taken when he was fourteen years old and seven feet five inches tall. He was regarded as an example of the type of gigantism which results from overstimulation of the pituitary gland at the base of the skull.

pitressin, and is known to raise the blood pressure as well as to stimulate the kidneys, and is thus used largely in shock and similar conditions. The other is called oxytocin, and is of superlative use to obstetricians, since by its local action is stimulates the uterine musculature to contract. When administered following delivery, oxytocin greatly lessens the danger of post-partum hemorrhage.

While it is possible to divide the diseases of the pituitary body into those which depend upon hyperpituitarism and hypopituitarism respectively, the symptoms are so intermixed and so dependent on other gland activities that few very clear types can be discussed, and these are possibly only in highly technical works for the most part. Nevertheless, there are one or two which show marked symptoms easily recognizable, and these may now be dealt with. It should be appreciated by all, however, that one outstanding evidence of pituitary trouble is the associated psychological abnormality, this being due to the functions of the gland mentioned above. So far we are only on the fringe of understanding a great emotional and functional controller, and much light is to be expected from researches now being pursued.

Acromegaly. There is no more striking example of the powerful influence of what are called the ductless glands of the body than that which is shown by acromegaly. The hands, the feet and the face, notably the bone of the lower jaw, become enormous, and a normal individual is transformed into an ill-proportioned giant. It has, in fact, been recognized that many circus giants are acromegalic, pituitary enlargement having been discovered after death in past examples. The nostrils, the ears, and all the soft parts of the face grow to an abnormal extent, and the eyelids become thickened. The skin is coarse and flabby. In the later stages of the disease curvature of the spine and wasting of the body occur. Women are more commonly affected than men, and it is, as a rule, about the twenty-fifth year that the symptoms are first noted.

There is no known cure, although in some cases, removal of a portion of the glandular growth by surgical operation has proved of value. This is especially so in cases where pressure symptoms

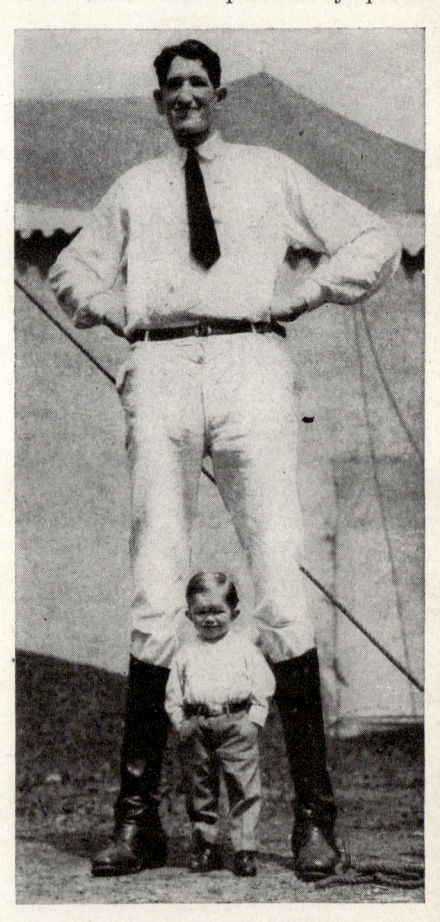

GIGANTIC AND TINY

These two circus performers are at or near the extremes of size in human beings. The giant, Jack Earle, is said to be eight feet seven inches tall; the small man's height is said to be twenty-three inches; he is known as Major Mite. Biologists and doctors find much valuable information, applicable to people of normal size, through the study of extraordinary individuals.
© *Ewing Galloway*

have developed. The progress of the trouble is slow, defects of vision are not uncommon after the disease has become well established, and headaches and general weakness are frequent accompaniments of the condition.

Gigantism. This term refers to an overgrowth of the bony skeleton that seems to have an intimate relationship with acromegaly.

About one-fifth of acromegalic patients may be regarded as giants, and many of the so-called giants described in literature were really sufferers from this disease. Though it has been assumed that these two conditions are really the same, and therefore that gigantism would be the acromegaly of youth before the ends of the growing bones have become united with the shafts, it is possible that gigantism may be due to some abnormal nutritional disturbance which creates a ready soil for the development of acromegaly.

Cushing's Disease. In this disease, due to excessive activity of the basophil cells of the anterior part of the pituitary body, the symptoms are such that once recognized they cannot be forgotten. There is an abnormal obesity affecting chiefly the face, which may be twice the usual size and very red owing to the presence of abnormal amounts of blood in the facial tissue. Blood pressure is raised, and abnormal genital conditions and unusual growth of hair may be

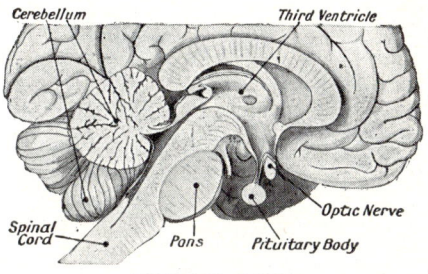

PITUITARY BODY

The pituitary body, here shown in section, consists of two main subdivisions connected by a third or intermediate part. The posterior part is a direct extension from the brain.

found. Generally there is sugar in the urine. Women begin to look like men, in a manner very similar to that of the diseases associated with overgrowth of the suprarenal bodies already discussed. The only treatment of any use appears to be that of deep X-ray doses.

INFANTILISM

This is an abnormality of development, the subjects of which bear with them into adult life the physical characters of childhood and usually some of the mental characteristics as well. Though infantilism has much in common with cretinism, dwarfism (whether rickety or achondroplasiac), and some types of imbecility such as "mongolism," the term is better reserved for special instances of arrested physical and mental development of different origin from the foregoing.

The arrest of growth may be due to one or more of several causes, may occur at any age of childhood, and may or may not prove amenable to treatment. While growth and development are inherent functions of all young tissues, this primitive "urge" may be adversely affected by many of the circumstances that influence the growing animal. Such influences include the provision and correct assimilation of necessary food substances, the subtle action of vitamins, the harmonious interaction of the ductless glands, and adequate exposure to the energy-producing rays of sunlight. When the condition of infantilism arises, a failure of one or other of these agencies can be blamed; the hope of cure lies in the detection of the harmful factor. Mention has already been made of progeria, and of other defects of growth due to interference with the concert of the hormones.

Thyroid Infantilism. Thyroid infantilism is one of the most common: its features are not those of gross physical and mental aberration such as are familiar in cases of cretinism and myxedema; rather are they a mere uniform absence of growth associated aften, but not always, with a retardation of mental development due to impairment of thyroid activity. The typical infantile person preserves, after the 'teens are passed, the physical stature and conformation of a young child in whom the secondary sexual characteristics have never appeared.

Renal Infantilism. Renal infantilism is due to the onset of chronic kidney disease in childhod; its victims are stunted physically and mentally, their skin is harsh and dry, they are delicate, and they are liable to succumb early to any infection.

Pancreatic Infantilism. Intestinal or pancreatic infantilism is due to diseased conditions of the bowel and of the digestive glands that interfere seriously with the adequate absorption of food; it is seen in quite young children of all classes and constitutes a very difficult problem in management. If appropriate measures are adopted early this form of infantilism is curable.

Frölich Infantilism. This is associated with defects of the pituitary gland. The outstanding sign is marked obesity in the young, especially in the pelvic and shoulder regions. Very often the sexual organs are rudimentary. Hair is scanty and the secondary teeth may be delayed. Treatment may be successful if pituitary extract is carefully given.

Sexual Infantilism. Lack of development of the testicles or ovaries may also bring about physical or mental infantilism or even both. The term infantilism is used by sexologists to refer to persons who, on account of organic deficiency of the sexual organs, are unable to carry out coitus or are unable to fertilize (male) or to be fertilized (female). They also use this term to describe that sexual abnormality in which sexual desire, instead of being directed towards mature persons, is directed towards children. This distressing, and for the community dangerous, abnormality may cause grave psychological harm to the child who is subjected to it. Persons suffering from this abnormality should be put under the care of a competent medical sexologist. A still further type of sexual infantilism is found in individuals who are only attracted by senile or senescent persons. This type is exemplified by some young men who marry old women, or vice versa, though of course some such marriages are due to such other factors as money or fame.

REJUVENATION

Attempts to find an elixir of life whose power will restore the failing vigor of the aging mind and body probably preceded civilization. With increasing knowledge of the subtle interplay of the various glands and organs of the body, the search has come to be concentrated upon essences and extracts of the glands whose importance is now so clearly recognized.

In the modern use of such substances mankind is following in the footsteps of medieval ancestors to whom concoctions of the blood and bodies of lower animals and reptiles were familiar and potent drugs. Whereas, however, the old remedies savored of magic and conscious or unconscious imposture, it may be said that at the present day animal drugs are given with some knowledge at least of their effects and in the legitimate hope that these effects may be forthcoming and prove of benefit to the patient.

Since the day of Brown-Séquard, who, experimenting upon himself, found that injections of testicular extract of animals renewed his mental and physical vigor after he had passed his three score years and ten, a vast amount of patient investigation and research has been done upon similar lines: much of it has been sterile, much has been inconclusive and disappointing, but a certain amount of truth has been revealed and appreciable progress has been made.

It is natural that search for a permanent invigorator should begin with the fountain of virility, the male generative gland. The cells of the testicle are of two kinds; the bulk of them line the tubules and discharge into them the sperm cells—the living elements of the seminal fluid; the others lie between the seminal tubes and play no part in generation. It is probable that these cells are responsible for the secondary sex characters, and that through their activity substances are discharged into the blood stream which excite the beneficial functions of the whole group of ductless glands. When the atrophic changes of age occur, the process is not necessarily equally progressive in these two types of cells.

Transplantation of Testicles. Upon this fact are based the transplantation methods which have been adopted toward off the general changes of old age. In Voronoff's method healthy testicles of a young and vigorous ape are grafted into the abdominal or scrotal cavities of a man. If the operation is performed under conditions of rigid asepsis such grafts may take; the implanted organ becomes permeated by new blood vessels and continues to live for a longer or shorter period. In these cases the germinal cells of the graft atrophy, but the other group of cells may retain their function. This is the much-discussed monkey-gland treatment. Its results are often nullified by failure of the graft to acquire a new blood supply. In successful cases its results are short-lived; for a time striking return of vigor may be seen, but gradually the graft, as is the fate of all tissue grafts in the body, is invaded by fibrous tissue and loses its function.

In Steinach's method, the gland which is transplanted is taken, not from an ape, but from a young, healthy, vigorous man. The graft has a much better chance of "taking," and the results are more favorable and more lasting. In women, ovaries may be grafted in a similar way.

Vasectomy and Vasoligature. A less serious operation has been devised with a somewhat similar aim. It has long been known that if the duct which carries the testicular secretion be divided or occluded, atrophy of the germ-producing cells takes place, while the internal secretory cells remain intact or may even increase in size and function. Steinach's operation of section and ligature of the testicular duct has now been performed in a large number of cases; its results in many have been encouraging.

While it must be said that neither of these operations has fully justified the hopes of their originators, they are of sufficient benefit in some instances to make their consideration worth while.

Medication. Drugs to be taken by the mouth or by injection under the skin are numerous; they are mostly combinations of organic substances formed in the healthy body by its glandular and other organs. Lecithin, a product of nerve activity, is an important constituent of most; spermin or didymin, derived from the testicle, is found in many. For the use of women, extracts of the ovary, the corpus luteum, or the mammary gland are obtainable, and their use is sometimes followed by striking improvement in the appearance, bodily vigor, and mental alertness of aging women.

It must be confessed, however, that treatment such as this is in the experimental stage. Those best qualified to express an opinion are least dogmatic in their statements and the first to admit that our knowledge of the nature of these extracts and of their mode of action is still very small. That longevity can be encouraged by attention to the simple rules of health is true, but that the appearance and attributes of vanished youth can to any extent be restored by drugs must be regarded as improbable.

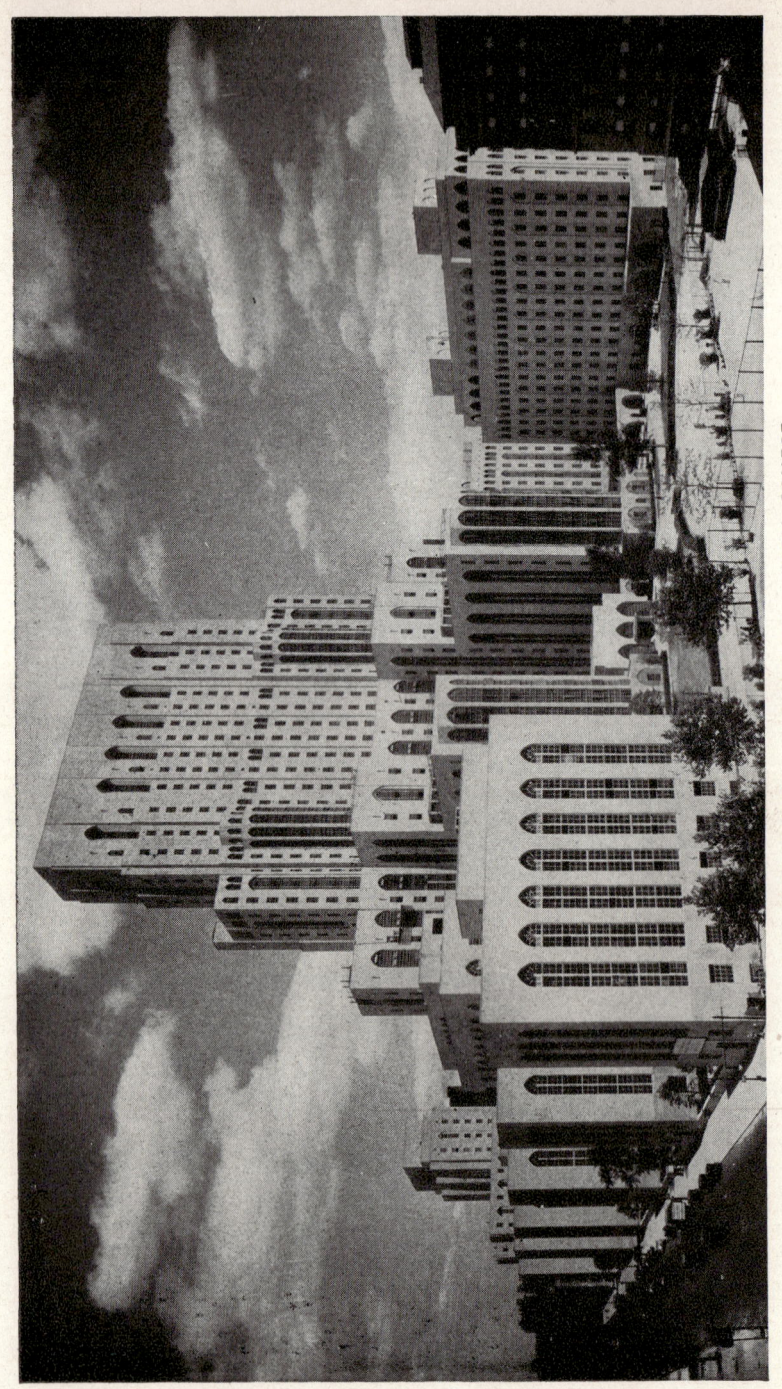

NEW YORK HOSPITAL AND CORNELL MEDICAL COLLEGE

Proper teaching of the arts of nursing and healing is furthered by the location of medical schools in large cities, where hospitals have a great number and variety of cases of sickness and injury. Thus Cornell University, at Ithaca in western New York State, maintains its medical school in New York City in connection with New York Hospital in these impressive buildings.
© *Ewing Galloway*

Section XIII | Infectious Diseases

CHAPTER 97

INFLAMMATION AND FEVER

Inflammation — Symptoms — Treatment — Fever — Manifestations—Course of an Attack—Management—Diet in Fever—Methods of Reducing Temperature—Use of Drugs — Artificial Fever.

THE subject of inflammation is one of the greatest importance, since the condition is met with so usually in all forms of disease. It is the reaction of the tissues of the body to anything that is irritating them, and is therefore one of nature's modes of defense against injury of any kind, infection by germs, damage by burns, etc.

Inflammation. The affection starts by being a purely local condition, characterized by the four symptoms of redness, swelling, heat, and pain, but after a time is liable to develop general symptoms affecting the whole body, and known collectively as fever.

All those conditions which lower the vitality of the whole body or any part of it, or interfere in any way with its healthy nutrition, must be considered as predisposing causes of inflammation, for they lessen its power of self-protection and render it vulnerable to the attack of any of the exciting causes. One of the best examples of a predisposing cause is that of exposure to cold, which may act either locally or generally. The exciting causes of inflammation are too numerous to mention, for they include all forms of injury and all sources of irritation. Among them are mechanical violence, chemical irritants, extreme degrees of heat and cold, and, more important than all, disease germs. The part played by microorganisms in producing inflammation has long been known, but the lessons learned in the First World War have had such an influence on the minds of scientists that some of them maintain that there can be no inflammation without the presence of germs. This has not, however, been proved, though it is considered by most authorities to be a true statement, with some few yet not unimportant exceptions. Germs are known to be present in the great majority of cases of severe inflammation.

Although inflammation must be looked upon as a disease, with definite causes and symptoms, it is most important to understand that, unlike diseased conditions in general, it has often a distinctly benign consequence, and is nature's method of repairing an injury, healing a wound, and bringing about a cure. No wound or injury can be healed without the occurrence of some inflammation: indeed, no bleeding can be permanently checked without it. When an artery is cut the loss of blood from it may be temporarily checked by the formation of a blood clot, or by the application of a ligature by a surgeon, but it is only by nature's reparative process, produced by a form of inflammation, that the recurrence of bleeding is prevented and the opening permanently sealed. The edges of a wound in the same way are fixed together, and the loss of structure caused by an injury is made good by the processes which follow inflammation.

The best way to explain what takes place in inflammation is to describe the cause of its four characteristic symptoms.

Symptoms. The redness is due to a great increase of the amount of blood in

Rapid flow of Blood, dilation of vessel

Exudation of Lymph

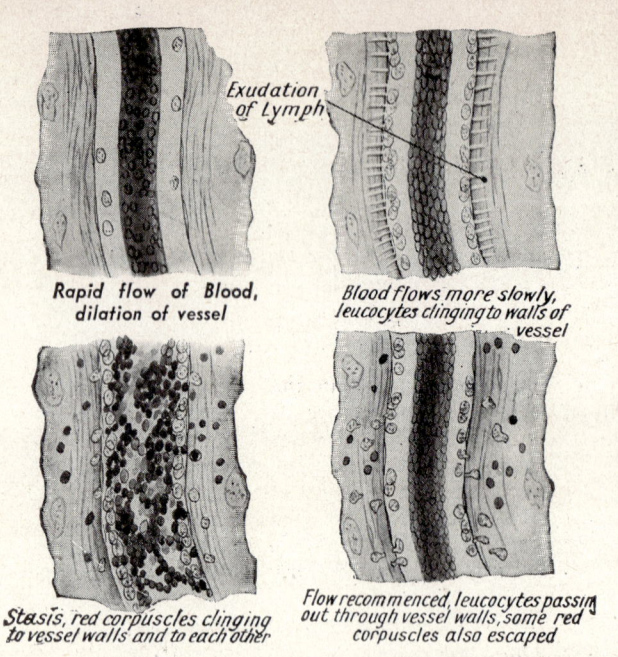

Blood flows more slowly, leucocytes clinging to walls of vessel

Stasis, red corpuscles clinging to vessel walls and to each other

Flow recommenced, leucocytes passing out through vessel walls, some red corpuscles also escaped

STAGES OF ACUTE INFLAMMATION

The blood vessel dilates as the circulation is quickened (above, left); the flow then slows (above, right), when white cells migrate and lymph oozes out. Next comes stasis (below, left), when migration ceases but red cells are squeezed out. The blood flows again (below, right) and there is migration and oozing of lymph.

the vessels of the inflamed part. The vessels dilate and become full of blood, a condition which is termed hyperemia, and the circulation is carried on more rapidly. But this is soon followed by a slowing of the flow of blood; the white blood cells, which have assembled in great numbers, appear to grow "sticky," and cling to the wall of the blood vessel, and the watery part of the blood soaks out of the vessel into the surrounding tissues. This is succeeded by a most interesting phenomenon, which is called diapedesis: the white blood cells clinging to the wall push out processes into and then through it, and finally follow the processes bodily and collect in large numbers outside the vessels. This oozing out of fluid and cells causes the next symptom, namely, swelling, and forms what is called the inflammatory exudation. The symptom of heat is due to the increased amount of blood in the part, and the pain to the pressure exerted on the small nerves by the exudation.

The course taken by inflammation varies. The exudation may gradually be absorbed, the blood supply become normal in amount, and the part affected resume its natural condition. This is called the resolution of inflammation, and is the course taken when the irritation has been slight or the wounds small and free from microbes.

If the inflammation has been more severe, or if microbes have entered the wound, a far larger number of white cells are called to the scene of action, and they collect in large quantity and, together with the débris and general wastage of the disintegrated tissues, form pus. The condition is then called suppuration, and the collection of pus is called an abscess. The pus has to find its way to the surface and discharge, or has to be let out after an incision has been made for the purpose.

In some cases the skin or the mucous membrane is the seat of inflammation, and the surface is destroyed; discharge is then formed which runs away, and the sore surface is called an ulcer, the inflammation being said to terminate by ulceration. New skin or membrane is gradually formed, and the ulcer heals, leaving a scar behind.

In severe injuries there is much destruction, the inflammation is excessive,

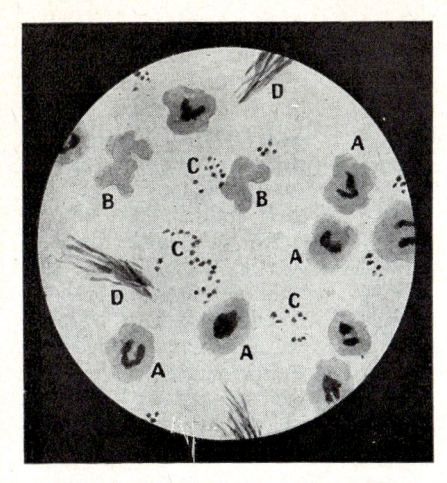

INFLAMMATION AND FEVER

PUS: MICROSCOPICAL APPEARANCE
Fresh pus when examined under the microscope is found to exhibit a large number of dead leucocytes (A); but one or two leucocytes (B) may be seen to manifest ameboid movements. Fragments of dead tissue, (D) and bacteria (C) may also be present.

of blood corpuscles, white and red, blood fluid or serum, and fibrin. It is called plastic lymph, because it forms new structures. It may break down into pus, or may form fibrous tissue or bone, according to the part injured. If the inflammation is in the pleura, pericardium, or peritoneum, the lymph sticks the opposing surfaces together and forms bands or adhesions; if it forms on the valves of the heart it produces little outgrowths, called vegetations.

Again, in inflammation of the serous membranes, of which the pleura is an example, the exudation is both solid and fluid, but the latter may be in great excess and cause a large collection, called an effusion. It is an effusion of fluid which causes the great swelling of joints when inflammation is set up in them by sprain or wound. This also occurs in and large portions of tissue die. This is called gangrene, or mortification. Gangrene is divided into two types: dry gangrene and moist gangrene. In the dry type, which is produced by interference with the blood supply to a part of the body, the dead part shrivels up and becomes dry, hard, and wrinkled. In the moist type, germs have entered into the weakened part, and it becomes inflamed and swollen; putrefaction usually sets in. During the First World War large numbers of wounds became infected and gangrenous, and it was discovered that the infecting germ was a bacillus which had been discovered by the late Dr. Welch, of Baltimore, and was called *Bacillus welchii* after him; it is also called the gasgangrene bacillus. This same germ is now known to cause acute inflammatory trouble in the various organs of the body when it is present in them.

There are a few more points of interest regarding the exudation which is formed around the vessels, and which consists

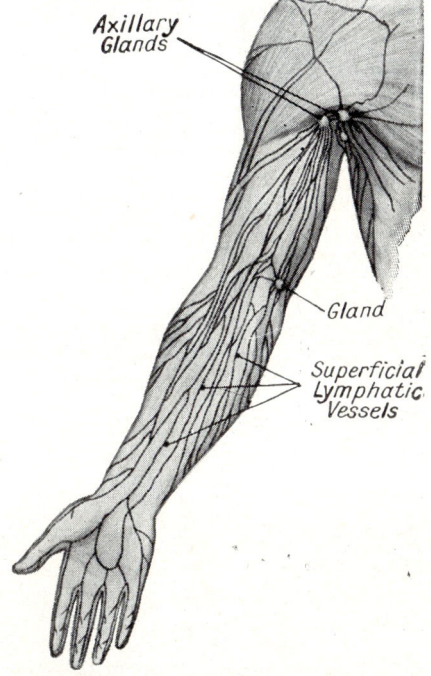

ADENITIS
Inflammation of the lymph glands, known as adenitis, may occur in the armpit by reason of poison from a septic finger traveling along the lymphatic vessels.

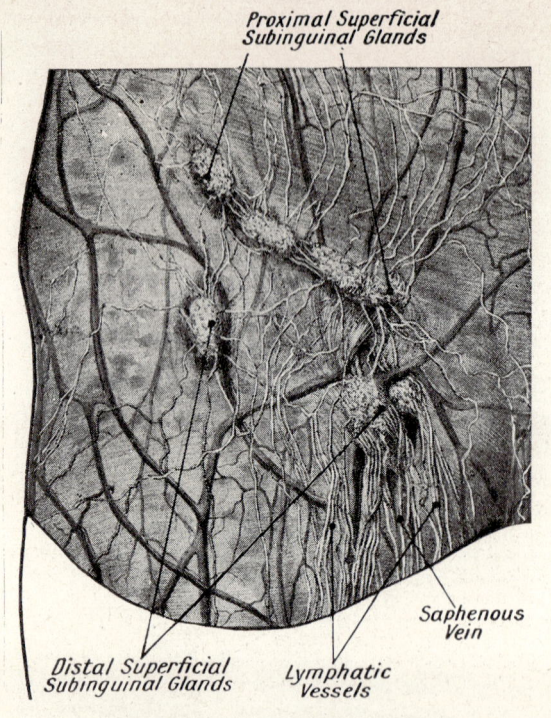

LYMPHATIC GLANDS IN THE GROIN

The lymphatic glands, a collection of which in the right groin is shown here, are widely distributed in the body. When inflamed they enlarge, and can be felt or even seen as definite swellings. Lymph brought to them by special vessels is filtered free of noxious substances.

inflammation of the mucous membranes, as in a cold in the head, but the fluid effusion then comes away in the form of discharge.

The activity of inflammation depends a good deal upon the extent of the irritation or injury by which it is set up, but it also depends upon the constitutional state of the person affected. In strong, full-blooded persons it is active and severe, but in the weak and debilitated it is less severe and more passive. It is important to recognize the difference, for the treatment required varies according to the form the inflammation takes.

Again, according to its mode of onset and the course it takes, inflammation is spoken of as acute, subacute, or chronic, but not infrequently the chronic inflammation is the result of an acute attack imperfectly cured.

Ulceration, the destruction of tissues in very small particles, may occur not only in the skin and mucous membrane, but in the bone, cartilage, etc. In the skin and mucous membrane it produces a sore place or ulcer, from which the particles mixed with matter come away as discharge. The discharge developed during suppuration (pus) is a thick, creamy, light-yellow, faintly smelling fluid which, under the microscope, is seen to be formed of a thin, clear, watery fluid with enormous numbers of round cells floating in it, the pus corpuscles, which are mainly composed of dead leucocytes.

In chronic inflammation the exudation neither undergoes resolution and disappears nor breaks down into pus, but becomes gradually changed into fibrous tissue and forms a firm, hard swelling.

In some cases of local inflammation, especially when it is set up by germs, as in erysipelas, the disease spreads very rapidly over the surface. It may also involve the lymphatic vessels and spread upwards along them to the lymphatic glands. These little organs act like filters, and for a time at least remove the poisonous substances and prevent their entry into the blood. The glands then become enlarged and inflamed, a condition termed adenitis, and may finally break down and form abscesses. They are situated at definite spots, and the lymphatic vessels of different parts of the body pass to distinct sets. Those of the calf run up to some glands in the

INFLAMMATION AND FEVER

hollow behind the knee, while all others of the lower limb pass to glands in the groin. The glands of the armpit receive all the lymph from the arm, except for a few vessels which pass to a small gland above the inner side of the elbow.

Along both sides of the neck, extending from the lower jaw to the collar bone, are situated important chains of glands which are prone to disease. They receive the lymph from the head, neck, tongue, and throat. When any gland becomes

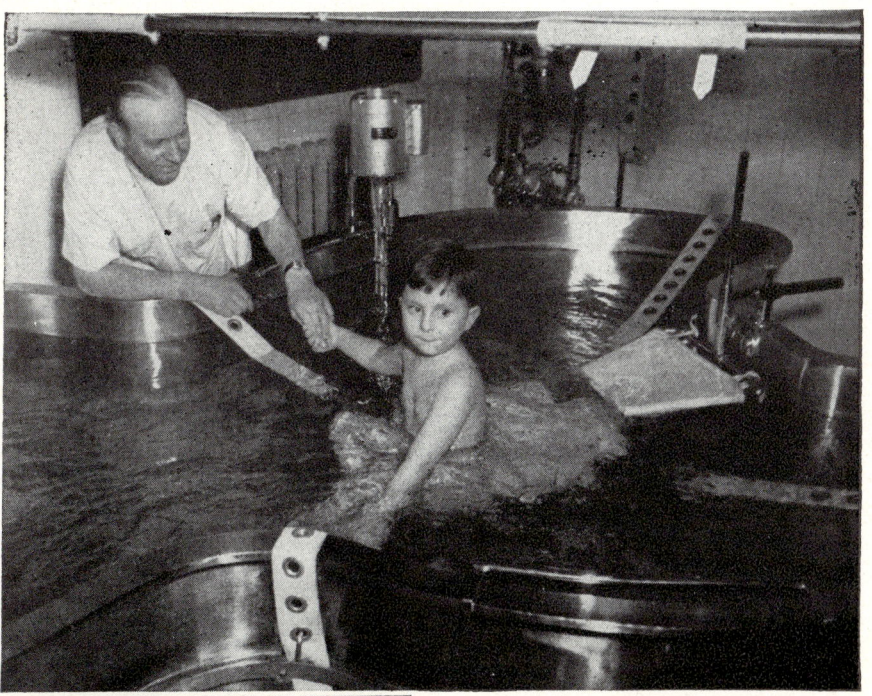

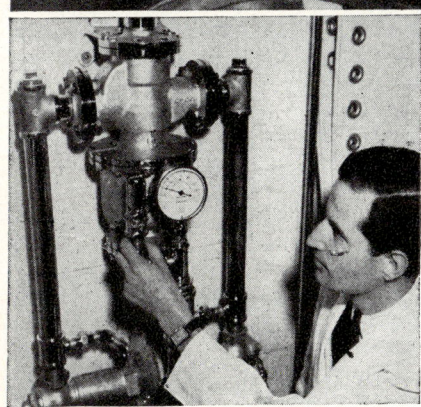

ADVANCED HYDROTHERAPEUTIC EQUIPMENT

The Hubbard-Currence tank at the New York Orthopaedic Hospital, here shown, is an enlargement and improvement over earlier and smaller types of whirlpool-bath underwater massage tubs. Either an adult or child can be completely immersed in reclining position for massage by streams of water. The velocity of these streams is governed by turbine pumps; the motor which drives one of these can be seen. The tank is large enough to allow the patient freedom of movement but is shaped like a dumbbell or figure 8 to allow of the technician's reaching all parts of the patient's body without entering the water himself; only one end of the tank is shown. Both the temperature and velocity of the water are controlled at a mixing valve, shown in the lower picture. Underwater massage of this kind has been found to be of help to patients seriously affected by arthritis, joint injuries, infantile paralysis, and some other diseases.

© *International News Photos*

enlarged and tender, it is of the utmost importance to find the source of irritation, to remove it at once, and also to subdue as quickly as possible any inflammation that has been set up in the gland. Wherever the adenitis continues to the stage of abscess, surgical interference will be necessary in order to prevent a general infection of the body.

Treatment. When inflammation arises in any part of the body the first endeavor is to discover its cause, and at once remove it. This is often easy in an external part, sometimes also in an internal part, but the definite exciting cause of many internal inflammations is beyond recognition or, if recognized, is incapable of removal mechanically. It is an important principle, generally received as true, that inflammation tends spontaneously to recover if its exciting cause is removed. Of mechanical causes of inflammation good examples are a piece of grit in the eye, a stone in the bladder, or indigestible food in the stomach.

But microorganisms constitute the commonest exciting cause, and these also have to be got rid of in order to carry out the first principle of treatment.

Antiseptic Applications. If the inflammation is in an open wound antiseptic dressings can be used. Of these there are a great number on the market and

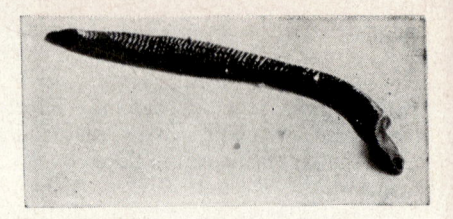

BLOODSUCKING WORM
The leech provides a natural method of withdrawing blood from the body. The mouth is at the end of the reader's right.

they are easily obtained in convenient strengths for external application. Phenol was for a long time first favorite, and is still greatly used, but like many other drugs it must be used carefully and not in too great a strength. Of mild antiseptics boracic acid is one of the most generally used. If the inflammation is under the skin, as in the case of an unbroken abscess or cellulitis, hot compresses or poultices or antiphlogistine are used to cover the area and bring the inflammation to the surface. The heat acts by increasing the blood supply at one point and thus increasing the numbers of white blood corpuscles and the amount of lmyph available to fight the infection.

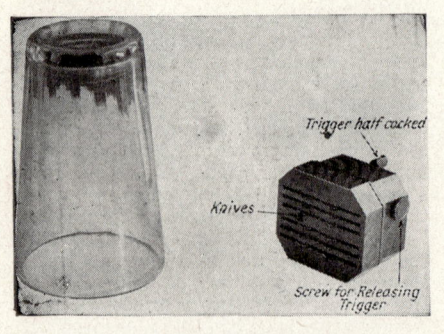

Inflammation in the internal organs of the body is more difficult to get at for the purpose of treatment, and in this case, if the inflamed part cannot be removed by operation, drugs must be used which have an antiseptic or curative action; vaccine treatment sometimes gives good results. Many organs can now be treated as external parts and can be washed out with antiseptics under skilled supervision, thus saving surgery, which a few years ago would have been considered the sole means of cure. For instance, stomach ulcers and especially duodenal ulcers are frequently cured by a course of lavage and rest. The Plombières system of washing out the further parts of the intestine which are not reached by the ordinary enema is often curative in cases of colitis or catarrhal inflammation of the intestines. The

SCARIFICATOR
The scarificator is an instrument consisting of a number of little blades operated by a spring and making small superficial incisions. A cupping glass is also shown.

INFLAMMATION AND FEVER

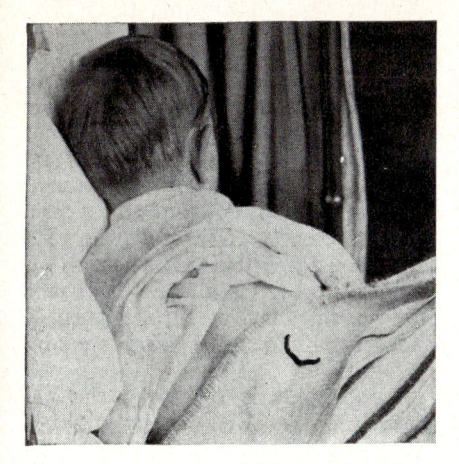

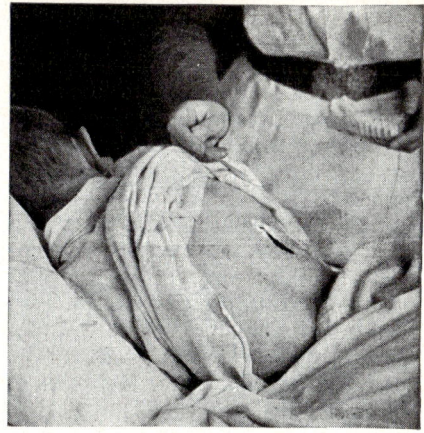

HOW THE LEECH IS USED IN BLOODLETTING
A refractory leech will sometimes bite more readily if it is made to crawl over the blanket. A leech usually drops off when satisfied, but if not, it can be dislodged by sprinkling some common salt over it. If there is any repugnance to the use of ordinary leeches, an artificial leech can be used instead.

maxillary antrum, connected with the nose on each side, can also be washed with antiseptics. The bladder is another part in which such treatment is sometimes useful. All these processes are carried out by or under the close direction of doctors who specialize in the treatment of the various regions affected.

Rest. The second cardinal principle is that an inflamed part should be rested. Pain may be looked upon as nature's call for rest. This may be carried out in many ways, according to the part affected. An inflamed eye should be covered up from all light, an inflamed arm supported in a sling, an inflamed knee fixed on a splint, an inflamed stomach relieved of the work of digestion. Further, if the inflammation is considerable or involves an important organ—as the brain, lung, or heart—a patient can escape from all external stimulation by resting in bed in a quiet, darkened room.

Rest is of essential importance when the body generally is affected or when the constitutional symptoms show themselves in the form of fever. The constitutional treatment is therefore that of

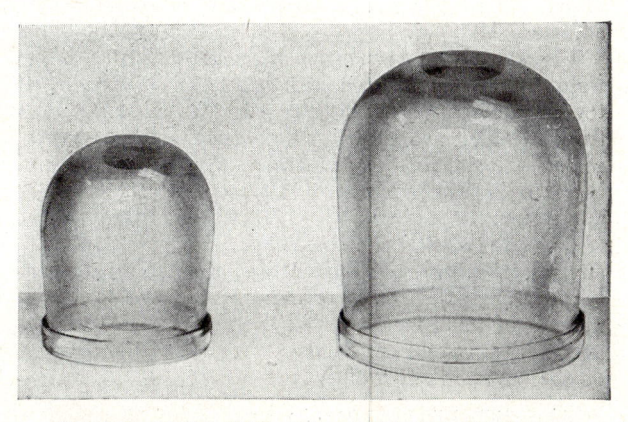

CUPPING GLASS USED FOR RELIEVING CONGESTION
Suction is procured in this type of glass by heating it before application and then allowing it to cool. One method is to burn a minute piece of blotting paper or cotton soaked in alcohol, in the glass. The air in the glass is thus used up, a vacuum is created, the flame is extinguished, and the skin is sucked up.

fever, and here we shall only consider the local measures.

Bloodletting. An inflamed part should be raised in order to favor the flow of blood from it. Local bloodletting also relieves the congested state of the blood vessels. It may be carried out in various ways, by cupping, by leeches—old-fashioned methods which are still useful—and by scarification in conjunction with cupping.

Cupping glasses are glass beakers having a capacity of about one-quarter of a pint, with ground edges which adhere closely to the skin. After the air in it has been heated, the glass is applied to the surface of the body. The cooling of the air then causes the formation of a partial vacuum, and blood is thus drawn up from neighboring parts into the skin under the cup.

In the operation of wet cupping, the blood is abstracted from the body by means of incisions made by an instrument called a scarificator. It consists of a metal box containing many small blades acting together. These blades are caused to emerge by releasing a spring which makes them revolve suddenly, and in so doing they protrude through slits to a distance which can be accurately adjusted.

The skin is first sponged with hot water and partially dried with a warm towel. A cupping glass is held over the flame of an alcohol lamp for a moment, so that the air in it becomes heated, and the glass is then applied to the smooth, damp skin.

When the skin is seen to be red and swollen, the cup is removed and the scarificator applied so as to cut a large number of small incisions. Without delay another heated cup is then clapped on the part and left until it is seen that three or four ounces of blood have been sucked into it.

Wet cupping is suitable only for those parts where the skin is thick and cushioned, such as the nape of the neck, the loins, or the front of the chest; it is used as a form of bleeding to relieve congestion of the brain and for inflamed conditions of the kidneys or lungs, such as acute bronchitis and nephritis.

Dry cupping is in effect the first stage of wet cupping. The scarificator is not used, and no blood is abstracted from the body. After dry cupping, a hard cherry-red mass is left beneath the skin. The condition is precisely similar to a large bruise. Within a few days the swelling turns black and it passes through the familiar purple, greenish, and yellow tints as the blood is gradually absorbed.

Dry cupping is free from the unpleasantness involved in wet cupping, and the pain caused by it is trivial, yet its effect is probably the same. It is useful in modifying the amount of blood supply to underlying organs by reflex action through the spinal cord.

Bier's Treatment. This is a method of treatment of acute and chronic inflammation introduced and advocated by

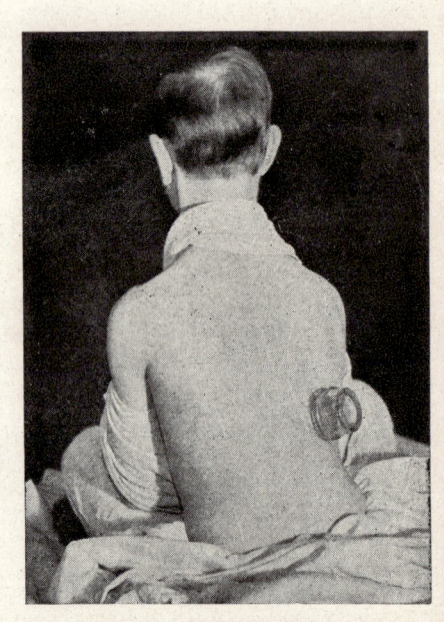

CUPPING AFTER SCARIFICATION

When the scarificator, illustrated upon page 1326, has cut the skin in several places, blood is drawn from the incisions by using a cupping glass, as shown here.

INFLAMMATION AND FEVER

Professor Bier. As already noted, nature's method of curing inflammation involves an increase of the blood supply to the affected part. This natural method is intensified by Bier's treatment, which increases the supply of blood by the application of heat (active hyperemia) or furthers exudation of serum by preventing the normal return in the veins (passive hyperemia).

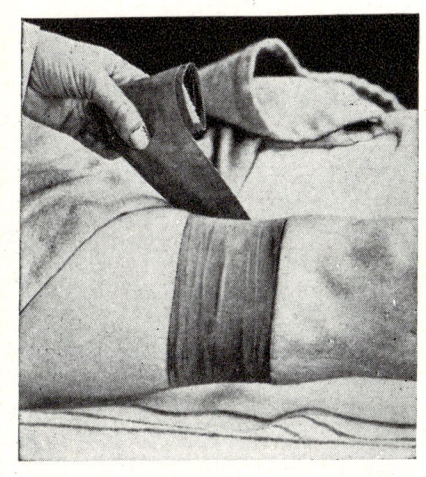

BIER'S TREATMENT FOR INFLAMMATION
The cure of inflammatory disease affecting a limb may be furthered by so constricting the limb above the site of the disease that while the blood can flow into the limb it is delayed in getting out. This may be accomplished by applying a soft elastic bandage firmly around the limb.

Active hyperemia can be produced by inserting the affected part of the limb into a hot-air bath or into a fluid bath at a temperature as hot as can be comfortably borne.

Passive congestion—and to this particularly the term Bier's treatment is applied—is produced by constricting the limb above the diseased part. This is best done by a few turns of a soft, thin rubber bandage applied firmly around the limb, on a segment nearer the trunk. The bandage should not cause pain nor cause the limb to become cold, and the pulse must still be felt below the site of constriction. The bandage is kept on for a period varying from a quarter of an hour to several hours, according to circumstances.

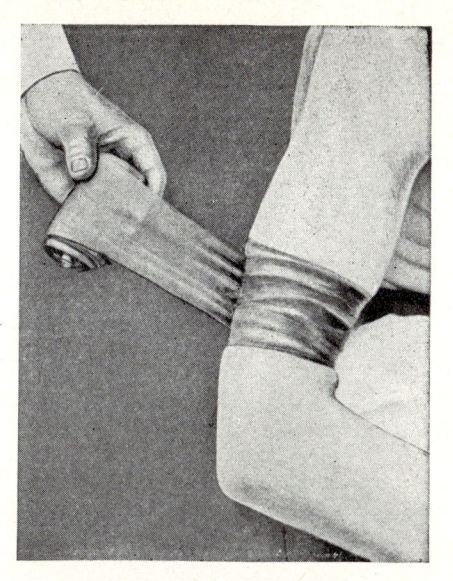

BIER'S TREATMENT OF THE ARM
Rubber elastic bandage applied to the arm to produce passive congestion in the affected elbow and parts below. These become blue and swell up.

The method is applicable for most types of inflammation of the limbs. When a bandage cannot conveniently be applied, for example on the back of the neck, the same effect can be produced by cupping.

Cold and Heat. The application of cold is frequently resorted to in order to subdue inflammation. It acts by constricting the blood vessels and thus driving the blood from the part. A bandage wetted in cold water, a piece of wet absorbent cotton, a waterproof bag filled with ice, or an evaporating solution (lead or alcohol lotion), are some of the means of carrying out this treatment. In other cases moist heat is more suitable. It may be applied in the form of poultices, fomentations, and compresses—to any of which such sedatives as laudanum, tincture of belladonna, or liniment of aconite may be added.

It is not always easy to decide whether hot or cold applications are the more suitable. First we may consult the patient's feeling, using whichever gives the more relief and is the more soothing. The effect depends also upon the nature of the part. When it is loose, and swelling can take place freely, heat is the better, but when it is firm and tight, and the swelling causes great pain, more relief is obtained from cold. Heat is better also when suppuration is inevitable and there are great heat and throbbing pain in the part; cold, on the other hand, checks swelling and often relieves the symptoms of a sprained joint. Methods of making cold and hot applications are described and illustrated in the section on Home Nursing, Chapter 86.

In the more chronic forms of inflammation, when there is little heat and pain but much thickening and stiffness of the part, stimulating treatment is advisable —very hot applications, strong liniments, and counterirritation with blisters or iodine paint. A method of applying heat which is found very useful in these cases is to douche the part with very hot water, which may be played onto it from a tap or poured from a height out of a pitcher. Great heat can also be applied by special apparatus in which the limb or other part is placed in a chamber or cylinder and subjected to high degrees of dry heat, or a bath of hot paraffin may be used.

Friction forms part of the massage treatment, which can be strongly recommended for removing the final results of inflammation. It increases the circulation through the part, improves its nutrition, lessens thickening and stiffness, and soothes pain. Treatment by hydropathy is sometimes found useful in chronic inflammatory conditions, such methods as douches, packs, and baths being employed, but all these are best carried out in special institutions. Highly specialized electrical methods may be employed by the physician in the office or hospital.

FEVER

Fever is a response of the body to infection. This response is so often associated with a rise of temperature that the term fever is often used simply to denote the heightened temperature. The body temperature may be raised from other causes than infection, but in what follows the term is used to denote response to infection of which the rise in temperature is only one feature. On the other hand, apyrexial forms of many infective fevers may occur when the other classical signs of fever are present.

The heightened temperature in infective fevers is often spoken of as pyrexia; when due to other causes generally of nervous origin it is best referred to as hyperthermia. Here the term is used in its broadest sense.

The pyrexia is now thought to be the most essential factor in the defensive mechanism of fever. The rise of temperature has been proved to be detrimental to the invading bacteria, although not powerful enough actually to kill them. Thus, when infection has occurred, pyrexia is by no means an unwelcome sign. The height of the temperature bears no definite relation to the severity of the disease. In most diseases a moderate temperature is a favorable sign, but very ill and debilitated patients may show no rise of temperature when infection is severe.

The temperature of the body in health is about 98.6° F., but in normal people it may vary between 96° and 99°. A diurnal variation occurs, the lowest temperature being recorded between 6:00 and 7:00 a.m., after which it gradually rises to reach its highest point between 5:00 and 7:00 p.m., and then slowly falls again. Those who work by night and sleep by day show a reversal of this temperature curve. In infants and young children the temperature tends to be higher, and variations are much more easily produced than in adults.

The rise of temperature which usually accompanies fever is due to a disorder of the heat-regulating processes brought about by the toxins produced by the invading organisms. These act on the heat-regulating centers and also increase the rate of the metabolic processes, the tissues breaking down too rapidly.

Manifestations. The manifestations of fever vary considerably with the diseases which cause it, but there are certain effects which are so universally associated with a rise of temperature that they may be classed together as significant of fever. The most important are as follows: A certain feeling of malaise is always present, associated with weariness and often with headache. Some degree of muscular pain and stiffness is felt, and the patient is usually constipated. Digestion is almost always impaired, the tongue being dry and furred and the appetite poor. Thirst is complained of, and the urine is markedly diminished in quantity and of high color, the so-called febrile urine. Albumin is often present. The skin is dry, hot and prickling, the patient is restless, feeling sometimes hot and sometimes cold, with frequent shivering attacks. In some cases sweating is profuse and the skin is moist.

The patient's sensations of heat and cold are thus no guide to his temperature. At the onset of fever there is usually a marked contraction of the arterioles of the skin. This causes the feeling of chilliness which is often associated with shivering and rigors. At this time the temperature of the skin is actually below normal while the temperature of the internal parts is greatly heightened. The pulse is usually rapid, but in some diseases, such as typhoid fever, the rise of pulse rate is not proportionate to the increase of temperature. The breathing is usually rapid. Nervous symptoms may be marked, and in some cases delirium is present. Many infectious fevers have a characteristic rash, which affords aid in diagnosis.

The severity of the disease determines in a large measure which of the above symptoms predominates, and in grave cases the patient may pass into what is called the typhoid state. It is characterized by extreme muscular weakness, with involuntary movements of the limbs. The tongue is dry and brown.

The blood shows important changes as the result of the infection. The white cells are increased in number in most febrile diseases, the most notable exceptions being typhoid fever and influenza. This increase in the white cells is a defensive mechanism whereby the germs are ingested and destroyed, and various protective substances known as antibodies are poured out into the blood to neutralize the circulating poisons (see Chapter 20). The blood pressure in most fevers is lowered, due mainly to a dilatation of the arterioles in the skin, together with the weak action of the heart. Wasting and loss of weight occur during prolonged fever. This is partly due to the loss of appetite and disordered secretion of the digestive glands and partly to the increased rate at which the tissues break down as the result of the toxemia.

The onset of fever is often sudden, the patient feeling in quite good health until a sharp rise of temperature to about 103° F. occurs. This type of onset is usually seen in pneumonia and in some forms of influenza. In typhoid fever and bronchopneumonia, on the other hand, there is often a more gradual onset, the temperature increasing by one to two degrees in the evening and falling by a smaller amount the next morning until the maximum is reached. The temperature may fall either suddenly (crisis) or gradually (lysis).

Crisis occurs in many specific fevers, for example, measles, typhus, and most typically in acute lobar pneumonia. The more marked and acute the onset of a fever, the more rapid will be the rise of temperature and the greater the probability of an early crisis. It is popularly known as "the turn."

The process of crisis occupies usually less than twenty-four hours. There is a rapid fall in temperature to the normal,

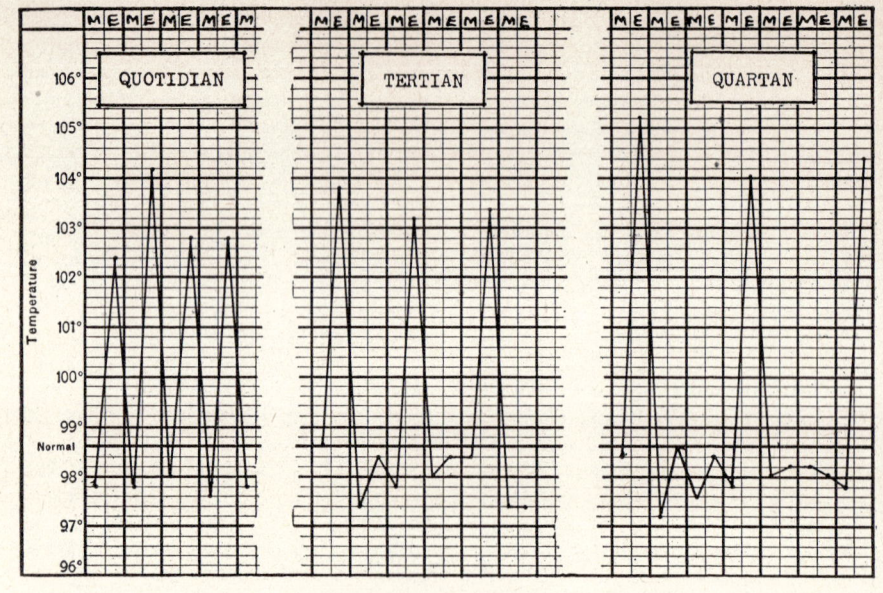

INTERMITTENT FEVERS

These are parts of the temperature charts of three malaria patients. The life cycles of the malaria parasites affect the intervals between high points in the fever. The temperature peaks occur in tertian fever on the first and third days of illness, in quartan fever on the first and fourth.

Courtesy of the Physicians' Record Co.

which coincides with a corresponding fall in the pulse rate; the tongue becomes moist, the skin resumes its normal feel and sense of warmth to the touch. These conditions are often accompanied by profuse sweating, occasionally by the passing of a large quantity of urine, and sometimes by diarrhea. Finally the patient falls into a quiet sleep.

In lysis the temperature falls a little each day until it reaches the normal. This takes place in the majority of illnesses and is usual in typhoid fever.

Course of an Attack. The whole period of fever can be divided into certain stages, namely, incubation, onset, fastigium, and decline.

During a febrile attack the temperature may assume one of the three following types: (1) continued, when the temperature remains high and there is only a slight daily remission; (2) remittent, when the daily variation extends over several degrees but the temperature never falls to the normal; (3) intermittent, in which the temperature is normal or subnormal at some period in the twenty-four hours. In certain fevers there are periodical rises of temperature, which remains elevated for intervals of three or four days and then falls to normal for a longer period. These are known as relapsing types, examples of which are relapsing fever, caused by a spirochete, and one variety of trench fever. The intermittent fevers may occur at regular intervals of every second or third day, as in tertian and quartan malaria.

Although in fever the temperature is usually highest in the evening, in some diseases what is known as the inverted type of temperature chart may be seen. In such a case the morning temperature is higher than the evening. This is especially the case in certain varieties of pul-

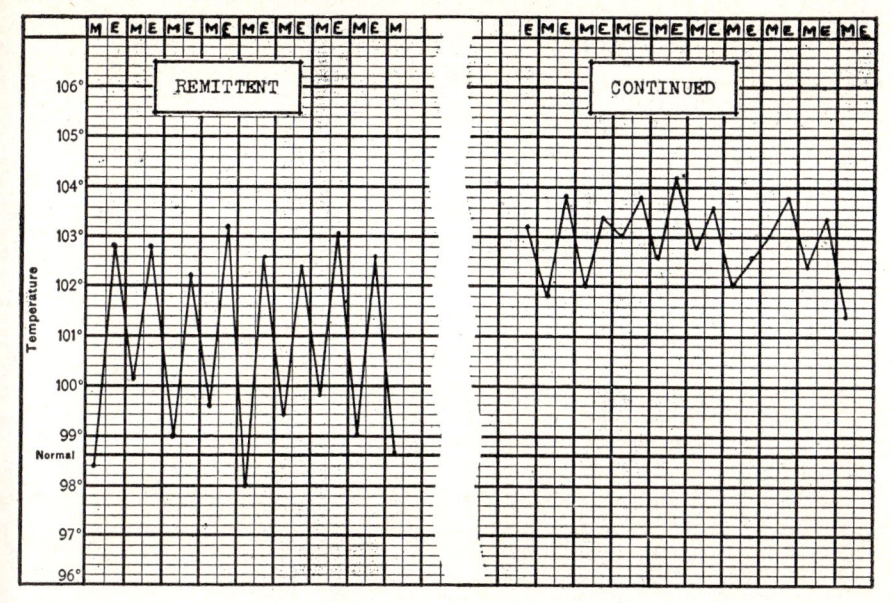

REMITTENT AND CONTINUED FEVERS

The temperature pattern at the left is of the sort that occurs in pulmonary tuberculosis (and some other diseases), returning toward normal in decided drops from peaks at regular intervals; that at the left is typical of typhoid fever, fluctuating daily but not dropping more than about two degrees until the beginning of recovery.

Courtesy of the Physicians' Record Co.

monary tuberculosis; it usually indicates that the disease is actively spreading.

Management. Fresh air is one of the most important factors in the treatment of fevers. The fever patient finds cool, fresh air very soothing, and it is also extremely valuable in promoting sleep. While the temperature is high the bed coverings should be light and a single sheet may often suffice. Eiderdowns and heavy blankets are unnecessary and harmful. One or two light blankets may be added as the temperature subsides. The room in which the patient is nursed must be large enough to secure adequate ventilation without a draft, and windows should be kept open in all weathers, fog alone excepted. The best aspect for a sickroom is southeast or southwest, in order that sunlight should enter the room at some time during the day.

The following points have already been mentioned in the section on Home Nursing, but it will be as well to recapitulate them here.

If the fever is one of the infectious diseases, the room chosen for the patient should be at the top of the house if possible, and in any case well away from the other occupants. An adjoining room should contain a table with the patient's medicines and toilet requisites. Here, too, unless a bathroom is close at hand for them, should be a basin, towel, nailbrush, and soap for the doctor, nurse, and visitors to wash their hands and faces after visiting the patient. Gowns should hang here, and must be worn when in the sickroom and removed when leaving. There should also be provision for washing up the patient's utensils so that no infected cups, etc., should go to the family kitchen. The old-fashioned custom of hanging a sheet soaked in phenol solution outside the sickroom door may not be as important as it used to be, but it is at any rate a pungent symbol of warning to children and others to keep away.

The bed should be placed away from the wall so as to facilitate nursing. It must not face the light; the light from the window should, if possible, fall on the patient's left.

The fever patient often sweats freely, and as the skin is the organ of excretion of certain waste products it is important to keep it functioning properly. This is accomplished by a careful daily washing all over with soap and warm water and frequent sponging of the face and hands. Prevention of bedsores is very important in cases of prolonged fever such as typhoid.

In all febrile conditions careful attention must be directed to the mouth. The salivary secretion is diminished and thus the mouth becomes an easy prey to the onslaught of bacteria. A condition of mild or severe stomatitis is liable to develop, with a coated tongue, foul breath, and marked discomfort. To obviate this the teeth must be cleaned twice daily or oftener and the mouth washed out with a mild antiseptic such as a weak salt or a weak phenol solution. Frequent drinks of water also have a marked cleansing effect.

Diet in Fever. The high temperature of a febrile patient and the fact that metabolism is occurring at a rapid rate indicate that the body needs an adequate supply of foods, so that if the feverish illness is prolonged the old adage "starve a fever" is proceeding on the wrong lines. The poor appetite, impaired digestion and dry mouth of the patient, however, render it difficult for him to eat adequately, and care, tact, and skill may be required to induce him to take an adequate dietary. All food must be given in small quantities and at fairly frequent

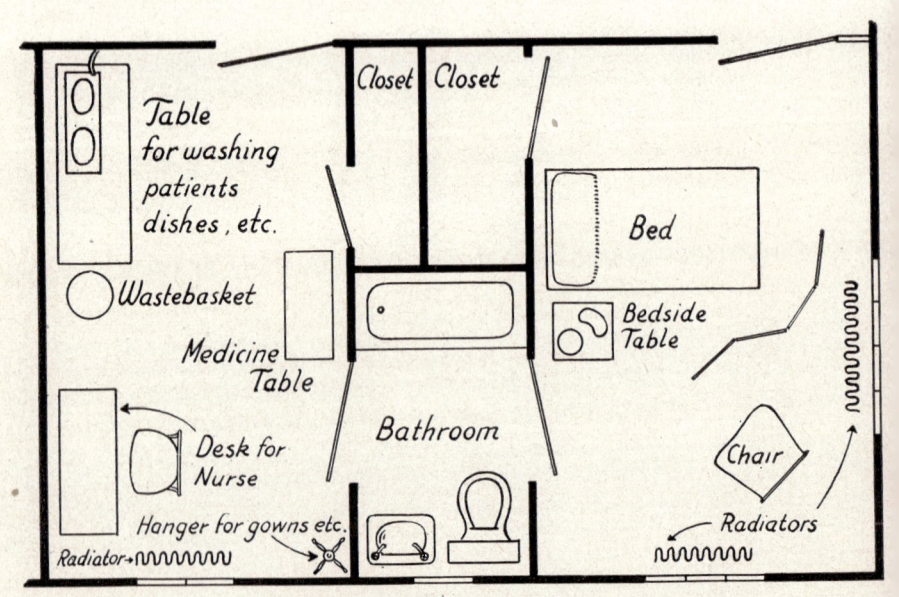

IDEAL ROOM ARRANGEMENT TO CARE FOR A FEVER PATIENT

If possible, the patient should have one of two communicating rooms at the top of the house. The patient will of course have the larger and better ventilated room; the smaller room is the nurse's workroom. The latter must be accessible without necessitating passage through the sickroom. A screen between the bed and the east or west window permits the window to be kept open and the shade raised without annoying the patient by glare.

intervals; every three hours during the day is not too often. For the first few days of fever, however, food is best abstained from, water and fruit juices such as orange and lemon drinks being given freely.

The impairment of digestion and assimilation necessitates the use of easily digested foods, and milk must form the basis of the diet in almost all cases of prolonged fever. It seldom gives rise to indigestion if diluted with one-third its volume of water. Sometimes, however, it causes some degree of flatulence, and in these cases a large part of it should be replaced by more solid food. A patient on a milk diet requires three pints a day, but this may usually be given partly as coffee, cocoa or junket with different flavorings, thus varying the monotony of the diet. Milk is a complete food, and patients can live on it for a long time, but it is not a perfect food, as the volume of fluid required is very large compared with the amount of nourishment obtained.

Unless the temperature is very high, light milky foods, such as bread and milk, milk toast, or arrowroot puddings made with milk, may be included in the diet, and bread and butter is usually well taken. Vegetable and meat broths form a pleasant change and are excellent stimulants; they also help to secure an action of the bowels, but their nutritive value is very low. They can, however, be made more nutritious by adding barley or rice or breakcrumb to them. Eggs are nutritious and easily assimilated. Fish and chicken are among the solid foods reserved for convalescence and are both nutritious and easily digested. Beef, mutton, etc., should never be given until convalescence is well established. Certain fevers connected with lesions in the alimentary canal need special diet, typhoid fever being the most important.

The fever patient is usually thirsty and fluids should be given in large quantities. Of these the best is cold water. Where this is not well taken, hot water or weak tea may be substituted. It is a good plan to give food at regular intervals and to have a glass of water by the patient's bedside so that he may drink between meals as much as he desires. The great need of the body for fluid in fever cases cannot be overstressed.

Water, particularly when cold, has a very beneficial effect on fevers. It allays thirst, cleanses the mouth and dilutes the poisons of the disease. Headache, so often a characteristic symptom of fever, frequently disappears after copious drinks of cold water, and delirium and sleeplessness often yield to this as to no other form of treatment. Fruit juices should be used freely both for their refreshing properties and their chemical action. Recipes for beverages suitable for fever patients appear on pages 1181-1184.

Methods of Reducing Temperature. Pyrexia, as has already been pointed out, is a defensive mechanism of the body in its attempt to overcome the invading bacteria with their toxins. Thus attempts to reduce the temperature of a febrile patient are mistaken unless such hyperpyrexia is present as may be dangerous to life, or unless the temperature is unduly prolonged and the patient is suffering from exhaustion. The aim in treatment should be to maintain the patient's resistance by securing him rest and quiet, suitable nourishment, and free eliminatory action of the skin, kidneys, and bowels.

Temperature may be temporarily reduced when necessary by hot, tepid, and cold sponging, or if necessary by cold packs (see page 1133) and even baths. These often soothe the patient, promote sleep, and prevent the exhaustion due to prolonged high temperature.

Use of Drugs. The use of drugs in the treatment of fever has but very limited scope. Quinine is specific in its action in treating malaria and the salicylates in acute rheumatic fever. Drugs such as acetate of ammonia, spirits of nitrous ether, and aspirin have an indirect influence in reducing temperature, and the indications for their

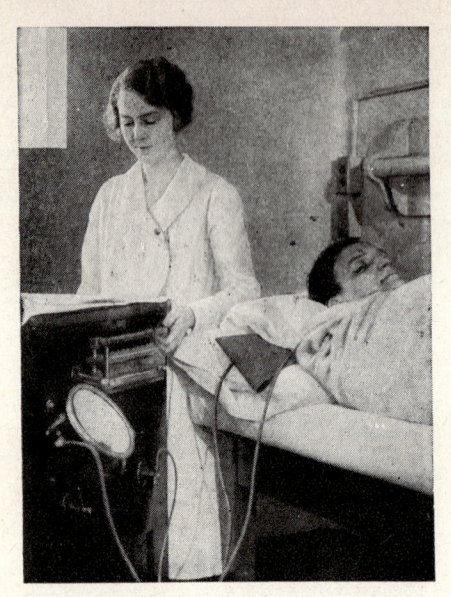

FEVER INDUCED BY ELECTRICITY
Fever being nature's method of combating acute infection, artificially raised temperatures are effective in chronic conditions. They are produced by controlled high-frequency electric currents which can raise the body temperature up to 106°.

use are similar to those for tepid sponging, cold packs, etc. They are suitable only in the early acute stages, and should not be given unless ordered by the physician.

The bowels must be kept freely open. This is almost always difficult to accomplish, as the rest in bed, milk diet, and diminished secretions all tend to give rise to constipation. Attempts should first be made to overcome constipation by means of diet, fruit and vegetable juices being given whenever permissible. The ingestion of large quantities of cold water acts as a stimulant to the intestine. Mineral oil, about one ounce for an adult and half an ounce for a child, may be given daily. If a more active remedy is required, one of the most useful laxatives for children during febrile attacks is syrup of figs in doses of one-half to two teaspoonfuls, while for adults senna tea infused from the pods, or tablets of cascara sagrada in two grain or four-grain doses, are usually effective. If constipation persists, a simple enema should be given on alternate days.

Sleep, more valuable to the patient than medicine, is best assured by skilled nursing.

Hypnotics are often called for and should not be withheld if sleep is markedly deficient. The following drugs may prove useful, subject to the doctor's instructions. Twenty grains of potassium bromide combined with ten grains of choral hydrate gives a quiet sleep. Paraldehyde in doses of one or two drachms sometimes works well, but is unpleasant to take. It is stimulating and has no after effects.

Artificial Fever. It has been known for some time that a number of disease conditions or nervous disorders, particularly those of a chronic rather than those of an acute nature, are improved or actually cured when fevers occur during the course of the disease. This has had its most striking application in the treatment of general paralysis of the insane by deliberately inducing malaria with its accompanying pyrexia. It has also been used in allergic disorders, such as asthma. The principle has now been developed by the use of diathermy, electric currents of very high frequency producing in the tissues temperatures similar to those of high fever. The method is applied to rheumatic conditions, gonorrhea, and in cardiac and nervous disorders, and it has obvious advantages including that of close control, over disease-induced fever.

CHAPTER 98

DISEASES CAUSED BY KNOWN GERMS: VARIOUS

Typhoid Fever — Paratyphoid Fever — Blood Poisoning — Sapremia — Septicemia — Pyemia — Erysipelas — Scarlet Fever — Cerebrospinal Fever — Influenza — Gonorrhea — Syphilis—Marriage and Venereal Disease—Tetanus—Animal Diseases Transmissible to Man — Glanders — Anthrax — Tularemia — Rocky Mountain Spotted Fever.

THE subject of infectious diseases, their source, mode of spread, and prevention has been considered from a general standpoint in Chapter 21, where regulations about notification and quarantine are also detailed. In this and the succeeding chapters it is proposed to consider separately certain of the infectious disorders which may attack adults. This rather arbitrary division has been made because the number of infectious diseases is very large, and some of them can be quite appropriately assigned to other sections of this work.

For instance, the section on Diseases of Children in Volume VIII includes detailed accounts of the following common infectious disorders: measles, German measles, diphtheria and membranous croup, chickenpox, whooping cough, infantile paralysis, encephalitis lethargica, and tubercular meningitis. Pneumonia, tuberculosis of the lungs (consumption) and the common colds are dealt with in the section on Diseases of the Respiratory System in Volume V. Cholera, plague, malaria, dysentery and certain other infectious diseases are described in the section on Tropical Diseases. The symptoms and treatment of puerperal fever are considered in detail in Chapter 192.

It must be borne in mind, of course, that infectious eruptive diseases may attack human beings at any age. For instance, mumps is more serious in the adult than it is in the child, and therefore it is included in this section. Similarly, measles may afflict adults, but as a general rule children are the victims of an epidemic, and so this disease appears in the section on Diseases of Children.

Again, dysentery occurs here and there in the United States, but we cannot say that it is anything but a rarity in these circumstances. The disease is therefore dealt with under the heading Tropical Diseases. Similarly for malaria, indigenous cases of which are known to occur now and then in regions other than those in which tropical swamps afford

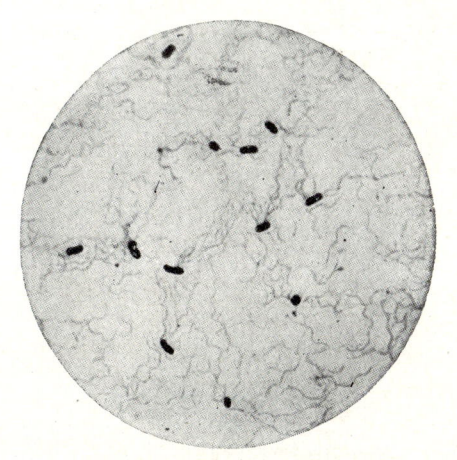

TYPHOID BACILLI AND THEIR FLAGELLA
This microphotograph shows clearly the flagella, the organs of motility. Paratyphoid and food-poisoning bacilli are similar in appearance to the typhoid germ.

TYPHOID FEVER

Typhoid fever is a prolonged illness affecting chiefly the intestinal tract and caused by the typhoid bacillus. It is closely allied to paratyphoid fever A and paratyphoid fever B, the three being classified together as the enteric group of diseases. The typhoid bacillus is a rod-shaped organism, resembling very

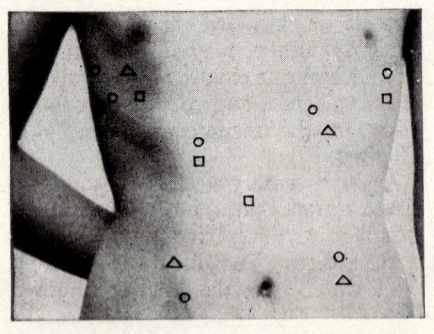

FIRST SITES OF RASH IN TYPHOID
Crops of small red papules appear on the abdomen and sides of the chest, successive crops being indicated here by different signs. The typhus rash comes out on the same sites but differs in character.

closely the colon bacillus, which is a normal inhabitant of the intestine. It may be found in the blood, urine, stools and skin at different stages of the illness, and it is also present in such internal organs as the spleen and gall bladder.

Mode of Spread. The disease is contracted by ingestion, or more rarely by inhalation, of the bacilli by persons attending on the patient, or by those to whom they are carried through infected water or other intermediate carrier. Nurses not infrequently contract typhoid from their patients. This may be acquired by partaking of food with soiled hands which have made contact with any of the patient's excreta such as dried fecal or urinal stains on the bed linen. Such articles as sheets, blankets, or clothes used by a typhoid patient may also spread the disease to anyone handling them. The most usual mode of spread is by water which has become contaminated by discharges from a case of typhoid fever. This contamination may arise by defective drains allowing the soil to become fouled so that water obtained from that soil may be infected with the typhoid germ. Epidemics caused in this way are likely to be very widespread in their distribution.

Infected Food. Milk is frequently the means by which typhoid is spread. The germs may enter the milk by means of the washing of the cans or the dilution of the milk with infected water; some person handling it may be a carrier of the disease or may be nursing a typhoid patient. Milk is an ideal breeding ground for the germs, and even if only a few gain entrance they may multiply and ultimately cause a large epidemic.

Food grown in infected water, such as watercress or celery, and ice cream made from polluted milk or water, are further examples of the means of spread of typhoid fever, while oysters, clams, and other shellfish which are derived from beds near the mouths of rivers are a serious menace to the community, since they are extremely likely to contain typhoid bacilli. Flies and other insects undoubtedly aid in the spread of disease. They pass from manure heaps to food, carrying germs on their hairy legs, and deposit them in the milk or on any article of food on which they alight.

Typhoid Carriers. Typhoid fever is one of the diseases in which carriers play an important part. Typhoid carriers have almost always suffered from the disease at some previous time, and still harbor the bacilli in their intestines, gall bladder, or urinary tract long after all symptoms of illness have passed away. Bacilli have been found in the excreta of carriers as long as thirty years after an attack of typhoid fever. Such people are particularly dangerous when their work is concerned with the preparation of food, and numerous epidemics have been traced to dairy workers and cooks who have been found to be carriers of disease.

The presence of a carrier should always be suspected when an epidemic arises, and if such be found he must be removed from any post where he is liable to spread infection.

Incidence. Climate plays little part in the incidence of typhoid fever, but in the United States the greatest number of cases occur in the autumn months. Babies are seldom affected, the disease chiefly attacking young adults, and men somewhat oftener than women.

The incidence of typhoid fever indicates the level of the hygiene of a community. Where this is bad, typhoid is apt to be rife, and the remarkable decline both in its incidence and severity is a tribute to the advance in public health in the United States.

The incubation period of typhoid fever varies greatly with the number of bacilli ingested, but it is usually between two and twenty-one days.

Formation of Ulcers. The typhoid bacilli enter the stomach and intestines, and then pass in the blood to the gall bladder, bone marrow, skin, and spleen. In the small intestine, particularly near its lower end, the Peyer's patches (small masses of lymphoid tissue) undergo very characteristic changes. They first become swollen and thickened, and later sloughs are formed which separate, leaving characteristic ulcers. These may be very shallow or very deep. The depth varies with the severity of the disease, and it may be taken that when the fever runs its course with a high temperature with only slight remissions, the ulceration is correspondingly deep. Deep ulceration is a serious factor in the disease, as it renders liable the two most dread complications, perforation and hemorrhage. In favorable cases the ulcers heal, leaving no cicatricial contraction. The toxins of the typhoid bacillus act directly on the heart muscle, causing it to be flabby and weak, and death from cardiac failure is by no means uncommon during the later stages of the illness.

Methods of Diagnosis. The early symptoms are vague and the onset gradual in all but a very few exceptional cases, so that the differential diagnosis of typhoid is sometimes a matter of difficulty. It is apt to be confused with influenza, lobar or bronchial pneumonia, miliary tuberculosis, pleurisy, meningitis, and tuberculous peritonitis. Appendicitis, colitis, typhus fever, and meningitis may at times also be mistaken for it.

The diagnosis may be made in most cases by a careful clinical examination, but chemical and bacteriological reactions are often used to confirm it.

Signs and Symptoms. At the onset of the disease the patient complains of headache and vague pains throughout the body, and there is generally some abdominal discomfort, with constipation or diarrhea. The tongue is furred. Sleep is generally fitful, and nose bleeding is very commonly met with in the early stages, while cough with some degree of bronchitis is almost always present. The temperature rises gradually, being higher each morning than the previous one, but lower than that of the night before. Early symptoms are thus so indefinite that the patient often keeps at work for six or seven days after the onset of the disease.

At the beginning of the second week the temperature is high, often about 103° F., and the patient takes to bed. The temperature remains at approximately the same level for ten days, or sometimes even longer, and the patient lies prostrated and weak. The face is often flushed, and the skin shows a characteristic eruption, best seen on the abdomen, back and chest; it may also appear on the limbs and face. It consists of a few pink spots, slightly raised above the skin, which disappear on pressure (see color plate facing page 1345). The rash comes out about the seventh to the tenth day of illness, and appears in crops, each of which may last three or four days. The tongue is dry and furred, and, if not properly cleaned, becomes swollen, brown, and cracked.

The abdomen is slightly distended and may be a little tender, the spleen being often palpable. Constipation or diarrhea is generally present, and the stools may be soft and loose, and resemble pea soup. They often contain sloughs from the ulcers and undigested curds of milk. When hemorrhage into the bowel occurs, blood is passed in the stools. The patient always complains of headache throughout the illness, which may be so severe as to resemble meningitis. Deafness is common, and delirium often occurs in severe cases.

So-called Typhoid State. In severe infections the third week of the disease may find the patient in a condition of profound toxemia known as the typhoid state. A patient in this state sinks down in bed, becomes semiconscious, picking at the bedclothes and muttering low in delirium. The tongue is dry and coated, and the mouth is kept in a partly open position.

Symptoms of heart failure threaten and abdominal complications are likely to occur. Death may ensue or recovery set in after a few days of severe illness.

Decline of the Disease. After two, three or four weeks, in favorable cases, the temperature begins to fall. This takes place by lysis, usually extends over a period of a week or ten days, and finally reaches a subnormal level. During this time the patient's general condition improves slowly, although the heart's action is very weak. Appetite improves and hunger is often bitterly complained of, while the abdominal distension and discomfort pass away.

The temperature is often unstable for several days after it has touched normal, and constipation or the addition of some fresh article of diet may be sufficient to cause a further recrudescence.

Relapses. Convalescence is interrupted in some cases by relapses. These are attacks very similar to the original disease, but are usually shorter and milder. They occur mostly when the temperature has failed to become subnormal after the original attack, but once this has become established the risk of a relapse is very small. Relapses are seldom fatal, but the patient usually suffers from toxemia, and cardiac weakness is often very marked.

Complications. The course of typhoid fever is often interrupted by one or more complications. The most dangerous of these are hemorrhage and perforation of the intestine, due to the erosion of an ulcer into a blood vessel or its extension through the wall of the bowel, giving rise to a hole at the base of the ulcer, through which the intestinal contents pass. These two calamities occur generally during the third week of illness, when the Peyer's patches are becoming necrotic.

The hemorrhage may be slight, the only indication of its taking place being the dark reddish color of the stools, which may also contain some clots. This may occur once or be repeated on several days, and in the latter case is always of serious significance. With a large hemorrhage the patient becomes very pale and suffers from severe shock. The temperature falls suddenly from about 103° F. to below normal, and the pulse becomes quickened and feeble and may be almost uncountable in severe cases. When once the hemorrhage ceases the temperature rises gradually to normal again, the pulse rate slows down and the general condition improves.

Perforation of the bowel is a rarer complication than hemorrhage, but is much more serious, as peritonitis always follows in its train. The first indication is severe pain in the abdomen accompanied by a sudden drop in temperature. The pulse rate rises and the patient assumes an anxious expression, while the

DISEASES CAUSED BY KNOWN GERMS: VARIOUS

abdomen is rigid and tender and often somewhat distended. The signs and symptoms of peritonitis follow within a few hours of the perforation, and death occurs within two or three days unless the condition is treated by operation.

Affections of the lungs are liable to appear in all cases of typhoid fever. Bronchitis is so often present that it may almost be looked upon as a symptom of the disease, and pneumonia is by no means uncommon.

Thrombosis of the veins is a very characteristic complication, the veins most effected being the femoral, popliteal, and internal saphenous. The thrombosed vein is painful, the leg edematous, and the temperature is somewhat raised. This condition occurs generally during convalescence, but after a week or two usually subsides.

Cholecystitis, or inflammation of the gall bladder, is seen occasionally during an attack of typhoid fever. This causes pain under the edge of the ribs on the right side, and there may be some degree of jaundice. Such cases are especially likely to become carriers of the disease, as the gall bladder is a favorite site for the growth of the typhoid bacillus.

Periostitis may affect any bone, but the tibia, ribs, and femur are particularly likely to be attacked. This complication arises chiefly during convalescence, and gives rise to pain and swelling around the bone and may go on to suppuration.

A rare complication, but one which sometimes persists for months, is an inflammation of the intervertebral disks of the spine, giving rise to pain and stiffness of the back. The condition is called typhoid spine.

Laryngitis, which only occurs in severe cases, causes much pain and hoarseness, and is always of grave significance.

Some degree of parotitis, or inflammation of the parotid glands as in mumps, is often seen, especially when the mouth is very septic or has not been properly cleansed.

When an attack of typhoid fever occurs during pregnancy, abortion generally takes place, the infant being usually either born dead or living only a few hours.

Treatment. There is at present no specfic cure for typhoid fever; the best form of treatment is to put the patient under the best conditions to combat the infection and treat the symptoms and complications as they arise. The disease is thus treated on the general lines laid down for fever. Good nursing is all-important in the prevention of many of the complications and discomforts that are apt to occur. It is safest, whenever possible, to send patients with typhoid fever to hospital for isolation and treatment.

The patient must be kept strictly lying down, but should be turned from side to side or on to his back every few hours in order to avoid bedsores, which are especially liable to develop in this disease. The bedclothes must be kept very clean and dry, and care must be taken that there are no creases or particles of food in the sheet on which the patient is lying.

The mouth must be cleansed frequently with water, boric glycerin, or listerine. A clean mouth adds greatly to the patient's comfort and well-being, and diminishes the likelihood of infection of the parotid gland.

As in the treatment of all fevers, the taking of copious amounts of water is very beneficial. It preserves the moisture of the mouth, assists in the elimination of toxins, and has a sedative effect on the nervous system. An adult should be induced to take at least three quarts of water daily.

The excreta should be broken up and mixed with a 5 per cent solution of phenol, and allowed to stand over for an hour before being poured down the drain. Bed pans must be kept clean and standing in weak phenol solution. Sheets must be changed immediately they are soiled, and fecal stains washed out, and they must be soaked in a 2½ per cent phenol solution for twelve hours before being washed. Nurses should wear gowns when attending their patients, and must wash and disinfect their hands thoroughly before their meals.

Rules of Diet. A diet high enough in calorie value to cover the energy requirement of the patient is essential for recovery. Milk in one form or another is the most suitable food, and it is best given diluted with water during the acute stages of the disease. A satisfactory diet when the temperature is high consists of three ounces of milk with one ounce of water, given at intervals of two hours during the day. The milk must be taken as a food and not used to quench the thirst during the intervals between the feedings. Sodium citrate in doses of one grain to each ounce of milk should be added. This renders the curd finer and more digestible and perhaps lessens the risk of thrombosis, which is thought to be due partly to the large amount of calcium in the milk dietary causing an increased tendency of the blood to clot. A little diluted lemon juice has a similarly beneficial effect. Milk, eggs, and cereals can be relied upon to replenish the nitrogen needs of the patient. Meat is not recommended until the second or third week of convalescence.

A diarrhea which persists is in most cases due to an improper diet. This is frequently due to an excess of cream or lactose and in practically all instances can be controlled by an alteration in the diet.

When a normal temperature in the mornings has been reached, bread and milk, steamed pounded fish, vegetable purées, and fruit juices may be given in small quantities, and, if these are well tolerated and there is no subsequent increase in temperature, chicken and mashed potatoes may be added. On these lines the dietary may be made up and slowly increased, but any food leaving much residue should be avoided. Some physicians favor a more varied diet in the acute stage and believe that it tends to prevent complications and shorten convalescence. They permit milk puddings, soft-boiled eggs, vegetable soups thickened with flour, finely minced tender meat or fish, and mashed potatoes to be given in small amounts at a time.

Digestive Troubles. Constipation must be treated by enemata, which should be administered on alternate days if the patient has no natural movements. Diarrhea can usually be checked by alterations in the diet; the milk may be diluted, and if this does not prove efficacious the administration of a starch and opium enema will probably produce the desired result.

Abdominal distension is treated by the application of turpentine stupes to the abdomen, and some modification of the diet may be necessary. Insomnia is often complained of, and is best overcome by tepid or cold sponging, the use of warm drinks, and, if necessary, the administration of a hypnotic preparation containing twenty grains of chloral hydrate and sodium bromide.

Drugs and Stimulants. Few drugs are required in the routine treatment of typhoid fever, and they should be withheld for special symptoms or complications. The bronchitis is rarely severe enough to require treatment. If delirium occurs and is severe, the continued use of hypnotics may be necessary. The physician may prescribe certain circulatory stimulants, the most reliable of which are alcohol, strychnine, caffeine, digitalis, and camphor.

Alcohol may be required if there is great exhaustion or nourishment is being badly taken, but it is better not to use it unless it is really necessary. Whisky and brandy are valuable during the acute stages of the disease and port wine is often useful in convalescence.

Treatment of Complications. When hemorrhage takes place the patient and the intestine must be put absolutely at rest. This is best effected by the administration of ten minims of tincture of opium and the cessation of all feeding and drinking for from twelve to twenty-four hours, after which time small amounts of water, and later of milk and water, may be given. The bowels must not be opened for four days, when an olive-oil enema must be used.

The only hope of cure in a case of intestinal perforation is immediate operation. The patient is generally very weak from toxemia, and even immediate operation offers only a slender hope of recovery.

Cold Baths. The treatment of typhoid fever by the cold bath has been found of great value, and is used a good deal, especially in America. When the temperature is above 102.2° F., the patient is immersed in a cold bath at a temperature of 60° F., where he is allowed to lie for fifteen minutes if his pulse remains good. He is then lifted out and rubbed dry all over and returned to bed. This may be repeated five or six times during the day, and has been found to give excellent results, diminishing headache, delirium, etc., and producing refreshing sleep (see Chapter 86).

The use of vaccines and sera in the treatment of typhoid fever has not been attended with much success, but vaccines have given the better results.

Prophylaxis. The prophylactic treatment of the disease consists in the notification of all cases to the health authorities for the district in which they have occurred, the isolation and careful nursing of the patient, the satisfactory disposal of all excreta, and the inoculation of all persons liable to infection. In addition, the water and milk supply and the source of all shellfish must be preserved from sewage contamination.

It is safest, whenever possible, to send all patients suffering from typhoid fever to hospital for isolation and treatment.

Prophylactic inoculation is of undoubted value. It is advisable that all nurses and doctors in charge of typhoid patients, and persons going to places where the water supply is liable to be tainted, should be protected by inoculation. Troops on active service should also always be protected. The typhoid vaccine is generally given in conjunction with paratyphoid A and B, the resultant preparation being called the triple typhoid vaccine. The usual dose recommended is five hundred million typhoid bacilli and two hundred and fifty millions each of paratyphoid A and B bacilli, followed at an interval of ten days by twice that amount. It is injected subcutaneously, and usually gives rise to some degree of malaise lasting for about twenty-four hours, with a sharp but short rise of temperature. The immunity conferred lasts for about two years, and if the disease is contracted it always takes a milder form than in the unvaccinated.

PARATYPHOID FEVER

This disease in most of its aspects very closely resembles typhoid fever. It is caused by two separate and distinct organisms, the Bacilli paratyphosus A and paratyphosus B. It was very prevalent among European soldiers in Egypt, Salonika, and Mesopotamia before the triple vaccine was introduced. This consists of the two para bacilli, A and B, together with the Bacillus typhosus; hence the name. The germs are borne by fecal-feeding flies, contacts, infected water, and carriers. Paratyphoid B is fairly frequently met with in the United States and in Europe, while paratyphoid A is more common in the tropics.

Diagnosis rests on the bacteriological examination of the stools and the agglutination reaction of the blood.

After an incubation period of ten days the onset is comparatively sudden with malaise, headache, and abdominal pains. Vomiting, shivering fits, pain in the back and limbs, and nose bleeding occur in the more severe cases. The temperature rises fairly sharply and continues up from ten to eighteen days. Even at the height of the attack, however, the patient rarely looks ill, and there is but little abdominal discomfort. Rose spots often appear on the trunk between the seventh and tenth days and some bronchial catarrh may be present. The outlook is good, although some of the less serious complications associated with typhoid fever may occur.

Treatment is the same as for typhoid fever. An adequate diet, good nursing care, and regard for complications are the principles. The patient must, of course, be isolated. This disease should be suspected in cases of acute prolonged fever without obvious cause.

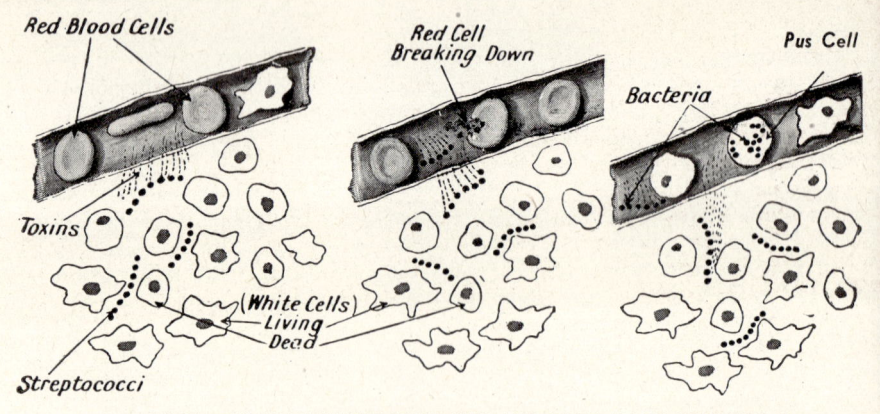

SEPTICEMIA: DIAGRAM ILLUSTRATING THIS AND SOME ALLIED CONDITIONS

Left: streptococci in the tissues are discharging toxins into the blood; clinically, this is sometimes described as septicemia, thought strictly a toxemia. Center: streptococci have invaded the blood stream, in which they are multiplying—septicemia; red blood corpuscles are being broken down, though some streptococci do not do this. Right: pyogenic bacteria, circulating in the blood stream, cause scattered abscesses, a condition called pyemia.

BLOOD POISONING

Blood poisoning is the popular name for the acute illness which arises when living germs, or the poisons produced by living germs, find their way into the blood stream. It is most often caused by those germs which produce suppuration (staphylococci and streptococci), but may also be due to other kinds. It is found in three different types called respectively sapremia, septicemia and pyemia.

Sapremia. This is the type which arises when the poison produced by germs and by the destruction of tissue finds it way into the blood. The germs causing this decomposition do not themselves enter the blood, but remain in the tissue which is undergoing putrefaction.

Sapremia is the type of blood poisoning which is, for example, likely to follow an injury, when dead pieces of bone or flesh have resulted. The onset is rapid, and there is pain and swelling at the seat of the injury, with general constitutional disturbance—chills, fever, and marked weakness. Diarrhea and skin hemorrhages may occur, while the typhoid state (see page 1340) is seen in many acute cases.

Treatment is directed to the removal of decomposing matter, for it is here that the poison is being manufactured. Wounds are opened and drained and dead tissues removed.

Septicemia. Micro-organisms or disease-producing germs may enter the circulation from some infected spot in the body and multiply in the blood stream. Such a condition is known as septicemia. It is most frequently met

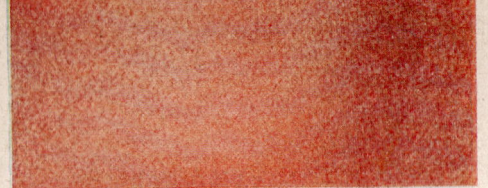

Scarlet Fever: dark red spots with pink skin around them

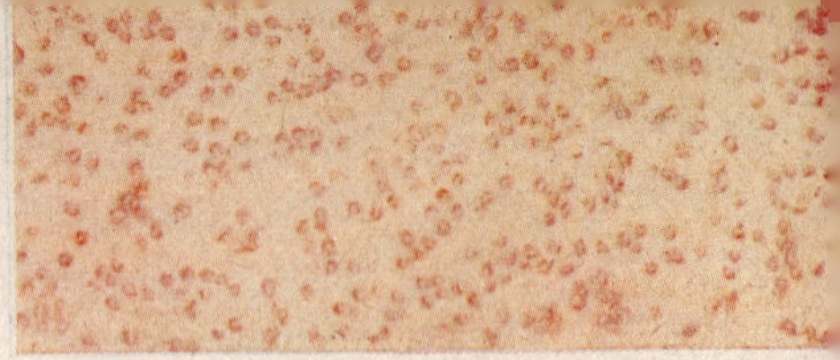

Measles: small red papules in patches, often crescentic

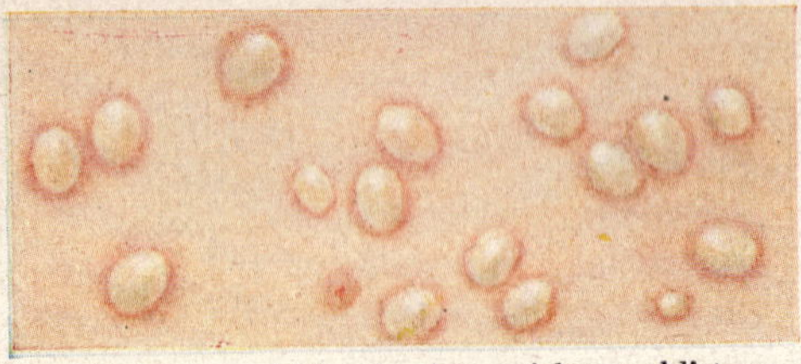

Chickenpox: little circular vesicles, or blisters, with clear fluid

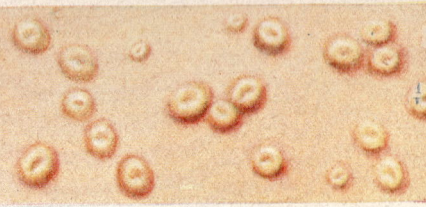

Smallpox: oval yellow blisters depressed or umbilicated in center

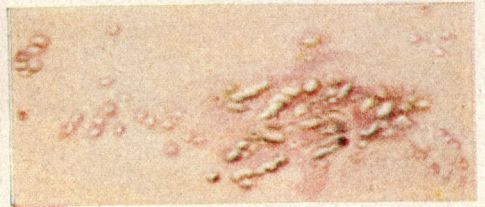

Herpes: crops of small clear, or yellow, vesicles which may coalesce

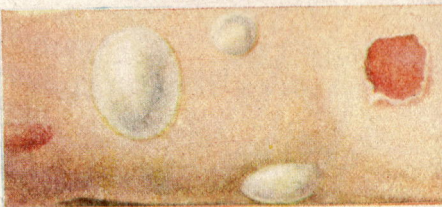

Pemphigus: large blisters, or bullae, with clear or turbid contents

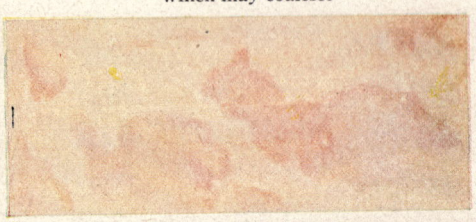

Hives: wheals and reddened patches, with great itching

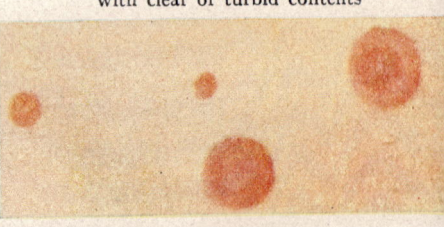

Antipyrine Rash: reddened circular areas with raised margins

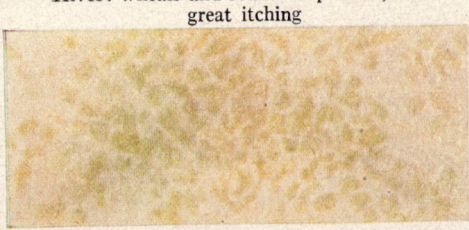

Pityriasis versicolor: greenish-yellow scales in irregular patches

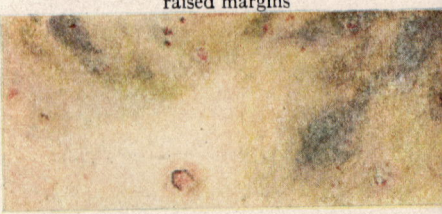

Purpura: large patches of livid discoloration from effused blood

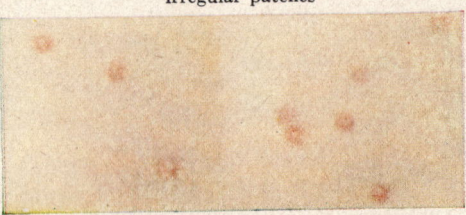

Typhoid Fever: red papules, size of lentils, occurring in crops

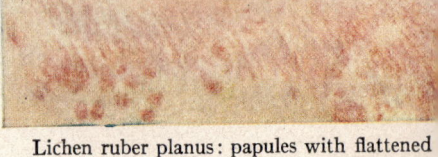

Lichen ruber planus: papules with flattened tops; very itchy

PLATE XI.   RASH IN INFECTIOUS AND OTHER DISORDERS

with in association with diseases of the throat and tonsils, sore places or wounds on the hands or feet or other parts of the body, or in connection with childbirth, when it is known as puerperal fever (see Chapter 192). In any of these conditions germs which are multiplying and giving rise to inflammation are present in the affected part or organ. In the majority of cases the germs are localized as just described under Sapremia, but in septicemia the zone of tissue which separates the diseased spot from the general circulation is penetrated by the germs, which pass into the circulation and multiply therein. If such germs merely enter the blood stream, but do not multiply there, a less serious state called bacteremia ensues. Such a condition is met with in pneumonia and typhoid fever during the early stages. If, on the other hand, the germs both circulate and multiply in the blood stream the condition is one of septicemia.

The germs which are most commonly found in the blood in cases of septicemia are the Streptococcus pyogenes and the Staphylococcus aureus. Other germs which are at times met with in the blood stream are the pneumococcus, gonococcus, meningococcus, the influenza bacillus of Pfeiffer, the anthrax bacillus, and the Bacillus pyocyaneus. The term septicemia is, however, properly only applied to the septic infections.

Signs of Septicemia. Patients who are suffering from septicemia present two groups of signs and symptoms, those due to the primary disease and those associated with the invasion of the blood stream with the germs which lead to the condition of septicemia. The signs and symptoms of the primary diseases with which septicemia is wont to be associated, such as tonsilitis, puerperal fever, wounds, etc., are described in their appropriate chapters.

In some cases, however, the primary source of entry of the micro-organisms into the circulation cannot be discovered, and such examples of septicemia are referred to as cryptogenetic. In some cases of true septicemia the organisms for one reason or another cannot be found in the blood.

The symptoms and signs of septicemia are very variable, but are generally of grave significance. The temperature usually rises and shows a considerable variation during the twenty-four hours, being high in the evening and low in the morning, producing a typical intermittent or remittent temperature curve (septic temperature). The pulse becomes correspondingly rapid. Attacks of shivering or chills are common and are a warning that some serious complication is developing. In some cases also the patient experiences frequent and drenching sweats during the night.

There is no actual pain associated with septicemia, but the invalid becomes progressively weaker and more obviously ill as the disease progresses. The abdomen may be distended owing to flatulence and the appetite and digestion are usually impaired. Examination shows a progressively increasing degree of anemia, owing to a diminution in number of the red cells. The white blood cells are usually increased in number, constituting what is known as a leucocytosis, but in very grave cases the number of white cells falls, and their enumeration therefore affords an indication as to prognosis.

In some instances a red rash appears upon the skin, first in one part and then in another, and minute hemorrhagic spots may develop. Fleeting pains in the joints are not infrequent, and the urine nearly always contains a small amount of albumin.

Septicemia may assume all degrees of severity, from a mild case which shows comparatively little disturbance and ends in a complete recovery, to a very severe one which simulates a very acute attack of typhoid fever. In these severe "typhoid" types the patient rapidly becomes prostrated and drowsy, and delirium is the rule. The pulse is very rapid, and it is difficult to distinguish between the individual beats at the wrist, so that it is called a running pulse. The skin is hot and dry and the temperature often gradually falls as the patient becomes worse, until finally it remains below the normal level. There are marked gastrointestinal disturbances with diarrhea and vomiting, and jaundice may be noted in the terminal stages. In addition to hemorrhages in the skin, blood may be passed in the urine or vomited from the stomach.

Diagnosis and Treatment. There is not usually much difficulty in diagnosing that a patient is suffering from septicemia when the symptoms of the condition develop during some other illness, such as in infected wound, severe sore throat, or ofter childbirth. In addition, certain special examinations should be carried out, in order to establish firmly the diagnosis. The most important of these are examinations of the blood.

When septicemia starts without any obvious source of entry for the germs, the so-called cryptogenetic variety, it has to be differentiated from other causes of fever which may occur without localizing signs, such as enteric fever, miliary tuberculosis and infective or bacterial endocarditis.

In the treatment of any case of septicemia attention should be directed primarily towards finding the source of infection from which the organisms have entered the blood stream.

Medical Treatment. Intravenous injections of various antiserums, such as meningococcus or pneumococcus serum, are of value, and if the nature of the infecting germ is known, injections of its corresponding antiserum are indicated. There have been striking advances recently made in the chemotherapy of diseases caused by the streptococcus, gonococcus, pneumococcus and several other organisms. In the case of septicemia caused by these bacteria the group of drugs included under the term sulfonamides (sulfanilamide, prontosil, etc.) have proven their value. Blood transfusion sometimes is of service. Vaccines are very unsatisfactory and may easily do harm. Water must be given freely by the mouth or by the rectum. Normal saline solution may have to be administered intravenously.

Apart from these special procedures, treatment is to a large extent symptomatic. Constant and skilled nursing is required in order to conserve the patient's strength. Food must be light and nutritious and not of a kind liable to cause digestive upsets, and sleep must be procured, if necessary, by the use of suitable hypnotic drugs. During convalescence, the anemia must be combated by the administration of iron, and if severe enough by transfusion. A careful watch must be kept upon the heart, as the cardiac muscle is particularly liable to be weakened in septicemia.

Surgical Treatment. Treatment of the source of infection calls for good judgment, since too early interference may easily serve to increase the general infection by opening up nature's barriers around the infected area. Provision must be made for the free escape of suppurative discharges. In many cases incision and drainage are sufficient. In some cases, as in appendicitis, the focus must be removed to avoid further spread. Very often provision is made for drainage following abdominal operations should pus later accumulate.

Incision and opening of the infected area is indicated when the pus is formed or when there is great local swelling and tension. A carbuncle or badly infected wound may be excised under these circumstances. An infected uterus must first be thoroughly explored and cleansed, and may even require removal.

Pyemia. Pyemia is really only a modification of septicemia. The bacteria, having invaded the blood stream, are distributed all over the body (septicemia). If they settle down in certain definite situations and there cause suppuration, the condition becomes one of pyemia. The focus of infection may be anywhere, as, for instance, a septic wound, middle-ear disease, appendicitis, a suppurating lymph gland, and so on. A very common situation is the lining membrane of the heart, resulting in endocarditis. The organisms concerned are usually the streptococci and the staphylococci, although a large number of other bacteria may similarly invade the blood stream and cause foci of suppuration.

Signs of Pyemia. The onset of symptoms is often sudden, and is usually marked by a severe chill during which the temperature may rise to 104° or 106° F. This is followed by a profuse sweat and fall of temperature. The whole process is repeated at intervals of a day or two, or several such attacks may occur during the course of a single day.

A good deal of constitutional disturbance is usually present. Loss of appetite, nausea, and vomiting are generally marked, and as the disease progresses there is great emaciation. When the lungs are involved the patient will suffer from cough and shortness of breath, often accompanied by severe stabbing pain in the chest and spitting of blood. The joints are frequently the seats of abscesses, especially when the gonococcus is responsible. Septic rashes are sometimes seen and are usually a bad sign. Anemia is nearly always present and it may be very profound. The spleen is enlarged and painful, and there may be intense pain in the left side. Blood may be seen in the urine.

The course of the disease varies greatly with the intensity of the infection and with the virulence of the organisms. In rapid cases the patient may sink into a typhoid state and die in a week or two from the onset of the illness. In chronic cases the disease may last for months. The general course, however, is usually downward, and the patient succumbs to exhaustion or to a septic pneumonia.

Difficulties of Diagnosis. When pyemia follows a wound, an operation, or a confinement, it is, as a rule, readily recognized, but in other cases the diagnosis is not so easy. It may be especially difficult to distinguish it from typhoid fever, since many of the symptoms are similar in both diseases. Malaria is excluded by an examination of the blood for the malaria parasite and by the action of quinine. Acute miliary tuberculosis and tuberculosis of the kidneys are other conditions difficult to distinguish from pyemia. The arthritis which occurs after scarlet fever is really an instance of septic infection and may end in pyemia.

Treatment. The general treatment is to give nourishment as liberally as possible; to give fluids freely; if sufficient water cannot be taken by the mouth it must be given by the rectum, or into a vein, or under the skin. Alcohol is generally recommended, and in severe cases may be given in large doses. Careful nursing will do much to keep up the patient's strength and add to his comfort.

Local treatment consists in free evacuation and drainage of the pus wherever the abscess is accessible. But the focus of infection is very often not accessible, and the treatment is then purely that of septicemia.

Vaccines have been recommended and are of most value when they are autogenous, *i.e.* made by cultures from the patient's own blood or pus. In other cases, however, a stock antistreptococcal serum has proved helpful. Treatment with the sulfonamides is assuming a role of increasing prominence.

ERYSIPELAS

Erysipelas is an acute inflammatory condition of the skin; it is characterized by serious toxic symptoms of high fever and great prostration. Acute erysipelas without fever is unknown.

The cause is always infection by the Streptococcus pyogenes, or erysipelatosus, a highly virulent type of streptococcus. The infection spreads in the epidermis, or freely movable part of the skin itself. The inflammatory reaction which results being limited to a definite plane, and the disease spreading eccentrically from a local focus, there is always a well-marked edge which can be both seen and felt as the process extends. The rate of advance is not reg-

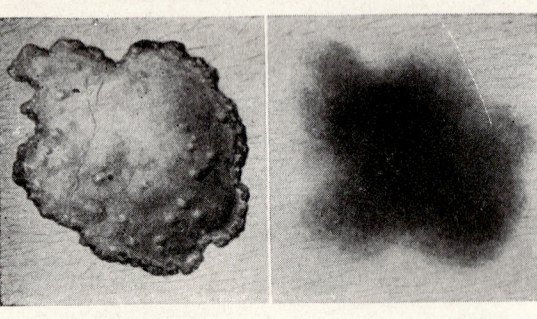

CHARACTERS OF THE ERUPTION IN ERYSIPELAS
Left, a spreading patch of erysipelas showing the raised and clearly defined edge; also little vesicles studded over the patch. Right, a patch of simple erythema, or inflammation, for contrast; the edge is not definite, but fades gradually into the healthy skin and is not raised.

ular, and the patches produced vary, therefore, in both shape and size, spreading rapidly in some parts and more slowly in others.

The color is usually rose-red, and the surface shiny from underlying tension. The fluid which is responsible for this may be exuded so rapidly that blisters may develop on the surface. The clear contents of these soon become opaque, and pus with subsequent crust formation adds to the difficulties of local treatment.

Symptoms. An attack of erysipelas is usually proceded by a feeling of malaise, which rapidly develops with shivering attacks and high fever. The climax is generally reached by the end of the fifth day if complications do not supervene. The evening temperature, which may previously have exceeded 103-104° F., drops to 100° or so, the local manifestations cease to spread, the swelling subsides, and the affected surface begins to peel, somewhat as occurs after scarlet fever. The feeling of tension, burning, or itching in the patch gives place to one of dryness or discomfort, which is easily relieved by suitable applications, and the patient is on the way to recovery.

The commonest site of an attack is on the face, usually at the junction of the skin with the mucous membrane of the mouth, the nose or the eye. Very likely there has been a small crack, fissure or irritable abrasion in one or other of these situations for a considerable time, and it is in such that the streptococcus flourishes and increases in virulence. In delicate and particularly in alcoholic subjects the resistance to streptococcal infection is often low, and when it breaks down erysipelas is apt to occur.

Erysipelas may also follow a mosquito bite on any part of the body, or occur round an infected wound or scratch in a susceptible individual. Accidental contamination from another patient with some streptococcal infection, or from a deep focus in the patient's own body, may be responsible.

Erysipelas occurs occasionally after childbirth, and before the proper training of midwives was responsible for many fatalities.

Complications. The complications of erysipelas are common and usually dangerous. They may be described as local and general.

The commonest local complication is infection of the deep cellular tissue under the skin and the production of cellulitis. When this spreads from the face to the neck there is a danger of involvement of the upper respiratory tract. The result of this may be exudation in the larynx and the production of edema of the glottis, so that the current of air is mechanically obstructed and no air can pass into the lungs. Such a patient is in imminent danger of death

DISEASES CAUSED BY KNOWN GERMS: VARIOUS

other's pencils, pens, books, etc.

Milk epidemics of scarlet fever were formerly of fairly frequent occurrence. They are generally due to some person concerned in handling and distributing the milk who is suffering from an unnoticed mild attack.

Domestic animals are thought to assist in spreading the disease, and even fleas have been suspected in this connection.

STRAWBERRY TONGUE IN SCARLET FEVER

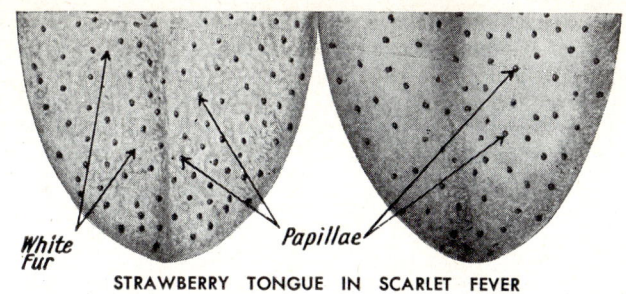

Two appearances of the tongue in scarlet fever which are described as strawberry tongue. Left: a thick white fur on the surface of the organ through which bright red papillae project. Right: raw red surface on which the bright scarlet papillae stand out.

Course of the Disease. The incubation period is short, being usually from one to eight days, and the symptoms vary considerably with the severity of the attack.

The most prominent early symptoms are headache, sore throat, which is often very severe, and vomiting, which occurs much more frequently in children than in adults. The other symptoms of fever, such as lassitude, lack of appetite, etc., are also present. The throat is red, the tonsils somewhat enlarged and the tongue badly coated. The temperature is somewhat raised, usually to about 100° F. On the second day of illness the characteristic rash appears, the temperature rises to 101° or 103° F., and the throat becomes more swollen and painful. The glands at the angle of the jaw are often enlarged and tender.

The rash (see color plate facing page 1345) appears first on the neck and chest, accompanied by a brightly flushed face with a white area around the mouth, which is very characteristic of scarlet fever, and is called circumoral pallor. The eyes are bright and the general appearance of the patient is one of intelligence, which contrasts very markedly with that of measles, where the patient looks heavy and stupid. The rash consists of scarlet dots on a flushed background of skin; it spreads downwards from the neck to the trunk and limbs, terminating on the feet and hands, the whole body being covered generally within one or two days. As it passes downwards it fades above.

The rash persists usually for three or four days. During this time, when the rash is at its height, the throat is very red and swollen and may show some yellowish exudation on the tonsils, resembling very closely a diphtheritic throat. The papillae of the tongue enlarge and show through the furred coating as red spots on a white surface, to which the name of white strawberry tongue has been given. About the third day the fur gradually peels off, leaving on the fourth day a raw, bright red tongue with prominent papillae, known as the red strawberry tongue. The tongue then gradually resumes its normal color.

In a straightforward case the temperature subsides gradually within a few days, and the patient feels quite well by the end of the first week. At this time the typical desquamation commences as a powdering of the face, and spreads downwards over the body in the same order as the rash appeared. The peeling is rarely completed by the end of the sixth week, and sometimes persists on the hands and feet for eight weeks or even longer.

Varying Types of Infection. Scarlet fever does not always pursue the simple course mentioned above, and various types of the disease have been described by medical men, the most important of which are the mild type, the septic type, and the toxic type.

Mild types differ from ordinary scarlet fever in that the patient is only very slightly ill. The throat symptoms are slight, and the rash may be so faint that it is overlooked. The infectious nature of such cases may not be realized, and so the disease may be widely spread.

Toxic or malignant cases are rare, but are almost always fatal. The general symptoms are most severe, while the rash is slight. The throat may be only a little red, but the temperature is usually very high, often 105° F. or more. The patient rarely lives more than four or five days.

Septic scarlet fever is much more common, and is not nearly so often fatal as the toxic type. It occurs generally in young children, and the fever is prolonged for about three or four weeks. The chief characteristics of the septic type are the severity of the throat symptoms and the height and prolonged duration of the temperature. The tonsils are usually ulcerated, and there is a profuse nasal discharge. From nose and throat inflammation spreads to the ear, and severe earache followed by purulent discharge is almost always present. Convalescence is slow and many complications are liable to intervene.

Complications. The most usual complications in scarlet fever are discharges from the nose and ears. The former is often very persistent, and is of importance largely because it is a recognized means by which scarlet fever spreads. The latter is much more serious and may, if not properly treated, lead to serious aftereffects. It arises from the spread of the infection from the nose and throat up the Eustachian tube, which passes from the throat to the middle ear. Inflammation of the ear is generally heralded by severe pain and a rise of temperature, both of which subside when the discharge is flowing freely. The infection may pass backwards and give rise to a mastoid abscess, when there is tenderness over the mastoid bone behind the ear, or it may pass inwards, giving rise to an abscess of the brain.

Adenitis, or inflammation of the glands, occurs in a large number of cases. The glands of the neck are most frequently involved, and become large and tender, and may suppurate, giving rise to large abscesses.

The most important complication is nephritis, or inflammation of the kidneys, which occurs usually at the end of the third week of the disease. There may be no symptoms of illness, but usually there is some rise of temperature with vomiting or headache. The urine becomes diminished in quantity and often contains blood, and there may be some edema of the face, hands, or feet.

Rheumatic manifestations occur in a large number of cases, giving rise to some stiffness, particularly in the hands and wrists. This sometimes assumes a serious character, and may be associated with affections of the heart, such as endocarditis or pericarditis.

Relapses are very uncommon in scarlet fever, but do occur occasionally, when the symptoms of the original disease are repeated, usually in a milder form.

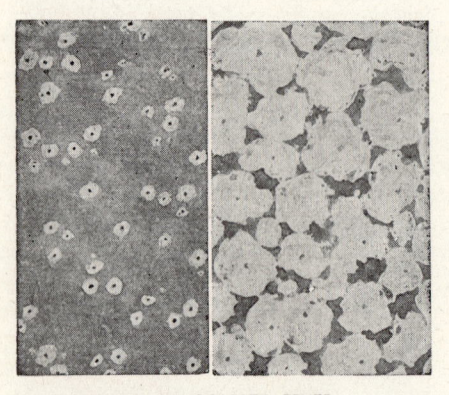

PEELING IN SCARLET FEVER
Peeling begins at the sites of the red spots of the eruption and at their edges, giving a pinhole appearance (left); later, the flakes are larger, making a semilacework pattern (right).

Patients suffering from scarlet fever are particularly liable to contract diphtheria; in other cases the diphtheria germ may be found in the throat, without the usual signs of the disease being present. It is unusual for a person to contract scarlet fever twice.

Treatment of a Typical Attack. The treatment of the disease must be considered under two headings — the treatment of the patient himself, and the means which must be taken to avoid the spread of infection.

The patient must be put to bed and kept there for three weeks, no matter how slight the attack may be. He must be warmly clad and the temperature of the room must be kept at about 60° F. This renders him less liable to chill and reduces the likelihood of nephritis and rheumatism developing. He should be well washed all over daily with soap and hot water, and hot baths are useful as soon as the temperature has subsided. This keeps the skin in good condition, helps to excrete some of the waste products of the body, and thus aids the kidneys. The diet at first should be restricted to milk, with copious drinks of water between meals. Later, when the temperature has subsided, light, solid food, such as bread and butter, milk puddings, fruit, etc., should be given, but meat, eggs, and soups must be withheld until after the end of the third week, as they cause increased work for the kidneys. The urine should be examined every alternate day so that kidney trouble, should it develop, may be treated early.

The mouth and nose must be kept clean and healthy, and all discharges carefully burned. Gargles and mouth washes of warm salt solution are useful, and the gums and teeth should be cleansed with absorbent cotton soaked in peroxide of hydrogen (five volumes) or phenol solution (one-in-forty). When the throat is much inflamed or septic, irrigation of the mouth with weak chlorine water gives good results. This is done by means of a douche can and tube. The latter is inserted into the patient's mouth while he leans over the edge of the bed above a basin. The douche can is held a little above the head, so that the water flows easily around the mouth and throat and out into the basin.

The nose must be swabbed with a solution of bicarbonate of soda (a teaspoonful to a pint of water) and anointed with a little carbolized vaseline. If very septic, peroxide of hydrogen (five volumes) will be found to be more effective than the soda solution. In some cases, such as the septic and toxic types, alcohol may prove a useful stimulant. Abundance of fresh air improves the appetite and induces sleep.

Antistreptococcus serum and convalescent serum are used in frankly septic cases.

Treatment of Complications. The various complications must be treated as they arise. When nasal discharge is present the nose must be syringed with saline solution and cleansed with peroxide of hydrogen. Discharge from the ear is treated by frequent cleansing with boracic lotion and the insertion of peroxide of hydrogen drops, which are removed after a few minutes by careful drying. Hot fomentations are useful for relieving pain in the ear, which, however, nearly always disappears when the

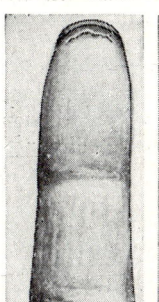

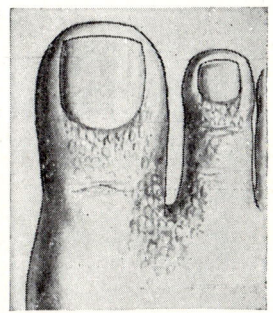

PEELING ON FINGERS AND TOES
Peeling on the fingers may begin as a crack parallel with the free edge of the nail (left), and may persist at the roots of the nails, fingers and toes, as shown on the right.

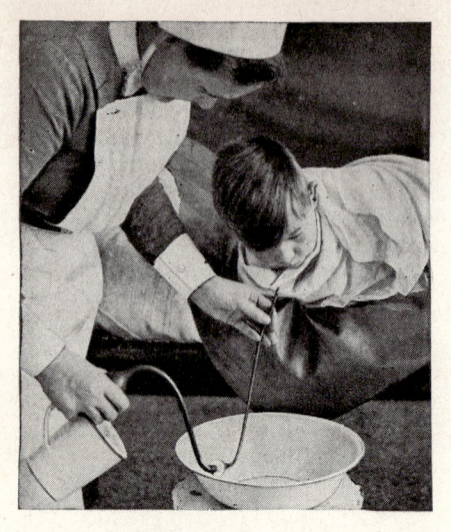

CLEANSING THE NOSE

Purulent discharge may be cleared out of the nose by gentle douching, using a syringe, to which is attached a piece of soft, narrow tubing, preferably a soft catheter.

drum perforates and the discharge becomes manifest. Whenever possible rupture should be anticipated by incision of the drum. Much pain and rise of temperature are sometimes caused by enlargements of the glands at the side of the neck. Hot fomentations should be applied to these at four-hour intervals, and the glands may require opening if they suppurate.

Nephritis is serious, and must be treated with the greatest possible care. The patient must sleep between blankets and avoid all risk of chill. Free action of the skin and bowels must be obtained by means of hot packs, hot-air baths, and frequent aperients, of which the best is jalap. Water must be drunk in large quantities, and the diet reduced to milk, and later supplemented by starchy and fat foods, and by fruit, vegetables, etc.

Rheumatic manifestations are relieved by sleeping between blankets and by the application of absorbent cotton to the joints. Salicylates are often of great use for joint pains, and if there is any affection of the heart the patient must be kept at rest on the back for a long time.

Preventive Measures. From the public health point of view the chief points to be considered in the treatment of scarlet fever are isolation of the patient, disinfection of his house, clothes, etc., quarantine of contacts, and prophylactic or preventive treatment. Scarlet fever is one of the reportable infectious diseases, and it is therefore the duty of the parent or guardian, and of the doctor, to report its occurrence at once to the health authorities of the district. The patient is then removed to a communicable-disease hospital or isolated at home, the latter being possible when there is plenty of accommodation and a responsible person in charge.

Isolation should be enforced for at least five weeks even in a straightforward case, and must always be prolonged until the patient is free from all discharges and the nose and throat are clean and healthy. Provided such is the case there is no risk of infection spreading from desquamating hands and feet.

The organism causing scarlet fever has not yet, in the opinion of some observers, been definitely isolated. Yet Dochez found a typical germ (in scarlet fever cases) in wounds, burns, uterine discharges, and in the milk during an epidemic caused by milk. Dick caused typical scarlet fever to appear in volunteers by injecting what he considered to be the Streptococcus scarlatinae. Infection undoubtedly spreads chiefly through the secretions of and discharge from the nose, mouth, and ear, or more rarely from the vagina. In the nursing of this disease, therefore, it is highly important that all such discharges should be burned at once, preferably in a fire in the patient's room. When free from infection he should have a bath, his hair should be washed, and he should sleep in a clean bed, and preferably in another room, for two days before mixing with other people. The bath and hair-washing should be repeated on the second day. The patient's room, clothes, bedding, etc., must

DISEASES CAUSED BY KNOWN GERMS: VARIOUS

all be disinfected, and toys and books should be burned.

Children in contact with scarlet fever should be quarantined for a period of two weeks. The milk supply should be investigated whenever an outbreak of the disease arises.

Susceptibility to infection and diagnosis of doubtful cases can be determined by the Dick reaction produced by inoculating the skin with a small quantity of an active suspension in broth containing the scarlet fever toxin. Protection of short duration can be given by further minute doses at intervals of four to seven days. Severe toxic cases can be treated by the administration of a specific serum.

CEREBROSPINAL FEVER

This is an infectious disease commonly known as spotted fever, because of a rash which frequently appears in the course of the disease. Epidemics appear more commonly in the spring and winter, but are not usually of an extensive nature. It is not highly infectious, and young people are most susceptible. Crowding seems to be an important contributory cause. The infective organism—the meningococcus—has been discovered. Though the disease is not highly contagious, infection may be transmitted by coughing and sneezing, since the organism enters and leaves the body by the membranes of the nose and throat. During an outbreak, therefore, the use of handkerchiefs and the question of kissing become important factors. Infected persons may become "carriers" though free from symptoms. Some cases crop up at times after or apart from any epidemic.

Symptoms. There are many different forms of the disease, so that when the disease picture presented is not typical, difficulties in diagnosis may easily arise, and the condition may pass unrecognized. In the commonest form the illness sets in more or less suddenly with headache, vomiting, and fever. The muscles of the neck early become stiff and painful, and in severe cases the head is drawn rigidly backwards. There is much irritability and undue sensitiveness to light and noise. Various bodily pains are often complained of, and there may be cramp and jerking spasms in the limbs. Squint is common, and some muscles of the eyeball may show paralysis. The headache is prominent and persists. Delirium may occur early. After a few days mental stupor sets in and the patient becomes difficult to rouse and resents disturbance. Fever continues high. More than one form of rash may appear, but purplish spots, variable but not uncommon, may cover the entire skin.

Course. The length and course of the disease vary greatly. If death takes place, it is generally after the first two weeks of the disease. In cases of milder severity the symptoms begin to lessen at the beginning of the second week, but improvement is not infrequently slow,

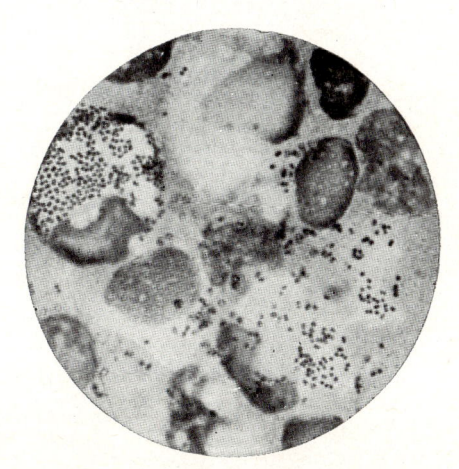

GERM OF CEREBROSPINAL FEVER
The causative agent in this disease (popularly called spotted fever and a form of meningitis) is the meningococcus, shown here, which produces inflammation of the meninges, or coverings of the brain and spinal cord.
Photo, Dr. W. R. Wiseman

and recurrence of fever and fresh complicating symptoms may arise during convalescence. Headache may persist for months or years after an attack, while pneumonia, pleurisy, joint troubles, and deafness may supervene.

In some epidemics very acute malignant cases occur which are very rapidly fatal. Other cases show a mild and long-lasting type of the disease.

When after death the brain has been examined it has been found that there has been an inflammatory condition of the pia mater and arachnoid membranes, and at the base of the brain, where the changes are most marked, there is a purulent exudation with much thickened membrances. Frequently there is an enlargement of the brain ventricles, which may contain a turbid fluid. The substance of the brain itself is more soft than it should be, and may show surface inflammation and points of hemorrhage. Many, if not all, of the cranial nerves may be found to have been involved in the morbid process.

Diagnosis. As already stated there may be difficulty sometimes in diagnosing the condition, and the disease is not seldom unrecognized or mistaken for other acute infections. Certain cases of typhoid fever especially present a picture similar to this disease. Influenza, pneumonia, rheumatic fever, and other acute infections may be accompanied by symptoms suggestive of this disease. Meningitis may also, of course, be due to other types of infection, especially tuberculosis. Points of importance to note are the severe headache, delirium, fever, the retraction of the neck, and the rigidity of limb muscles. Certainty of diagnosis rests on examination, by lumbar puncture, of the cerebrospinal fluid. It flows out under increased pressure when inflammation of the brain membrane is present, is commonly turbid and perhaps contains pus or blood, and the causative organism is found in it.

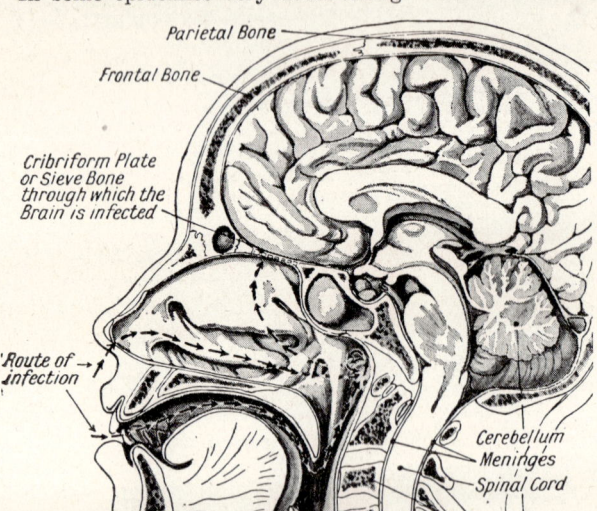

ROUTE OF INFECTION IN MENINGITIS
The route of infection of the brain coverings by the meningococcus which causes "spotted fever" is not definitely known, but the organism infects the nasopharynx in the first instance, and possibly reaches the skull through the roof of the nose.

Treatment. In treating the disease, since the central nervous system is involved, the patient should have absolute rest and quiet and freedom from all sources of external irritation. The hair of the head should be clipped close and an ice-bag should be placed lightly on the skull. The bowels should be kept freely open and copious fluid allowed. Sedatives may be necessary to ease the severe headache or alleviate a delirious condition. Much relief to these symptoms is derived by drawing off cerebrospinal fluid frequently by means of a needle puncture between the fourth and fifth lumbar vertebrae. This procedure, which should be carried out in every suspected case, is specially indicated when the head symptoms are marked and therefore much increase of pressure of the fluid within the cerebral ventricles is suspected. A curative serum has been introduced by an American physician, Flexner, the use of which has greatly reduced the mortality rate in some, but not all, epidemics and enhanced the chances of recovery. The sum and substance of Flexner's discovery is that whereas a few years ago the mortality rate was 75 per cent it is now less than 25 per cent. The antiserum should be given early in the illness and injected into the spinal canal frequently after withdrawal of some cerebrospinal fluid.

Serum may be given both intravenously and intrathecally in severe cases and if the appropriate serum is employed a cure is almost certain. Several doses at twelve to twenty-four hour intervals may be necessary.

Prevention. The provision of ample space, good ventilation, good food in plenty, and hygienic conditions for the community do much to prevent "spotted fever." Careful hygiene of the nasopharynx is a rational precaution against contracting the disease. Cases should be isolated with proper care and attention to disinfection. Carriers should be searched for by examining bacteriologically all contacts and suspects. Such cases should, if possible, be isolated, and have their throats disinfected with 1-in-1000 potassium permanganate until two negative results from the throat and nose swabs have been recorded. The disease is reportable.

INFLUENZA

At intervals of years epidemics of influenza have swept over the world, the last two occasions being in 1889-90 and in 1918. Beginning in some particular country — in the case of the 1918 epidemic it was said to be Spain, though it would appear that the epidemic started earlier in southern France and in Italy — the disease quickly crosses frontiers and moves with ships in their tracks. Each epidemic appears to occur in waves, which vary in severity, but as time goes on the disease becomes less formidable, though mild epidemics recur for years — as well as devastating waves. Here let it be said that although sporadic cases of influenza do occur between the pandemics, there are many cases of coryza, chill, tracheitis, and mild bronchitis, glibly referred to by an uninformed laity as "flu," but such illnesses do not resemble influenza, nor should they be mistaken for it.

Very little is known of the influences determining the occurrence and character of the epidemics. Age and climate and previous attacks confer little or no immunity. Influenza is cer-

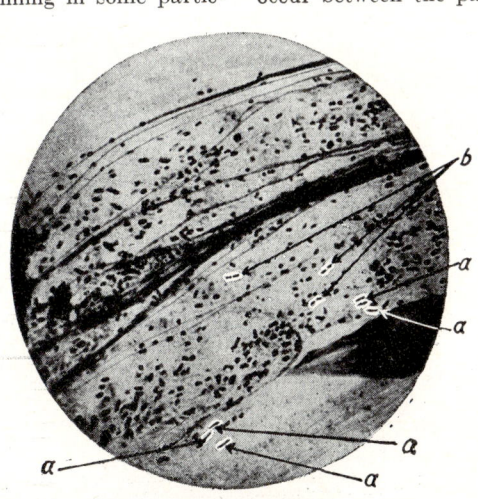

BACILLUS OF INFLUENZA

In this microscopical preparation the rodlike structures (*a*) are the bacilli of Pfeiffer, which are closely associated with influenza; the pneumococcus (*b*) often occurs with the influenza bacillus.

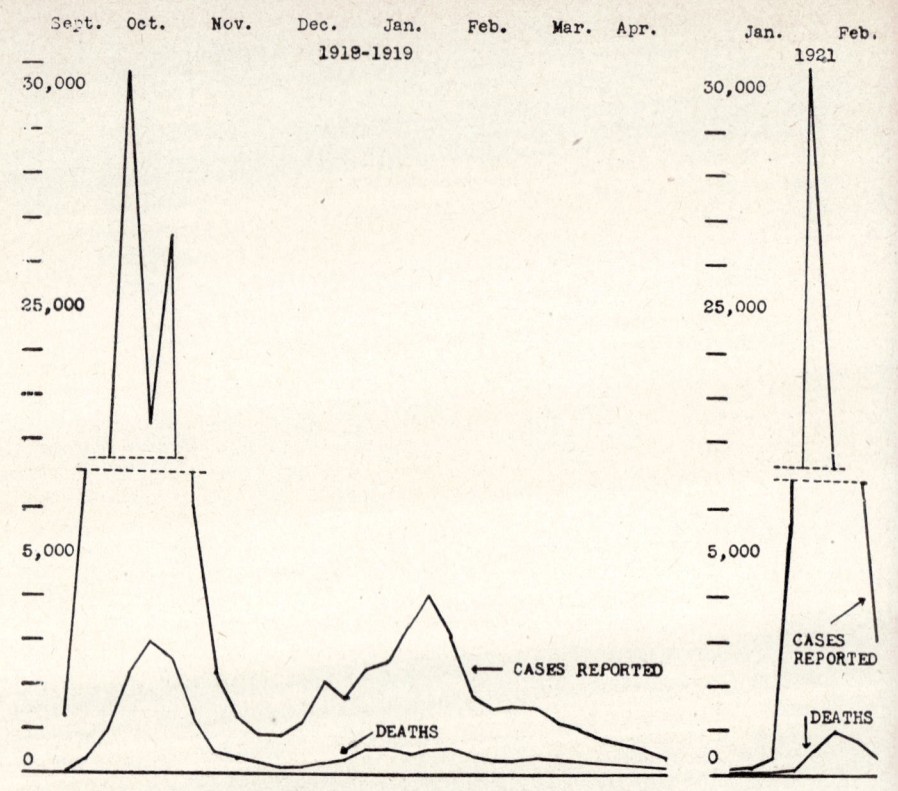

CASES REPORTED AND DEATHS FROM INFLUENZA

This and accompanying illustrations suggest the terrifying problem which a major epidemic brings. The graph shows figures by weeks for the months indicated, during the epidemics of 1918-1919 and 1921 in New York City, the lines being broken because if they were drawn complete the height of this page would not accommodate them.

Figures taken from records of the New York City Department of Health.

tainly highly contagious, the infection being disseminated when a person suffering from the disease coughs, sneezes, or even talks loudly. The breath is charged with a fine spray which carries the infective agent — it may be to a distance of six feet (see page 279). Infection may also be harbored by the handkerchiefs and clothes of the patients and continue in the rooms occupied.

It is not yet known what is the real nature of the infective agent. There have been found minute bodies which are able to pass through a porcelain filter, streptococci, the influenza bacillus of Pfeiffer and the pneumococcus. It is clear that the last three cause some of the complications of the disease. Of these a virulent streptococcus is responsible for many severe and fatal cases. In 1933 certain research workers by inoculation of the virus succeeded in establishing the disease among ferrets. It is also thought that the distemper of dogs may be due to infection with influenza organisms.

Symptoms of an Attack. The incubation period in influenza is relatively very short, perhaps about forty-five hours. The onset is very sudden, so much so that people who did not feel partic-

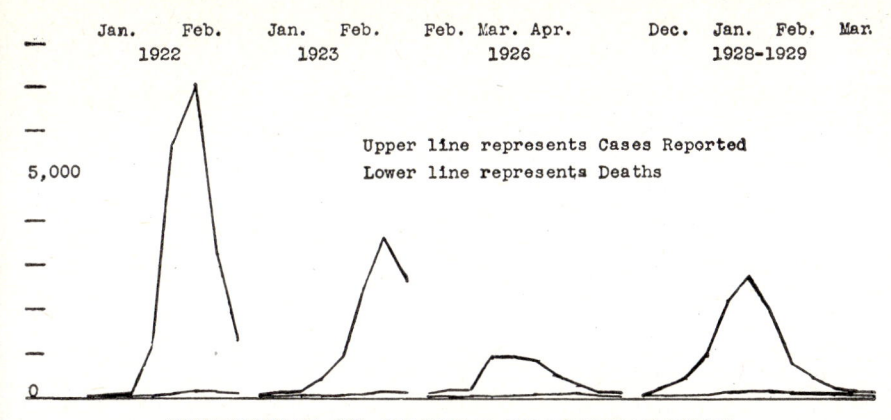

HOW INFLUENZA FELL OFF DURING THE NINETEEN-TWENTIES

These graphs provide an almost amazing comparison with those for the two great epidemics, shown on page 1358; scales are the same. Figures from the New York City Department of Health, used to prepare these graphs, are typical of those for most large cities of Europe and America, in proportion to size.

ularly out of sorts have fallen unconscious in the street. As a rule, there is severe headache and pains in the back and limbs; the temperature rises rapidly, the pulse, however, remaining relatively slow; the tongue is coated with a thick fur, and there is a dry, irritating cough. Running at the eyes and nose and a sore throat are often present and suggest a bad cold. Sometimes the patient is delirious from the outset.

There may be some sickness, pain in the abdomen, and slight diarrhea, and there are cases in which these symptoms assume such prominence that they overshadow all other symptoms, and the disease may be mistaken for some kind of food poisoning. A disagreeable feature of some of the cases of gastric influenza is that the patient may hiccough almost continuously for hours, and perhaps for several days. It should be noted, however, that sleeping sickness is known to manifest itself as epidemic hiccough. It is characteristic of influenza that the patient feels very depressed in body and spirits, and even after aparently mild attacks this may prove a very distressing feature. After remaining up for three, four, or five days the temperature falls, usually gradually.

Complications. The disease may not take this favorable course. In the malignant type of the disease the patient becomes rapidly and profoundly poisoned; there is a peculiar heliotrope cyanosis and rapid development of heart failure. The breathing may become rapid, the temperature rise again, if it has fallen, and the patient begin to spit up a sticky substance, colored bright red with blood, perhaps, or at other times of a greenish hue. The meaning of this is that the lungs have become involved and pneumonia, generally the lobular type, has set in. In the 1918 epidemic cases in which the lungs became waterlogged from secretion were very common and often rapidly fatal.

A sharp pain in the side may indicate the presence of pleurisy, and this may go on to empyema or the accumulation of pus in the pleural cavity.

In some cases when the urine is examined it is found to contain albumin and other substances, indicating the presence of inflammation of the kidneys or nephritis. The heart muscle may become weakened and a dilated heart may result. Cases are frequent in which after recovery from acute illness palpitation, undue rapidity of the heartbeat, and a

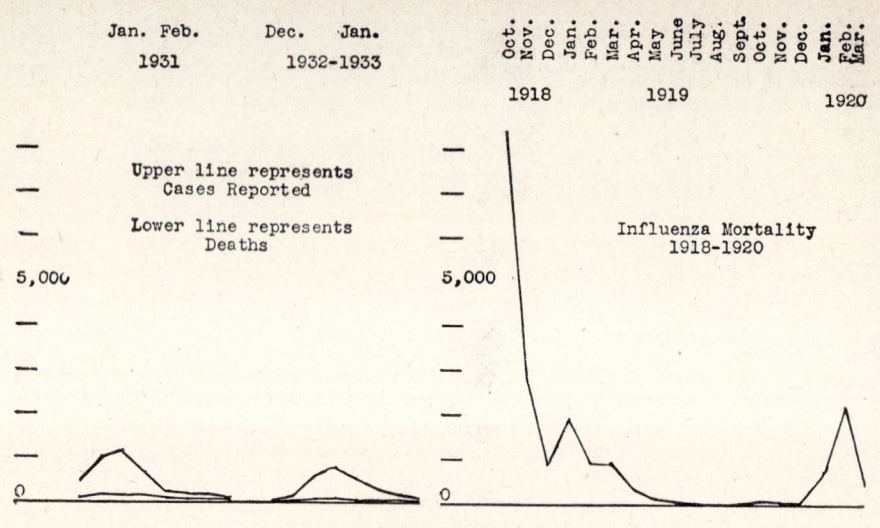

INFLUENZA STATISTICS

These graphs, together with those preceding, illustrate how influenza incidence and mortality fluctuate. At the left are the records for the critical months of 1931 and 1932-1933, extremely low in comparison with 1922, 1923, or 1928-1929, shown on page 1359 on the same scale as these. At the right is a month-by-month graph of deaths from influenza for eighteen months during 1918-1920. Note how few deaths occurred during the summer months. In view of the observed cyclical character of influenza outbreaks (see page 1249), this seasonal tendency may enable public health authorities to forecast the possibility of virulent epidemics. Figures are for New York City, from the Department of Health.

feeling of distress on the last exertion point to damage to the heart.

Many other organs and tissues may be affected, either during the first outburst of the disease or in the days that follow. The throat may be very sore, and along with this, perhaps, there may be swelling of the glands of the neck. Suppuration of the middle ear is not uncommon. Skin eruptions may appear.

The disease appears to predispose to other types of infection, so that some of these results are not directly due to the specific infection. Thus an attack of influenza may be followed by manifestations of tuberculosis of the lungs.

Convalescence from influenza may be very slow, and unwise attempts to shorten it may be followed by protracted ill-health. For months there may be a sense of lack of energy, both of body and mind. The mental depression may in some cases amount to melancholia, and suicidal attempts are not infrequent. Usually the nervous depression amounts to no more than a state of easily induced fatigue, mental, or bodily. Frequent attacks of neuralgia may also follow.

Treatment. In view of the considerable tax on the system imposed by even apparently mild attacks of influenza, and the serious complications of the disease, it is wise to procure medical advice. An attempt to ignore an attack of influenza and go on with one's work is extremely likely to be followed by disastrous results.

Where the attack resembles a bad cold, treatment is often commenced with a hot bath or a hot mustard foot bath, after which the patient goes to bed. The sooner this is done the better the chance of a quick recovery. It is important to isolate a case of influenza as far as possible. The bedroom should be kept at an even temperature of about

65° F., but must be thoroughly ventilated. Drafts may be obviated by using screens. If a cough is troublesome, the air should be kept sufficiently moist by steam from a kettle. If there is much fever the bedclothes must be light. The patient should be bathed each day with warm water and should have his mouth cleaned morning and evening.

Should the disease be severe, as when pneumonia supervenes, trained nursing should be secured if possible. The patient should abstain from all food except fruit juices, weak tea, and vegetable soups while there is much fever during the early days of the attack. Liquid must be taken freely in the form of lemonade, orangeade, or plain water.

As fever subsides, milk and milk foods and meat soups may be followed by well-cooked vegetables, eggs, and white fish as convalescence is established.

Drugs have no direct influence on the disease, but five grains of aspirin taken every four hour during the daytime relieves discomfort. Sleep may be promoted by the use of ten or fifteen grains of potassium bromide. A mild aperient should be taken at once and the bowels kept duly active by the use of mild laxatives is necessary.

Measures to Relieve the Cough. The cough may be lessened by using steam inhalations, either from a bronchitis kettle (see page 1142) or from a jug of nearly boiling water. The good effect of the steam is much improved by adding a teaspoonful of compound tincture of benzoin to the water. A spray, made up for example from the compound solution of thymol mixed with two or four parts of water, may help the cough and sore throat. A cold compress to the throat is often successful. This may be made by lightly wringing a double layer of lint of an appropriate length out of a mixture of three parts of cold water and two parts of alcohol, applying to the throat, and covering with gutta-percha tissue or oiled silk. The protective covering should overlap the lint about a quarter of an inch. The compress is fixed by a bandage or handkerchief. The cough may also be relieved by putting a linseed poultice over the front of the chest and another between the shoulders, and a poultice will usually be of use for pain in the chest or abdomen.

Complications are treated along the lines laid down in their special sections (*e.g.*, use of antipneumococcus or antistreptococcus serum for pneumonia.) When the patient is cyanosed or dusky from defective aeration of the blood the inhalation of oxygen may be helpful.

Aids to Convalescence. The patient must remain in bed until the temperature has remained normal for forty-eight hours. He may then sit up for a few hours, and if the weather permits go out for a short time after a further two days, provided there are no complications.

If the circumstances permit of a change to the country or to the seaside or to a milder climate, it is highly desirable to have it after influenza of any severity, and, in any event, it is necessary in such cases to have time to recuperate thoroughly.

The victim of influenza loses his infectiousness three or four days after the disappearance of fever, provided that bronchitis or other catarrhal conditions do not persist.

The room which has been occupied by a patient suffering from influenza should be disinfected, at least by widely opening the windows and allowing the air to blow through for two or three days.

Prevention of Infection. The prevention of influenza would be greatly furthered if all cases could be isolated, but so long as people in the early stages of influenza or throughout the disease in mild cases go about their business as usual there will be ample opportunity to become infected. It is probable that the liberal use of good dairy and vegetable produce and fruit juices tends to increase resistance to the infection.

Those who suffer from the disease should endeavor always to cough or sneeze into a handkerchief, and cloth handkerchiefs should be put into a disinfectant when discarded for washing. Paper handkerchiefs are to be preferred since they can be burned before they accumulate.

Definite value as a prophylactic must be assigned to the use of appropriate vaccines. These act by building up the resistance of the body to the microbes from which they are prepared, and while in the absence of exact knowledge of the causative agent this treatment cannot be relied on, it helps to protect against the complicating secondary infections.

The clinical picture of cases reported as influenza in recent years differs markedly from that prevailing during the pandemic of 1918-20 and the mortality is far lower. Considerable advances are being made in the study of this disease as a result of the successful transmission of human infection to ferrets.

GONORRHEA

Gonorrhea is a contagious venereal disease which appears to have existed from remote times, as it is mentioned in the book of Leviticus. It is an inflammation due to a small bean-shaped microbe, the gonococcus.

It may occur in either sex at all ages, babies and female children being particularly prone to infection. In men it is acquired, almost invariably, after promiscuous sexual relations; prostitutes are known to harbor the gonococcus in the vagina in many cases, and they are careless about disinfection, because they may have very few signs of the disease. In women gonorrhea is often contracted innocently in marital relations, or from unclean sanitary accommodation, or contaminated towels, etc. In children infected sponges, thermometers, towels, bed linen, underclothing, are the almost invariable sources of gonorrheal infection.

Symptoms. Symptoms appear from three to twenty-one days after infection, the average time being five days. These symptoms vary greatly according to the primary site of infection and the sex and age of the patient; but they are all characterized by a purulent urethral or other discharge, in which the gonococcus can be found, if pus is examined under the microscope.

The primary site of infection is usually in the genital region; but not uncommonly the eyes may be the first area involved, and so occasionally may the ears, mouth, or anus. In the male the usual first signs are a purulent discharge from the penis, associated with pain on passing urine. This discharge, if untreated, tends to spread backwards to the bladder, causing cystitis, or to the kidneys, causing nephritis. A warning that such spread is imminent is given when the patient finds that he is troubled with a constant and urgent desire to pass urine, even though the bladder is practically empty. A very common complication at this stage is inflammation and swelling of the testicles —epididymitis.

In addition to spreading locally, the germ may get directly into the blood stream and spread rapidly through the body, producing one form of blood poisoning (septicemia), or causing some particular organ of the body to bear the brunt of the infection. This latter is the more common accident. Inflammation of the heart (endocarditis) may thus be caused. Pleurisy, pneumonia, or inflammation of the joints, causing painful swellings in such places as the knee, ankle, wrist, or hands, may occur. Some of the most intractable types of so-called rheumatism are due to this disease.

In women the urethra is infected in most cases, and extensions to the bladder and kidneys may occur, but the main brunt of the disease is almost invariably borne by the uterus; and the chief symptom noticed, therefore, is a profuse yellow discharge from the vagina. Extensions of the disease in women tend to produce inflammation inside the lower abdominal cavity (pelvis), where the tubes leading to the ovaries, and the ovaries themselves, may become involved. This is a common cause of sterility in married women; but, in addition to that, it is calculated that 40 per cent of the pelvic operations done on women have been necessitated by pus and adhesions which have formed around the ovaries in patients who have previously been inadequately treated for gonorrhea. Early treatment, therefore, is essential if spread to these organs is to be prevented. Women, in addition to the special risks associated with the presence of an infected uterus, are liable to all the heart, lung, joint, and other troubles noted as occurring in men.

In small girls the inflammation of gonorrhea is confined mainly to the external genitals, with very little extension even into the vagina. It might be thought, therefore, that in these children cure would be easily produced. Such a happy sequence does not, however, occur. Children are notoriously difficult to cure, and relapses are very common after apparent success.

Newborn babies get the disease in the form of acute inflammation of the eyes, owing to infection from the genital passage during labor. It is calculated that 20 per cent of the total blindness in the world today is due to this cause. It is obvious, therefore, that in any case where the mother is known or suspected to be harboring the disease, the child's eyes must be treated immediately after it is born. Better yet are uniform laws requiring the instillation of silver nitrate into the eyes of all newborn babies.

Prevention. Unfortunately there has arisen an acrimonious controversy over the question as to whether or not the public should be instructed beforehand in the most efficient ways of preventing infection, even if this has been risked deliberately. The bulk of medical opinion is in favor of circulating this knowledge, in spite of the quite definite possibility that thereby vice may be made more safe. It is not so much the individual that the medical man is thinking about as his helpless future offspring or innocent relations; it is iniquitous that they should suffer for indiscretions or negligence over which they had no control.

There has in the past been too much secrecy about these diseases, and many patients have married without appreciating the fact that, if not cured, they may do irreparable damage to their life's partner, besides dangerously affecting the health of such children as may survive birth.

No one who has acquired gonorrhea should marry until assured that he or she is free from all traces of contagion. It is not enough that there should be no obvious signs of the disease. A complete examination and certain tests should be submitted to. This is a complicated and difficult investigation which cannot be undertaken except by an expert. All venereal clinics and genito-urinary specialists are constantly carrying out these tests, and in this way any patient should be able to discover whether or not he or she is a suitable candidate for married life. Such examination is not usually obligatory for gonorrhea although there are several states which require the applicant for marriage to verify a statement that he is free from infection from any venereal disease. An examination is required in the state of New York if either party has been infected with a venereal disease within five years. The feeling of the American mind is against any such coercion. But an increasing number of people, in all classes of life, have come to appreciate the often unsuspected ramifications of venereal disease and have voluntarily undergone such examinations.

Treatment. The first essential in the treatment of gonorrhea is to seek a doctor's care as soon as possible. All forms of self-treatment must be abstained from (unless specifically ordered by a doctor) and a patient should receive proper medical attention irrespective of his own estimate of the severity of the illness;

some patients are mistakenly inclined to think of an episode of gonorrhea as no more serious than a "bad cold." Any person who suspects after exposure to infection that he or she may have this disease should at once seek the care of a physician—and if the diagnosis proves to be gonorrhea, treatment should be continued until the patient is really cured. The disease is not necessarily arrested when the discharge from the penis, urethra, or vagina ceases.

While the patient is under treatment he should abide by the following suggestions to minimize the dangers involved and hasten recovery. It is important to cut down on physical exercise as much as possible, particularly dancing and riding, cycling, or any other form of exertion which might cause pressure on the buttocks. All forms of sexual excitement must be avoided, as this greatly aggravates the disease and, moreover, intercourse results in spread of the infection to the other party. The patient should make sure that at least one bowel movement occurs daily. Only plain food should be taken and all spicy dishes avoided. Abstinence from all forms of alcohol is essential, until infection has ceased. Coffee at night should be eliminated.

Cleanliness is most essential. The hands should be washed frequently with hot water and soap, particularly every time the genital organs are handled. The patient should also bathe frequently. All gauze, cotton, bandages, or any dressings should be burned after use. The patient should see to it that no one uses his towel, washcloths, or toilet articles.

A male patient may wear a cotton bag with clean cotton in it, changing the cotton frequently. Care must be taken not to let the cotton close the opening of the canal and dam back the pus. A pad may be worn by a female patient and this likewise should be changed frequently.

Under the appropriate medical treatment an average uncomplicated case, in the male, clears up in three to six weeks; but when complications occur treatment has often to be carried out from six months to two years before the patient can be declared cured.

The cure of gonorrhea in either sex may be and often is extremely difficult, and it is disastrous for anyone who contracts the disease to attempt to treat himself or herself. A crippling arthritis, sterility, and stricture are some of the likely complications in these cases.

The treatment which the physician carries out varies with the stage of the illness and the organ affected. In some instances antiseptic irrigations will suffice. In more advanced stages in the female, particularly when the Fallopian tubes are involved it may be necessary to use diathermy or surgery. The sulfonamides have been found to be of great value in the treatment of gonorrhea.

It is illegal for any unqualified person, such as a pharmacist, to prescribe treatment.

In every case a doctor should be consulted. Happily, there is no necessity for anyone, however poor, to be without adequate treatment. The various state health boards have established venereal clinics throughout the country. Every large general hospital also has a venereal outpatient department, and in several cities there are special hospitals for the treatment of venereal diseases only.

SYPHILIS

A highly contagious disease, syphilis is caused by the Spirocheta pallida, or Treponema pallidum, a germ resembling a tiny thread twisted like a corkscrew. This is communicated by contact with an infected surface, which is generally brought about by sexual intercourse, but may occur in kissing, suckling, or touching syphilitic sores. Sometimes the contact is indirect, as in drinking from a glass that has been used by an infected person and not washed.

The disease was at one time thought to be peculiar to man, none of the lower animals being considered susceptible. But it has now been found possible to inoculate monkeys and rabbits artificially; and it is known that the llama, or Peruvian sheep, can acquire it naturally—indeed, it is now thought possible that it was from this source that the disease originally spread to the human race.

The time at which the first symptoms of the disease occur is on an average twenty-five to twenty-eight days after the date of infection, but it may be delayed as long as eight weeks. This latent period is known as the incubation period. No signs, either on the skin or in the blood, can be discovered until this period is over.

Primary Symptoms. The first symptom is known as the primary sore or hard chancre. It occurs generally on the genitalia, but may be found on the lip, tongue, tonsil, finger, nipple, or any other area where small abrasions are liable to become infected with the virus. Typically this sore, or chancre, is a small buttonlike ulcerated area rather hard to the touch, not painful, and not discharging much pus. This primary sore is generally a solitary one, but in 20 per cent of cases it may be accompanied by one or more satellites.

When such a sore is scraped gently with a fine scalpel, the causal organism, the Spirocheta pallida, can be found in the scrapings in large numbers when viewed by dark-field illumination with the microscope. Any suspicious sore can thus be examined readily, and it is a routine procedure to do so now in cases of slowly healing sores outside the genital areas which do not seem to respond to ordinary surgical treatment. This is all the more important because an examination of the blood by the Wassermann reaction, the recognized diagnostic test for syphilis, generally discloses nothing in the primary stage.

Secondary Stage. Some six weeks after the primary sore or chancre has appeared, the secondary symptoms begin to show themselves, that is, if the patient has not been put under active treatment during the primary stage. There is a general enlargement of the lymphatic glands all over the body. These glands can be felt as hard, shotty nodules in such situations as the groins, above the elbows, in the armpits, and at the back of the neck.

Various rashes begin to show themselves, of which one resembling measles is the earliest. This may be followed by brown spots, or small flat papules, or pustules.

Sore throat is often complained of, and on examination mild grayish-looking ulcers, the so-called snail tracks, may be found on the tonsils and sodden whitish papules (mucous patches) on the tongue, inside the cheeks, or on the lips, generally at the angle of the mouth. These ulcers are particularly dangerous, as they are a frequent source of infection to others by kissing, or from innocent people using spoons, cups, towels, pipes, etc., which have belonged to or been used by the infected person.

An inflammatory condition, known as iritis, may occur in one or both eyes, causing redness, pain and swelling of the iris, the colored membrane which surrounds the pupil.

Sudden paralysis, with delirium, may occur from inflammation of the brain or spinal cord; and there are other rare complications which need not be set down in detail here.

The secondary stage lasts, off and on, for about two years in untreated or badly treated cases, and at this period large superficial curvilinear ulcers may occur all over the body (the great pocks which were noted in medieval times), causing marked scarring.

Tertiary Stage. After about the second year the secondary stage gradually fades into the tertiary, and this may last, off and on, for the rest of the patient's life. The characteristic peculiarity of the tertiary stage is the liability to gummatous formation. A gumma,

1366 THE CONCISE ENCYCLOPEDIA OF HEALTH

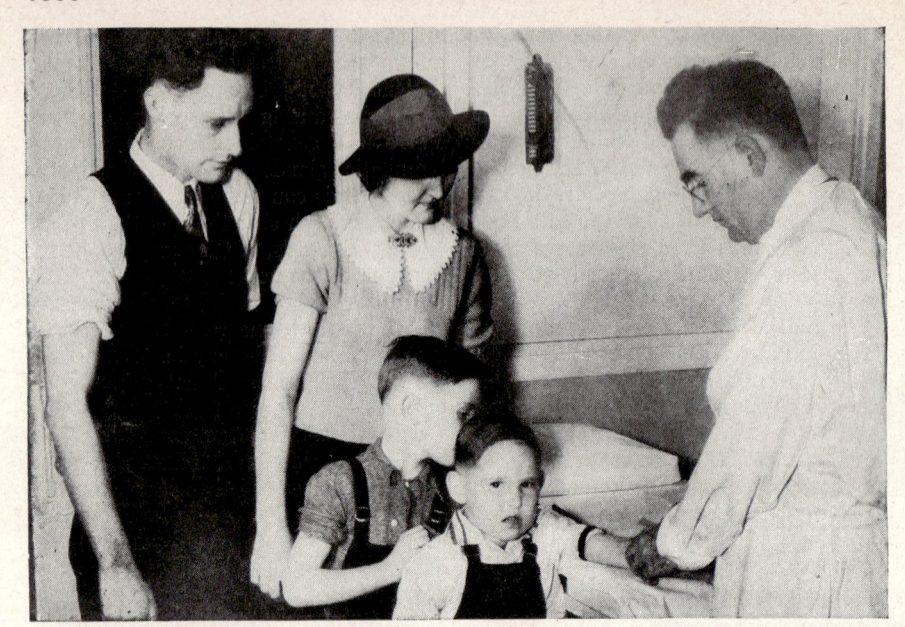

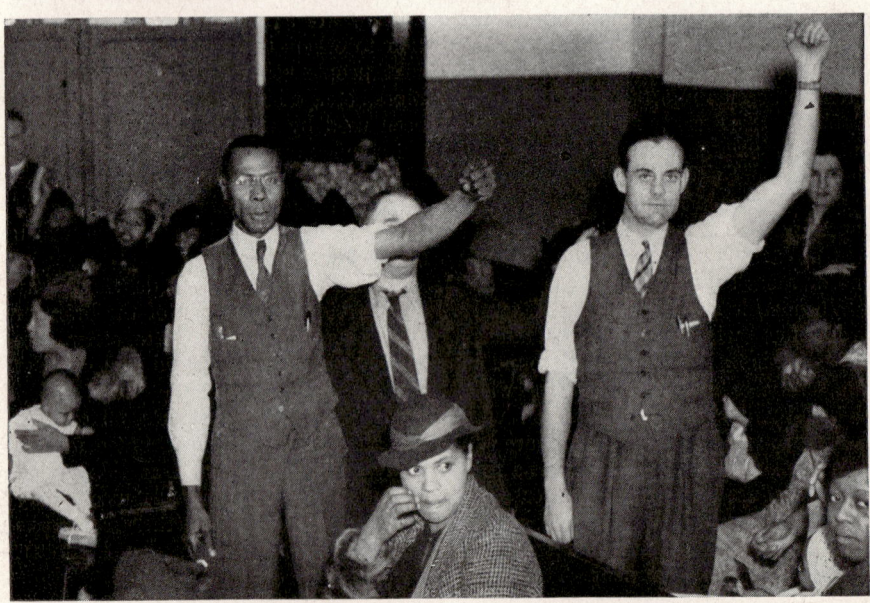

PUBLIC HEALTH CAMPAIGN AGAINST SYPHILIS

The vast majority of the American people were shocked to learn, during 1936 and 1937, that responsible experts estimated that from one in ten to one in three in the country's population had syphilis in one form or another. Cleanup campaigns were widely instituted, in the effort to find and cure the victims and to protect those who were not infected. Free examinations were offered, and entire families accepted and

—Continued at foot of next page

which is a soft form of tumor, may occur anywhere in the body, affecting bone, muscle, brain, skin, testicle, palate, joints, lungs, liver, kidneys, spleen, intestines, etc., causing symptoms peculiar to the organ implicated. It is in this stage that the vascular system often shows signs of the disease in the form of aneurysm, inflammation of the aorta, or aortic valvular disease.

If there is the slightest doubt about some obscure symptom, it is often quite easy to discover whether or not it is due to an old underlying syphilitic taint. All that is necessary is to obtain less than a teaspoonful of the patient's blood, send it to any reputable clinical laboratory, and ask for a Wassermann test. If this test is returned as positive, one can be quite sure that syphilis is still potentially active in the body. Even if the test is negative, syphilis cannot be definitely excluded as a possibility. Many patients are completely unaware that they had ever had the disease, the early signs having been so mild as to be overlooked, or misinterpreted.

A most important manifestation of tertiary syphilis occurs as a result of damage to the nervous system. Here the symptoms are confined mainly to the brain and the spinal cord. The two main diseases caused by nerve syphilis are locomotor ataxia or tabes, and general paralysis of the insane (dementia paralytica).

In these two diseases, which are described in Chapters 125 and 126 respectively, if the fluid from the spinal canal (cerebrospinal fluid), is examined, it gives certain definite signs, the most characteristic of which is a positive Wassermann reaction similar to that found in the blood of secondary or tertiary cases. Women are not nearly as liable to either of these two complica-

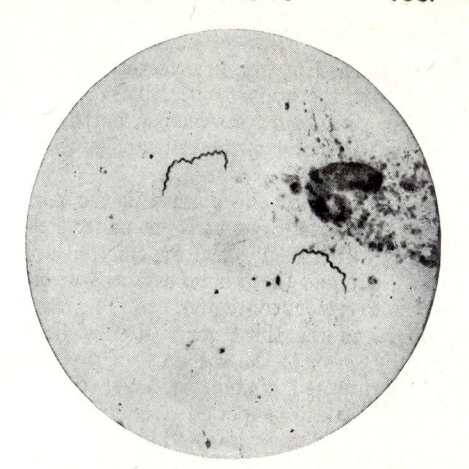

SPIROCHETA PALLIDA

The tiny spiral organism which causes syphilis is communicated by an infected person or some utensils, for example, a drinking vessel, used by such. At its point of entry into the body it produces a small buttonlike ulcerated area, generally referred to as the primary sore.

tions as men. The same immunity is also found among natives of tropical countries, both male and female. Wassermann tests of the spinal fluid are sometimes negative although the patient has or had central nervous system involvement.

"Inheritance" by Children. The children of parents suffering from syphilis may be born with all the signs of the disease on them. As a rule, however, when the parents are still in the earlier stages of the disease, such children as they may beget are born dead, and only as the condition regresses in the parents are live babies obtained. Such children may live, thrive, and show no signs of the ravages of the virus until they reach the age of puberty; but, as a rule, certain stigmata are present which indicate the disease to the initiated. The

---

Continued from preceding page—
had their blood tested. These two scenes are from the Chicago Health Department clinic, directed by Dr. Herman Bundeson. The family above was found free of the disease. Below is the clinic waiting room, with citizens who co-operated in the campaign waiting to be tested or to get reports on their tests.
© *International News Photos*

most characteristic of these is what is known as Hutchinson's teeth. In this condition the upper central incisor teeth of the permanent set have a notch cut out of the center of the biting edge which is absolutely characteristic.

Gradually, as the disease in the parents wears itself out or is got under control by treatment, healthy children are obtained, and there is no evidence whatever that the contagion can be transmitted to the third generation without a reinfection in the second.

An infected woman is never during her childbearing period free from the risk of bearing an infected child, though the risk diminishes as time goes on and as the result of treatment. Even if treatment is first begun during pregnancy it will be of great value as far as the child is concerned.

The mother may give a negative Wassermann reaction and herself show no sign of the disease. She may even have given birth to healthy children since she became infected.

If a woman becomes infected during pregnancy, infection of the child will depend on the stage of pregnancy at which infection occurs. Before the fifth month infection of the child is certain, unless immediate therapy is instituted. After the seventh month it will escape unless it acquires accidental infection from the mother during or after birth. For this reason she should not suckle her child. Where there has been any suspicion of the woman having been infected at any time, suckling should not be allowed unless both mother and child show a negative Wassermann test, or both show a positive one. Milk may be drawn off and given in a bottle, since the milk itself is not capable of carrying the infection.

Treatment. Obviously in a disease so protean in its manifestations, and liable to be so long-drawn-out in its various stages, treatment will depend largely on the stage in which the disease is first recognized, the severity or otherwise of the symptoms presenting themselves, the age and sex of the patient, and the presence or absence of other diseases which might bias one in favor of or against any drastic or radical line of procedure. Syphilis can be cured if treatment is given early enough and over a long enough period. The patient may have to remain under the constant care of a physician for from one to three years before a cure can be expected.

For optimal results, treatment must be continuous. Over a two-year period it may be necessary to administer between twenty and thirty injections of an arsenical preparation such as arsphenamine and a similar number of injections of a bismuth compound.

Arsphenamine is a yellowish powder which is dissolved and injected very slowly into a vein. The injections are given at weekly or shorter intervals as the case requires. A ten- to twelve-week course of arsphenamine is usually alternated with a four- to ten-week course of bismuth. The latter is a metal more or less akin to mercury which was formerly very widely used in the treatment of syphilis. It is, however, less poisonous and more powerful against the spirochete than mercury. It is given by intramuscular injection into the buttocks. One or more injections are given in a week, utilizing alternate buttocks for the injection. The pure metal in an oily suspension can be used, or one of the salts of the metal, such as the hydroxide, or a combination of the metal with quinine or iodine, such as iodobismuth-quinine. The drug is used in the treatment of syphilis in conjunction with arsphenamine. The progress of the case is judged not by the disappearance of symptoms, but by the condition of the blood, as shown by the Wassermann reaction. As long as this remains negative all is going well. After two years' treatment the blood should be examined twice a year for the next two years, and if it has been negative all the time the patient can be told that he or she is cured as far as human probability goes, though a woman may still produce syphilitic children. It is always worth

DISEASES CAUSED BY KNOWN GERMS: VARIOUS

while, however, to have a blood test made at intervals of two years for the next six years, as cases do occur where it again becomes positive. Before he grants the patient a rest period the doctor will usually advise a lumbar puncture for examination of the spinal fluid.

A woman who has once had syphilis should be treated throughout pregnancy. If, in spite of treatment, she has a persistently positive Wassermann reaction she should not attempt to bear a child.

When a patient is seen in the secondary stage of the disease the same treatment is required as for the primary, but more arsphenamine must be given, and the course of injections of that drug must be repeated once or twice according to symptoms. It is also advisable to keep the treatment up for at least two or three years. In this way the chances of curing the patient are very much increased, but it cannot be denied that these chances are not as good as if the disease had been tackled in the primary stage. When tertiary symptoms show themselves, that is an indication that the original treatment was inadequate, or has failed to cure the condition. One cannot then hope to be able to eradicate the disease. All that can be done is to treat symptoms as they arise. Many people, however, have tertiary symptoms without much discomfort other than that produced by the gummata as they arise. It does not mean that they are doomed to an early and painful death, or that they will develop other manifestations.

On the other hand, tertiary lesions often manifest themselves when it is too late for treatment to be effective. This is especially true of syphilitic disease of

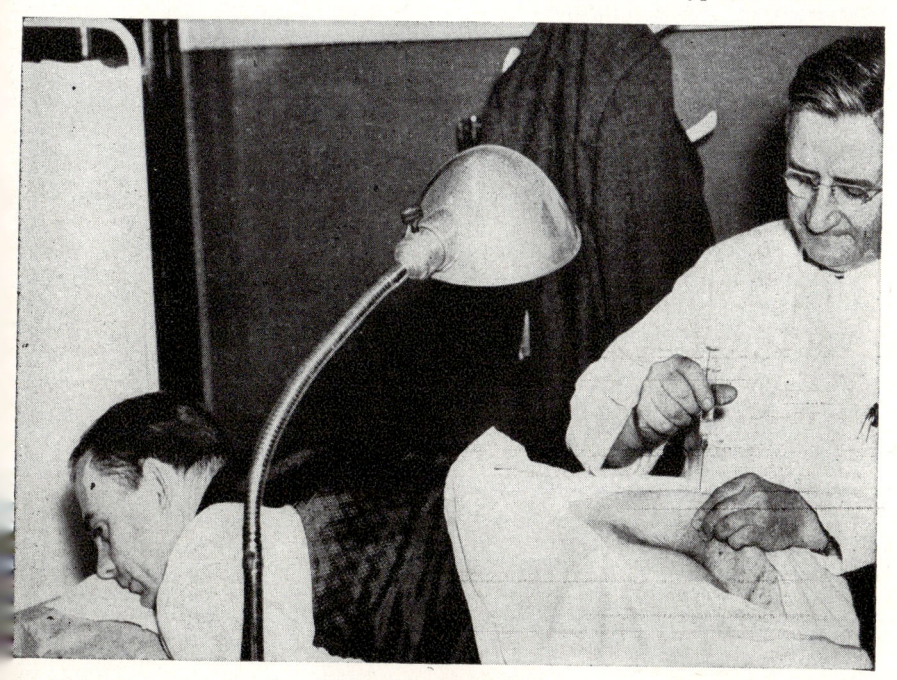

TREATMENT FOR SYPHILIS

When a person has contracted syphilis and undertakes to be cured, he begins a long series of visits to the doctor or clinic, with repeated hypodermic injections as a prominent feature of the treatment. These are often made into the large gluteal muscles. This picture was taken in the Chicago Board of Health clinic during the famous campaign to clean up syphilis.

© *International News Photos*

the circulatory system. Central nervous-system syphilis is often very resistant to treatment. The arsenicals, bismuth, and potassium iodide are the drugs most commonly used. Malarial and artificial-fever therapy have given beneficial results in cases of general paresis and tabes. Under malarial therapy, bouts of high fever are induced by injecting into the patient's blood carefully controlled doses of the malaria organism.

Treatment of Children. Infants with congenital syphilis are usually treated with intramuscular injections of suitable arsenical compounds. Bismuth has largely replaced mercury for use between courses of arsenical treatment. If they get over the first two years of life they usually survive, and no further symptoms of the syphilitic infection may appear until puberty.

At this time, however, they are liable to an eye trouble called interstitial keratitis, and it has been found unfortunately that it is not possible to guard against this complication by giving them a course of treatment before it is likely to appear. Instead it must be treated energetically when it does appear, and with arsphenamine and bismuth the condition can be cured.

Congenitally syphilitic children are liable to tertiary syphilis. This shows itself usually as feeble-mindedness, or juvenile general paralysis, or juvenile locomotor ataxia, and is incurable. If, however, congenitally syphilitic children escape the various complications to which they are liable, they may turn out quite brilliant afterwards, the disease in some way stimulating their brains. Some most distinguished men have been congenital syphilitics.

The conditions under which persons with acquired syphilis may marry are explained below.

MARRIAGE AND VENEREAL DISEASE

A man who has been unfortunate enough to acquire gonorrhea may recover completely, marry, and bring up perfectly healthy children. Before such a man, however, undertakes the responsibilities of matrimony he should have a thorough examination made, either in private or at one of the centers for the treatment of venereal disease which are now widely distributed; and unless and until he is declared clear of the disease he should not marry if he has any love for his prospective wife or thought for his potential children. If he is not clear he will assuredly infect his wife, and, if she is not thereby made sterile, his child, when born, will inevitably get ophthalmia neonatorum unless the mother's condition is known and precautions to protect the child's eyes at birth are undertaken.

Infantile Blindness. Ophthalmia neonatorum is a contagious inflammation of the eye in the newborn children of women who have gonorrhea. It is responsible for 20 per cent of the total blindness of the world, and it is criminal for anyone to expose children to such a risk. If, however, the baby's eyes are protected, according to the Credé method known to all doctors, the fact that the parents have gonorrhea will not otherwise affect the child's health in the future, provided it is not infected later. In this respect gonorrhea differs essentially from syphilis, where the taint is carried in the blood and may show itself a decade later.

Syphilis in the Male. In syphilis the conditions that should govern marriage are much more complicated. A man who contracts syphilis, if unmarried, should go through a complete course of treatment extending over two or three years, and should not marry for at least five years after becoming infected. After he has ceased treatment he should still have his blood tested by the Wassermann reaction at intervals of six months for another two years, and only then, if all his tests show his blood to be what is called negative and no signs of the dis-

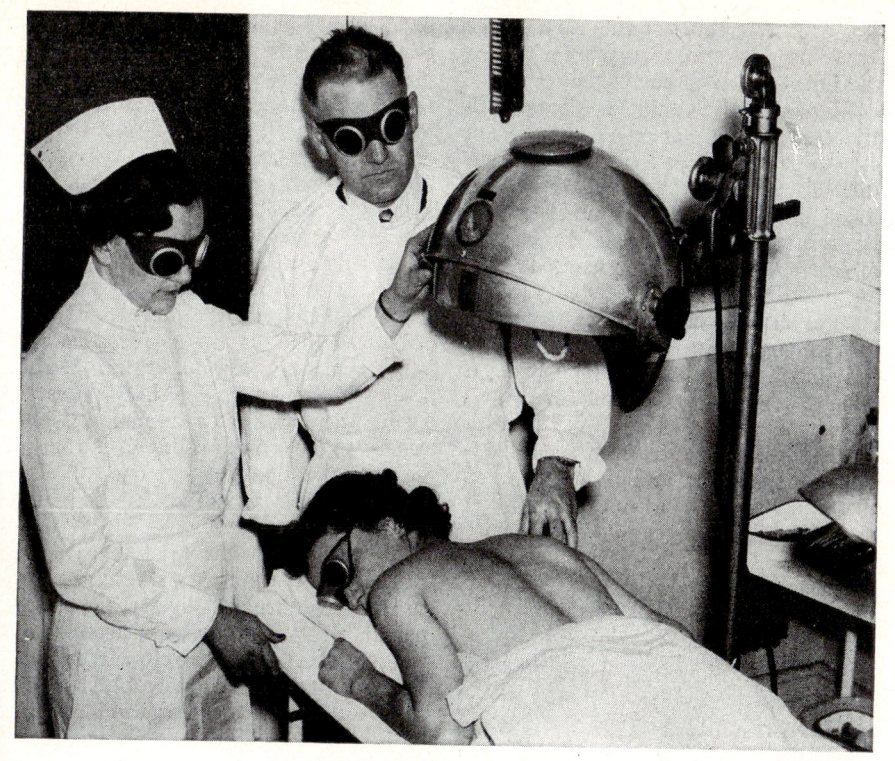

TREATMENT FOR SYPHILIS
Skin eruptions are usually present with syphilis. A therapeutic light treatment is used to help clear these up, after curative internal medication has been begun. This is in the Chicago Board of Health clinic during the famous clean-up campaign.
© *International News Photos*

ease have recurred, should he consider the question of marriage. This may be taken as a general safe limit, but, owing to the insidious nature of the disease, no guarantee can honestly be given by his doctor that he will not have recurrences later. All that can be said is that if he has fulfilled the above conditions the chance of his transmitting the disease to the wife he may marry is small, and to the children he may beget the risk is almost negligible.

A man who is already married should take all the precautions one takes with a contagious case, especially while he is in the early and communicable stage of the disease. His most important duty is to his wife. Sexual intercourse, even after the contagious stage is passed, must be totally interdicted until after two years of negative tests following the conclusion of treatment. If he neglects this warning and begets children while still uncured he exposes his wife to the risk of contracting the disease and in turn bearing syphilitic children.

Such children will be stillborn, or may live for only a few days, or be congenital idiots, or grow up to puberty and then show signs of the disease for the first time at the ages of 12 to 18, just when they ought to be developing into happy maturity.

No infected man, therefore, who hopes for healthy children, should risk the chance of bringing offspring into the world for five years or until his blood has been "negative" for two years after his treatment has been completed.

Marriage of Syphilitic Women. In the case of the woman conditions are still more complicated. It is sometimes difficult to detect an early syphilitic lesion in a woman as the chancre may be internally situated (on the cervix) and not be evident. A woman may thus go for a number of years and never suspect that she has the disease.

With regard to marriage women are in a much worse position than men. A woman who has had syphilis may produce syphilitic children at any time during her fertility period even after she is apparently cured; and if her husband dies and she remarries she may produce these syphilitic babies to a second husband who is himself free from the disease. This is a fact of enormous importance, because many war widows infected by their husbands have thus unwittingly carried on the strain to the children of innocent men.

If a woman knows that she has had syphilis or finds she has once produced what is called a congenital syphilitic baby, it is useless for her to rely on the fact that her blood may be negative when examined. That unfortunately does not prove that she will not produce another syphilitic baby in future. If she wishes to remarry, she has no safeguard, therefore. If she is married, and wishes to have more children, she must face the risk that the next one will also be a congenital syphilitic. But it is not quite an impasse.

A woman who has been infected, if she finds she is pregnant, should arrange to have treatment throughout the entire period of pregnancy, irrespective of whether she has any symptoms or not. In this way she can considerably increase the possibility that her baby will be born healthy.

This has been proved quite definitely by the work done at the London Lock Hospital for Women, where, of 680 babies born in the wards during a period of four years from mothers who were so treated, 669 were found free from the disease, the others being from cases not completely treated, or dying from other causes.

A widow who has had syphilis, knowing these facts and wishing to marry, should put them before her prospective husband. If he is willing to marry her under these conditions, she should arrange to have treatment as soon as she finds she is pregnant, and there will be a fair probability that her children will be as sound and healthy as those of a noninfected woman. If the childbearing period is over, of course, this necessity does not arise, and she will only require treatment if gummatous symptoms occur, as they frequently do at about the change of life. Tertiary syphilis is not

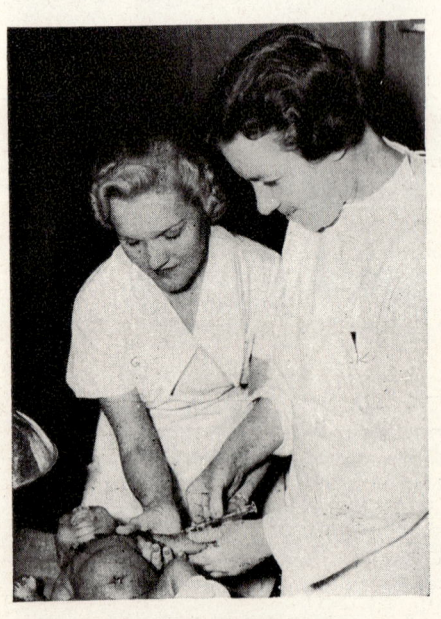

TREATMENT FOR SYPHILIS
This is perhaps the first of a series of treatments which this baby received to cure a syphilis infection discovered during the Chicago cleanup campaign. The taboo on public mention of syphilis was challenged after 1937, and thousands of unsuspected and innocent cases were discovered and treated in the large cities of the United States.
© *International News Photos*

considered contagious, however, and her husband runs no special risk therefrom.

Premarital Blood Tests. Wassermann tests, or other standard laboratory blood tests, are required for both brides and bridegrooms before marriage licenses can be secured in many states. Those which had such legislation in effect in January, 1941, were California, Colorado, Connecticut, Illinois, Indiana, Kentucky, Michigan, New Hampshire, New Jersey, New York, North Dakota, Oregon, Pennsylvania, Rhode Island, South Dakota, Virginia, West Virginia, Wisconsin, and Puerto Rico. In Tennessee, a law already passed was to take effect in July, 1941. Similar legislation is under consideration in other states; many of the latter have laws requiring evidence of freedom from syphilis from the male license applicant.

Importance of Sex Knowledge. In this general survey it will be seen what an important part the incidence of venereal disease plays in the hygiene of the sexes, and how essential it is that everyone, especially young people, should be warned against the dangers that may be produced thereby.

Owing to the complexities of modern civilization the age at which marriage is possible for the majority of young people is being pushed back later and later, and even late marriage is sometimes unlikely. This naturally tends to an increase of sexual intercourse outside marriage and to the continued propagation of venereal disease. The First World War started a wave of venereal trouble all over the world, forced the hands of governments and of all thinking people, and caused the matter to be ventilated in the light of day in a manner that had never previously been possible. As the result of the publicity and the preventive treatment advocated, the number of fresh cases in this country dropped appreciably, but the problem is still one of large proportions. The controversy which this policy of facing facts has unfortunately provoked is referred to on page 1363). But it is certain that with increased knowledge of the risks, and a higher demand by the public for adequate treatment, venereal diseases ought speedily to be reduced to a small residuum, and one of the greatest curses of humanity thus nullified.

TETANUS

Lockjaw, or tetanus, is an extremely serious disease, resulting from infection of a broken surface of the skin by a special organism—the tetanus bacillus. This is a rod-shaped germ bearing at one extremity a spore from which fresh germs can develop. This spore is very resistant to the effects of heat, cold, and ordinary antiseptics: it can withstand drying for years and when replaced in suitable surroundings can develop afresh into new bacilli. Such powers of resistance make the eradication of tetanus a difficult problem.

The bacillus is present in the gut of adult horses and cattle; it can be found in manured soil, such as that of gardens, and its spores are present in earthy dust. Development of the germ can take place only in the absence of oxygen. Such conditions are present in deep wounds, especially if other germs or liquefying tissues at the same time make demands upon the scanty store of oxygen available.

Tetanus bacilli are dangerous to life through the toxins they form in the wound which they have infected. The bacilli themselves do not spread widely through the body, but at the site of infection they form poisons that are carried along the fibers of the motor nerves supplying the muscles of the part. Along the path of these nerves tetanus toxin passes up to the brain and spinal cord, where it combines with nerve cells and produces their destruction.

For the development of tetanus it is necessary that there should be first a wound of some kind, cutting, crushing

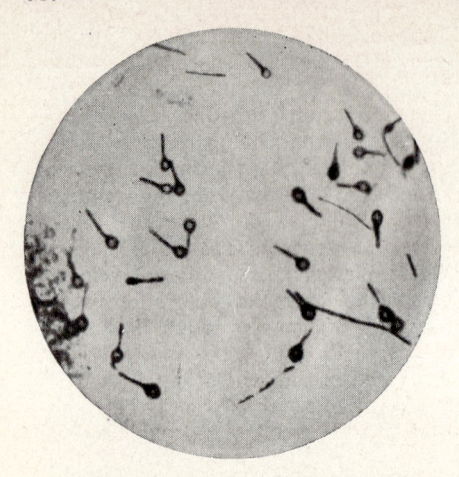

TETANUS: THE CAUSATIVE BACILLUS
The germ of tetanus is often called the drumstick bacillus on account of its shape; it is only active in the absence of air and when there is earth pollution of the wound.

or merely chafing, and that this wound should be or become infected with tetanus bacilli or spores. Its occurrence is made more likely if there is at the same time infection with other organisms and mechanical destruction of tissue, with formation of matter in the wound.

One form of tetanus which is now rarely seen is tetanus of the newborn infant, from infection of the stump of the umbilical cord.

Conditions Governing Recovery. The mortality of tetanus is very high; it may be taken as roughly 50 per cent of all cases, but the outlook is much influenced by the length of time which elapses between the time of infection and the onset of the first symptoms. It also depends to a great extent upon the promptitude and intensity of the treatment.

Should symptoms appear within ten days of infection the chances of recovery are 40 per cent; their appearance between the eleventh and twenty-first days raises the chances of recovery to 65 per cent; if they are delayed longer than three weeks the chances of recovery rise to 85 per cent. When symptoms have appeared the prospect of cure increases rapidly for every day that life is maintained after the tenth day of illness.

There is a tradition that wounds of the ball of the thumb are especially liable to set up lockjaw, but this has no basis in fact except in so far as gardeners and agricultural workers are more liable than others to scratches and abrasions of the hands, and to their contamination with infected soil or manure.

Symptoms of Infection. Spasm of the jaw muscles is merely one of many results of infection with the tetanus bacillus, but as it is one of the most constant it has been seized upon as a convenient label for the disease.

In view of the urgent importance of early treatment of this disease, it is imperative to watch carefully for anything that can be regarded as a warning symptom of its onset. Such premonitory symptoms may be any one or more of the following: sleeplessness or broken sleep disturbed by terrifying dreams, giddiness, frequent yawning, stiffness of the throat muscles with difficulty in swallowing, trembling of the tongue, sometimes with inability to put it out straight, watering of the mouth, lateral movements of the eyes (nystagmus) and transient double vision. Some symptom in this list may precede by a day or two the onset of spasm of the jaw muscles and inability to open the mouth which constitute typical lockjaw.

Developed tetanus presents one of the most distressing pictures of disease in man. The victim lies with jaws tightly clenched, rigid neck, head drawn back, face distorted in a fixed snarl or grin, displaying the teeth, this condition being sometimes referred to as *risus sardonicus*; his abdominal and back muscles are in a constant state of rigid contraction, his limbs bent and fixed; the slightest stimulus, such as a touch, a strong light, or the sound of a closing door, sets up violent and agonizing spasm of the muscles, with the result that rupture of these may occur. During the whole course of the disease consciousness is never lost; the patient throughout is fully alive to the seriousness of his condition, and, except from drugs or anesthetics, he obtains no relief from his constant pain and recurring agony. Profuse sweating, some rise of temperature and a quickening of the pulse usually occur, but these are trivial matters in comparison with the intensity of the spasms and convulsions.

Modified Forms of Tetanus. As a consequence of the institution of preventive inoculation as a routine in all cases of wounds during the First World War, certain modified types of tetanus came to be recognized; these took the form of mild attacks of the disease in its general features, or of localized tetanus. This consists in a spasm of the muscles in the neighborhood of the wound without spread to other parts. Its onset is sometimes delayed for many weeks, and it must be regarded as an evidence of incomplete immunization. The mortality is notably diminished, of course, by delaying the onset of the malady. Improvement in the method of dosage necessary has resulted in more complete immunization.

It cannot be too clearly recognized that any breach of the skin, however trivial it may seem, may open the way for tetanus. In order to be safe, all wounds should be thoroughly cleansed, treated with tincture of iodine and dressed with an antiseptic; and if there is reason to suspect contamination by soil or dust an injection of serum should be given. In many hospitals antitetanic serum is given as a routine in all cases of street accident.

Were such methods adopted as a routine, the deaths of schoolboys from tetanus following minor injuries in the football field, and of the amateur gardener from scratches by his rose bushes, could be prevented. In three out of four cases of tetanus due to hand wounds caused by toy pistol accidents in one month in 1932, fatal lockjaw oc-

curred because, although the serum was used, it was not injected when the wound was first dressed.

Value of Serum Treatment. In order to assess serum treatment at its proper value it is necessary to realize that the poison of tetanus germs is produced by them at the seat of the wound, that by the time symptoms have appeared the combination with the nerve cells of the poison carried to the spinal cord and brain has already taken place, and that it is unlikely that injection of serum into the blood can disturb the vicious combination.

For these reasons it is advisable that at the earliest moment after lockjaw is diagnosed big doses of serum should be injected into the spinal canal.

The serum used is prepared from the blood of horses which have been gradually immunized to the poison of tetanus by increasing doses. It is available in two strengths, 150 and 800 units per cubic centimeter. The unit is the amount which will preserve the life of a guinea pig for four days after it has been given 100 times a fatal dose of toxin. Very

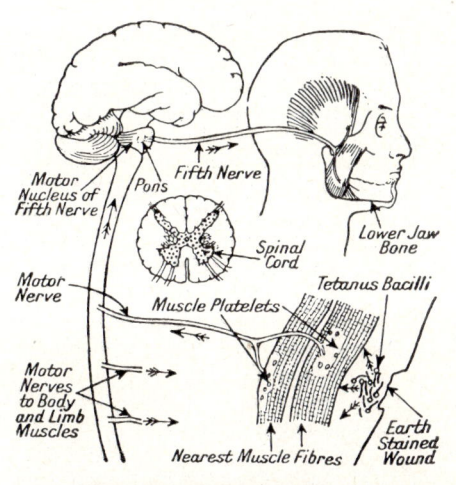

SCOPE OF TETANUS INFECTION

Germs of tetanus in an earth-soiled wound discharge a poison which enters the end plates of motor nerves and passes via the nerves to the spinal cord and nuclei of cranial motor nerves.

large doses of serum are necessary in treatment; 30,000 units may be given daily for a week, followed by weekly doses of 1000 or 2000 units if progress is good.

Treatment also includes general measures to secure seclusion, silence, and darkness, with the use of heavy doses of morphine or the administration of chloroform anesthesia to allay the intense irritability and facilitate the giving of adequate nourishment without inducing the characteristic and agonizing convulsions.

ANIMAL DISEASES TRANSMISSIBLE TO MAN

It is an ascertained fact that the contact of man with domestic animals leads to the communication of disease not only from animal to man, but also from man to animal. Rabies in a dog may give hydrophobia to a child. Tuberculosis in the lungs of a man may be conveyed to the lungs of his pet animal. But, in spite of the fact that investigation into the cause of disease in animals has not as yet proceeded very far, so that definite proof is not yet available, it seems probable that communication of disease from animal to man is not very common.

The appearance of a disease in an animal may have the semblance of a disease well known from its frequent occurrence in man. The cause of these similar appearances may be ascertained to be the same. Even so, there will remain to be proved whether the agent causing the disease in the animal can produce the same disease in man, or whether only a modified form of the same disease, or even another disease.

Rabies, glanders, and anthrax are communicable to man in the form in which they occur in animals. Rabies is a disease which occurs chiefly in dogs, although cats, cows, and horses have been known to develop it. The virus is still undefined, and therefore rabies is dealt with in a later chapter.

Glanders, or farcy, is a disease which occurs in horses. It is caused by a bacillus, the irritation of the presence of which in the system results in the growth of little nodules inside the nostrils or under the surface of the skin. If the nodules spring up in the nostrils, the disease is called glanders; if under the skin, farcy. Contact of the human skin, especially if an abrasion of the skin be present, with one of these nodules will communicate the disease to man.

Anthrax is the most widely spread of all infectious fevers among sheep and cattle. It may occur among horses. The disease is virtually never conveyed to man by mouth, but shepherds, butchers and tanners receive the infection through an abraded skin surface from the living, or even the dead, animals. The occurrence of glanders and anthrax in man is considered at greater length below.

In respect of other diseases of animals, the same certainty as to their communicability to man has not yet been established. Distemper in puppies may resemble measles or influenza; pink eye and megrims in horses may resemble influenza and epilepsy respectively in man; mange in dogs may resemble itch in the human subject. But the scientist will not allow himself to be misled by appearances, nor presume as to the communicability of these diseases to man, or vice versa. Actinomycosis, described later on, is a well-known disease in man. The communication of the disease from animal to man may occur, but it has not yet been proved.

Foot-and-mouth disease is a disease which spreads with the utmost rapidity among cattle, sheep, and pigs. It is known to be transmissible to man, but the method and degree of its communicability are uncertain. The causative agent is a virus and is found in the vesicles which characterize this disease. Ringworm and favus are other diseases which may be acquired from animals.

Certainty as to the noncommunicability of certain animal diseases has, how ever, been arrived at. It can be stated that tuberculosis in birds is not transmissible to man. Also that the diphtheria of calves, cats, and fowls is not identical with diphtheria in man, and is not communicable to man. Psittacosis, a virus disease of parrots, has been transmitted to human beings.

There are two diseases occurring in animals whose communicability to man, though well known, is of great importance to the community. These are cowpox and tuberculosis. Cowpox is a condition found in cows, or calves, which is due to a filtrable virus. There is a slight fever, and the development on the skin of pocks similar in all respects to those arising in man as the result of vaccination. Vaccination is, in fact, the intentional communication of cowpox to man. Tuberculosis (see Chapters 99 and 110) occurs in all animals and may be transmitted to man by cows' milk.

Animals sometimes pass on the insects attacking them, or the parasites living on them, to man. Ticks, fleas, and lice are good examples of this.

Animals in ill-health may lead to disease in man in yet another way. The excreta of dogs infested with the eggs of small intestinal worms may contaminate the water supply, and if such water be drunk the minute eggs may find their way into the human bowel. There they develop and result in a condition of ill-health known as hydatid disease. It is not a common disease in the United States, except among persons who have lived in the tropics. Cases have, however, occurred in which the disease has been acquired from pet dogs by the obviously unhygienic and dangerous habit of kissing them.

Finally, it must not be forgotten that disease may be communicated from man to animals, though not always. Smallpox in man may be given to cattle—human tuberculosis to animals. On the other hand, human influenza does not appear to be communicable to animals.

Glanders. The disease more commonly known as glanders is also called

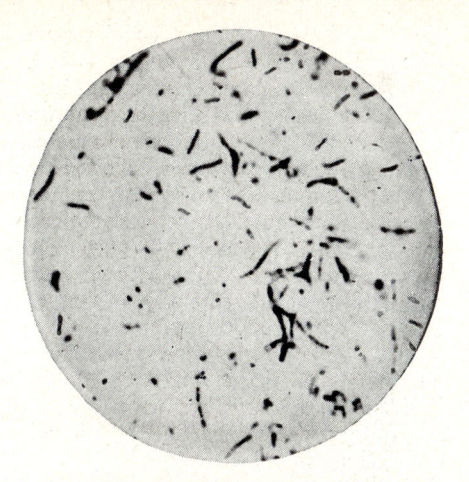

CAUSATIVE GERM OF GLANDERS
The Bacillus mallei, shown here, which may attack the lining of the nose (glanders) or the skin and glands (farcy), resembles somewhat the bacillus of tuberculosis. A disease of horses and asses, glanders also attacks man.

farcy, from the term farcy buds, applied to the nodules appearing under the skin and in the muscles, one of the characteristic signs of this disease. Glanders is due to the Bacillus mallei. The bacillus is found in the nodules.

The disease, which is most dangerous and fatal to man, is contracted by people who are in charge of any of the equine species, such as horse, donkey, etc., and by slaughters, and can be transmitted by one human being to another. Infection usually takes place through the nasal discharge or saliva of the diseased animal coming in contact with an abrasion or cut on the hand or arm, or by a bite; or the conjunctivae may be infected by rubbing the eyes with soiled fingers or by the animal sneezing on the face of the subject.

This disease occurs in two forms, the acute and the chronic. The former is usually fatal in about three weeks; it starts in two to seven days after infection, with malaise, headache, pain in the joints and muscles, and with a surrounding area of inflammation very similar to erysipelas in appearance at the site of the infection; nodules soon appear in the skin and muscles, which at first are painful and rapidly turn into papules or bullae, and then break down and ulcerate. The mucous membrane of the nose becomes reddened, followed by a discharge; ulcers may form in the nostrils, causing extensive destruction; the pharynx, larynx, and even the mucous membrane of the bronchi may be infected, and finally a condition of general pyemia supervenes.

The chronic form lasts about four months and is characterized by ulcerations and abscesses in the joints accompanied by pain, swellings in the skin and muscles, and often a cough.

The treatment is purely palliative, as unfortunately there is as yet no known specific for the disease; abscesses are opened and treated antiseptically. In the chronic form iodide of potassium and arsenic are used.

Anthrax. Anthrax, a Greek word meaning carbuncle, is the term applied to a disease produced in certain animals and in men by the growth in the body of a germ known as the anthrax bacillus. The microbe, which is illustrated on page 289, is one of the largest germs known, and can be seen by a fairly low power of the microscope. It can easily be destroyed by heat or by antiseptics, but is liable to form spores which are very resistant to conditions which would kill the germ itself. These spores may remain for a long time inactive, yet alive, in materials which are transported long distances, so that infection sometimes occurs in the most unlikely places. The disease commonly attacks sheep and cattle and other grass-eating beasts.

In countries where the disease is rife among cattle (known then as splenic fever), graziers and butchers may be infected, but in the United States and other countries where infectious diseases of animals are kept well in check the disease is more likely to attack those who handle imported wool and hides, *e.g.* tanners and woolsorters. There are certain countries in Asia from which the wool has always to be more carefully examined and dealt with because of the possibility of its being tainted with anthrax. Special hygienic precautions are in use among woolsorters to prevent the inhalation of possibly infected dust particles.

Anthrax may show itself in three ways, affecting either the skin, when it is termed malignant pustule, the lungs, or the intestines.

When the skin is affected it is usually on the face or arms, since those parts are exposed and likely to be scratched. A rare way in which infection has several times occurred is by the use of a shaving-brush in which anthrax spores have lain dormant. In these cases the bristles must have come from the hide of a diseased animal—an occurrence which would be impossible in any reputable factory. The infection of the skin leads to the formation of a red inflamed area, not painful at first but rather irritating and looking something like a boil. If the condition progresses, watery blisters form and the swelling spreads considerably. At this stage the patient begins to feel ill and becomes feverish. If his system is strong enough to overcome the microbic infection, the swelling may now gradually subside and the blister shrivel up, but sometimes no improvement occurs and there is serious risk of the microbe getting into the blood stream (anthracemia), with fatal result.

The lungs may be infected by the inhalation of infected dust. This form of the disease is known as woolsorter's disease. The symptoms are those of pneumonia with grave constitutional disturbance.

The third form shows itself by intestinal symptoms, such as abdominal pain, diarrhea, and vomiting.

The diagnosis of anthrax affecting the skin should be easy if it were suspected, for the microbe can readily be seen if a little fluid from a blister is examined under the microscope. The reason why the condition is overlooked in the early stages is that it is commonly taken for a pimple or boil. It should be an invariable rule for any worker in raw hides or wool to report to the doctor on the appearance of any irritating pimple, especially in cases where a small blister develops.

The majority of cases of malignant pustule recover either spontaneously or under treatment. The more serious pulmonary and intestinal forms, both of which are difficult to diagnose, give little hope of recovery and, apart from the injection of serum, all that can be done is to maintain the strength by general treatment and good nursing.

Tularemia. Cases of tularemia have been reported in forty-six of the forty-eight states. It is an acute infectious disease caused by a bacterium, Bacillus tularense, and transmitted to man from lower animals, especially wild hares, rabbits, and squirrels. Skinning or dressing these animals causes many cases. Infection also commonly results from the bite of a tick or fly which has fed on diseased animals.

The clinical picture is very variable and many different types have been described, depending on which particular organ system is most involved and the location of the primary lesion. The onset is about three days after inoculation and is usually sudden with fever, chills or chilliness, nausea, and vomiting. Weakness and, in severe cases, prostration occur. Occasionally a rash appears. Convalescence is slow so that the patient does not return to work for two or three months.

The diagnosis is established on the basis of history, clinical findings, and bacteriological tests. Treatment is symptomatic. No drugs or serum have been found which exert specific effects. Rest in bed is most essential.

Rocky Mountain Spotted Fever. This is a disease occurring for the most part in the West and Midwest in regions infested with the wood tick. It is endemic in thirty-seven states and is sometimes referred to as tick fever.

The causative agent belongs to the group known as Rickettsia bodies, a group of bacterialike bodies which can be found in the blood of patients with Rocky Mountain spotted fever and in other conditions, notably typhus and trench fever. Infected ticks are transmitted to man through contact with rodents such as the rabbit or squirrel. The peak of cases occurs in the spring and early summer.

After an incubation period of from two to seven days the disease begins with an acute onset resembling influenza. There are chills, fever, nausea, vomiting and sometimes jaundice. The spleen is enlarged and edema may develop. The rash appears about the third day. It is rose-colored, beginning on the forearms and spreading over the entire body. After three or four days it becomes purplish and sometimes hemorrhagic. Gastrointestinal complaints are frequent. There may be upper abdominal pain, constipation, or diarrhea. Sometimes the pain is so severe as to simulate an acute surgical problem.

The temperature varies from 101° to 105° F. and comes down by lysis in three or four weeks. The mortality from this disease is as high as 90 per cent in some regions and as low as 10 per cent in others. One attack does not always produce an immunity. Serum injections, however, produce immunity for a year.

Adequate nursing care and complete bed rest are the two essentials of treatment. Drug therapy has not been uniformly successful.

CHAPTER 99

DISEASES CAUSED BY KNOWN GERMS: TUBERCULOSIS

Two Strains of Bacilli—Incidence—Infection by Inhalation—Infection by Absorption—Tuberculous Enteritis—Inoculation—Childhood Tuberculosis—Prevention of Tuberculosis—Public Control—Treatment of Tuberculosis—Surgical Tuberculosis—Bones and Joints—Excision—Ankylosis—Glandular Tuberculosis—Skin Lesions—Genitourinary Organs—Varieties of Tuberculosis—Miliary Tuberculosis—Lupus—Pott's Disease.

DESPITE the centuries that tuberculosis has been recognized as a special disease, it was not until comparatively recently that it was shown experimentally to be a contagious disease. In the year 1882, Koch showed that tuberculosis is due to a parasite called the tubercle bacillus, which is a slender rod, straight or slightly curved, and non-motile.

The parasite lives and grows naturally only in the bodies of certain animals and in man. Outside such hosts the germs are rapidly destroyed by sunlight, but if protected by a mucinous covering, as is the case when they are present in sputum, they may survive for eight or ten days in sunlight. In dark and dusty rooms the length of life of tubercle bacilli is somewhat doubtful, some authorities saying that they can rarely live for longer than ten days and retain their power of provoking disease in a susceptible animal, whereas others maintain they may prove pathogenic after as long as ten months outside the body in the dust of dark rooms.

Two Strains of Bacilli. There are two main types of tubercle bacilli which are capable of producing disease in mammals, known respectively as the human and bovine strains. The bovine type rarely causes chronic forms of pulmonary tuberculosis in adults, but tuberculous glands and the acute infections of childhood are sometimes due to this variety of organism. The bovine bacilli are met with in cows, and the source of infection for man may be the milk or milk products from tuberculous cows, or tuberculous meat. The danger from the latter source is far less than from the former, owing to the meat being cooked before consumption.

Bird, fish, and reptile types of tubercle bacilli are also described. It is interesting to note that tuberculosis has never been found to occur in wild birds, but only in domesticated and captive ones.

Incidence. Tuberculosis is never directly inherited through the germ plasm. A child can become infected in utero from an infected placenta, and this probably accounts for authentic cases of "congenital tuberculosis."

What is inherited is a special tissue susceptibility to infection existing in certain families. There is no difference in the degree of susceptibility in the two sexes. Some races are more prone to the disease than others, Europeans being especially liable to infection. It is in general much more prevalent in cities than in country districts, and it is probable that at least 90 per cent of adults in the large towns of Europe have been infected at some time in their life with the germs of the disease, although they may never have shown signs of ill health. Pulmonary tuberculosis is more com mon in males than in females, and the effect of occupation on the incidence of the disease is well recognized.

In Asia tuberculosis is also very prevalent, owing to the denseness of the population, especially in the large towns. In Africa and America it has followed in the wake of colonization and civilization, and has often produced devastating effects upon a population which has previously been free from infection. Such races as are free from tuberculosis are not therefore naturally immune to the disease, and the only immunity that exists is in those peoples who have been repeatedly and almost constantly exposed to mild degrees of infection without showing obvious signs of the disease.

Twenty-five years ago tuberculosis was the greatest single cause of death in the United States, and especially in the city of New York: today it has fallen to seventh place for the nation, and to the fifth place for New York City. The tuberculosis death rate in the latter metropolis has been cut to less than half. (See chart, page 1383.)

Although there has been a growing feeling that the Negro will react to tuberculosis quite similarly to the white, nevertheless there is a striking difference in the tuberculosis death rate among Negroes as compared to the whites. This is undoubtedly closely related to the generally low economic status of the Negroes, and the consequent overcrowded and hygienically poor living conditions. In 1937, of the 4264 tuberculosis deaths in New York City, 3148 occurred in the white population, 1055 among Negroes, and 61 among other colored; the proportion of Negro deaths being 25 per cent.

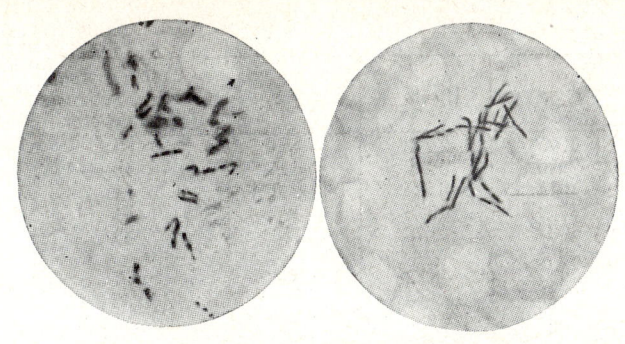

TWO TYPES OF TUBERCLE BACILLUS
Left: Section of the udder of a cow showing the bovine type of tubercle bacillus. This is found in cases of tuberculosis at all ages, but is much more common in children. Right: Human type of bacillus in a specimen of urine, pus cells also being present. The length of a tubercle bacillus is about half the diameter of a red blood cell.

This tremendous fall in the tuberculosis death rate throughout the United States may have been due in part to a lessened degree of virulence of the disease, but undoubtedly much of it may be attributed to improvements in sanitation, better housing and feeding, the partial elimination of slums, and advances in medical treatment.

Occupations involving the inhalation of dust and carried on in badly lit and ventilated rooms increase the liability to lung infection. Debility from any cause will increase a natural susceptibility and set up the disease in those who are not disposed to it. It is doubtful whether in nonsusceptible persons other forms of lung disease increase the liability to tubercular lung infection. Such infection is, however, frequently a terminal event in chronic disease.

Infection by Inhalation. The methods by which the germs gain access to the body are of importance. There are three main routes of infection: by inhalation, by absorption from some part of the alimentary tract, and by inoculation through the skin.

The first is by far the most important. In order that infection may occur by inhalation, it has been shown experimentally that large numbers of bacilli

Tuberculosis (All Forms) Deaths in New York City

Year	White	Negro	Other Colored: Chinese, Japanese, Indian, etc.	Total	Per Cent Negro
1905	9,173	450	39	9,662	5
1910	9,507	522	45	10,074	5
1915	9,555	653	41	10,249	6
1920	6,486	596	53	7,135	8
1925	4,679	743	53	5,475	14
1930	4,072	971	46	5,089	19
1931	3,849	999	74	4,922	20
1932	3,535	952	53	4,540	21
1933	3,553	967	57	4,577	21
1934	3,408	955	57	4,420	22
1935	3,267	1,034	70	4,371	24
1936	3,439	1,076	70	4,585	23
1937	3,148	1,055	61	4,264	25
1938	2,982	904	47	3,833	24

	White	Negro	Other Colored	All Races
Population:				
1905	3,945,066	74,251	6,425	4,025,742
1937	7,066,197	351,496	16,653	7,434,346
Death rate per 100,000:				
1905	233	300	607	240
1937	45	606	366	57

must be inhaled. The risk to a healthy person from inhaling a few tubercle germs floating in the air does not therefore appear very great, although there is little doubt from clinical evidence that tuberculosis may be contracted by sleeping in a room which has been previously occupied by a pulmonary tuberculosis patient.

Infection from sputum or dried sputum, often through the agency of flies which have touched such sputum and transferred the germs on their feet to articles of food, is a very real and potent source of danger. Infection by inhalation may also occur by means of the spread of germs in droplets of saliva expelled from the mouth of a coughing consumptive. It has been shown that a patient may expel from his mouth during coughing as many as 20,000 germs in half an hour.

The organisms which enter the mouth by inhalation in these ways may be carried direct to the lungs in the inspired air, or may reach them indirectly by absorption through the lining membrane of the mouth, pharynx, or intestines, or through the tonsils. Further, the germs may enter the body through the skin or the covering membrane of the eye, and produce disease in the lungs.

A monograph by J. W. S. Blacklock supplied one theory of the means by which tubercle infection occurs. His researches, based upon 1800 post-mortem examinations of children, led to the conclusion that the pathway of infection to the lungs and lymphatic system is the air, and that all the children who died from a primary lung tuberculosis died "by direct infection of the lungs through the air passages by bacilli derived from other human beings." So far as primary abdominal infections, as opposed to pulmonary tuberculosis, are concerned, death was mainly due to the bovine bacillus.

DISEASES CAUSED BY KNOWN GERMS: TUBERCULOSIS

The greatest number of cases of primary abdominal infection was found in the second year of life—that is, at the time when children are taking large amounts of raw milk. Clearly, this type of infection is due to infected milk, a risk which can be considerably lessened by pasteurizing the milk.

It cannot be too widely realized, however, that, despite the dangers of infected milk, it is the human source of infection which represents the greatest danger in childhood. More than two-thirds of the fatal pulmonary cases in infants and young children examined by Dr. Blacklock were due to human infection.

Infection by Absorption. In very many cases the tubercle bacilli enter the body through that part of the alimentary

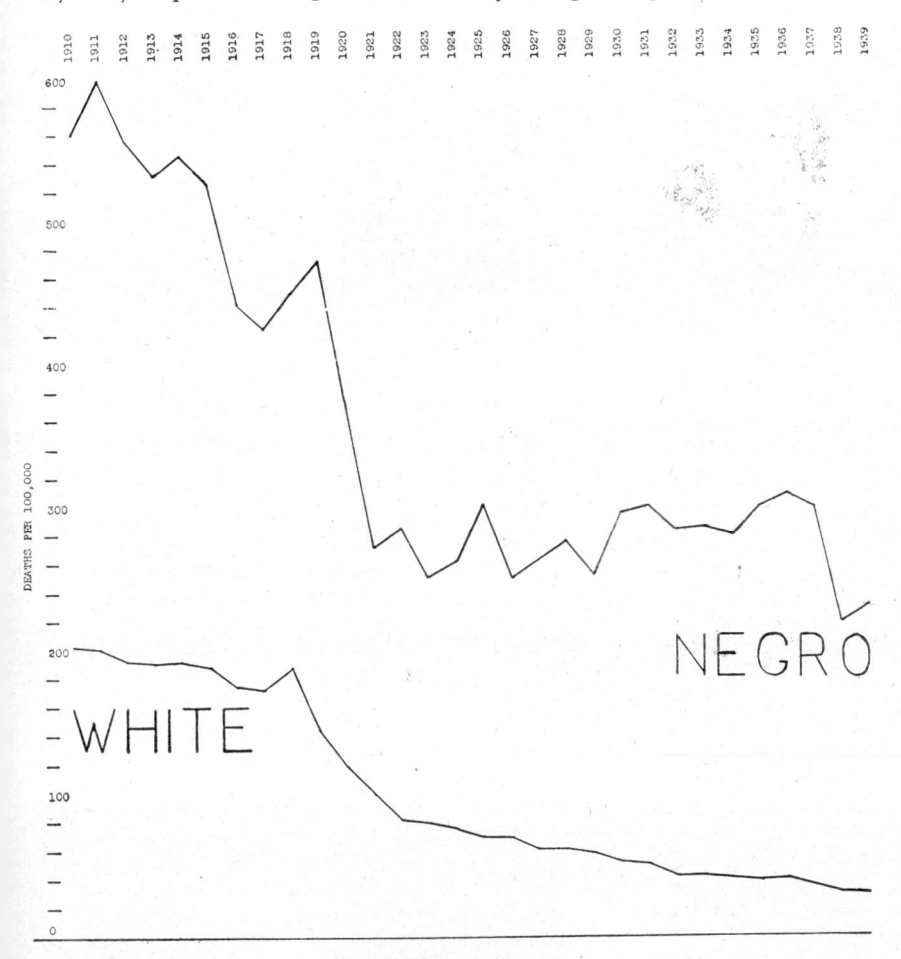

TUBERCULOSIS MORTALITY

This graph, prepared from New York Department of Health figures, shows the death rate from pulmonary and other forms of tuberculosis for the thirty-year period 1910-1939, inclusive. The greater susceptibility of Negroes as compared to whites appears dramatically; many sociologists ascribe this to the poverty of New York Negroes rather than to any racial peculiarity. Note the sharp drop in the death rates for both races from 1919 to 1921.

tract whose function it is to absorb food material.

By experiments upon animals it has been demonstrated that if tubercle germs are mixed with their food in sufficient numbers tuberculosis results. In young animals, thereupon, the disease affects chiefly the abdominal glands, corresponding with that form of tuberculosis which occurs in children and is

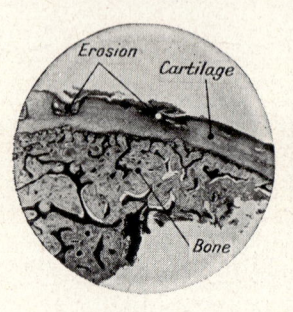

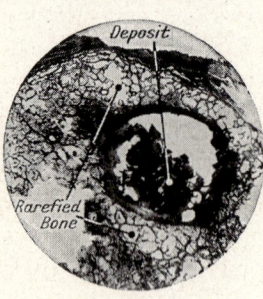

TUBERCULOSIS IN BONE AND CARTILAGE

Left, tuberculous process in cartilage; the tissue is thickened and softened and is eroded at various points. Such erosions give rise to exquisite pain when the joint is moved. Right, a tuberculous deposit in bone; by degeneration of the cells in the nodules a cheesy mass is formed, liquefying into tuberculous pus.

Courtesy of National Association for Prevention of Tuberculosis

known as tabes mesenterica. In older animals, however, the disease is first noted in the lungs; this again corresponds with the relative frequency of pulmonary tuberculosis in adults and its comparative rarity in children.

In cases of alimentary infection the organisms are absorbed in the small intestine, and may pass through the walls without causing any appreciable lesion. It has also been found, when the glands in the chest and neck are enlarged owing to tuberculosis, that tubercle bacilli have been present in the glands in the abdomen. It is possible in such cases that the infection has entered the body through the intestines.

Tuberculous Enteritis. Local tuberculous lesions (miliary tubercles) may occur in the intestinal wall due to the swallowing of tubercle bacilli in food or in the sputum where the lung is infected. They may develop into ulceration owing to secondary infection by septic organisms.

Symptoms may be entirely absent in the case of a simple tubercular infection, but if the condition proceeds to inflammation and ulceration there will be diarrhea with fever, abdominal distension, anemia, and wasting. Tubercle bacilli and septic organisms will be present in the stools. Bleeding from the rectum is very significant in association with the other symptoms.

Treatment is that of tuberculosis in general, with a diet suitable to intestinal inflammation.

Inoculation. There are various skin lesions which are due either to local infection by the tubercle bacillus or to the action of the toxin or poison produced by these germs. In lupus, tuberculous lesions appear on the skin, usually on the face, neck, hands, and feet. Tuberculous ulcers of the skin may be met with upon the lips or around the anus, and are usually due to infection from the germs excreted from the body in the sputum or the feces. In a similar way, by local infection, wartlike growths may be seen upon the hands, especially in butchers who have handled tuberculous meat and in those doctors who carry out post-mortem examinations. Tuberculous granulation masses may form beneath the skin and, gradually breaking through, cause ulceration. Such a tuberculous infection affecting the skin is known as scrofuloderma.

Certain skin lesions are believed to be produced by the action of the toxins liberated from the germs located in some other part of the body or circulating in the blood and are known as tuberculides. Among these may be mentioned such diseases as lichen scrofulosorum and lupus erythematosus.

Childhood Tuberculosis. Tuberculosis is in most cases acquired in childhood as result of contact with an open case. The earliest manifestation is a comparatively benign pathology of the tracheobronchial lymph glands, accompanied by a tubercle in the lung tissue—the source of infection of the glands. The most common symptom is a tendency to tire easily, but more often than not symptoms are absent and the child may appear in good health. This first infection in most cases heals completely.

In a certain number of cases, however, progression occurs. This may result in further lung damage or blood stream infection as a result of breakdown of the lymph glands with rupture into a blood vessel. In either case serious consequences will follow. Dissemination by way of the blood stream results in a condition known as general miliary tuberculosis (page 1389). The bacilli may be discharged into the blood from infected glands at varying intervals of time and result in isolated tuberculous lesions in distant organs, for example bone, joint, or meningeal involvement.

Tuberculous meningitis, dealt with in Chapter 195, is a disease which may also have a sudden onset in children. In other cases, tuberculosis may start insidiously and the symptoms be confined to one part of the body, such as the abdomen or the glands. There is little doubt that the chest glands are the part of the body which is most commonly affected with tuberculosis in children, the lungs being comparatively infrequently involved.

The germs may reach these glands in a variety of ways, but usually they do so by inhalation or ingestion. Abdominal tuberculosis is rarely met with in children under one year; it is commonest in the second and third years, and then gradually diminishes.

Tuberculous glands in the neck are very common in children, but they are rarely found under the age of three years. The germs in such cases usually enter the body through the tonsils, but the eyes, the nose, the pharynx or a wound in the skin may be avenues of entrance.

Tuberculosis of the bones and joints has its highest incidence between the third and fifteenth years. The spine is frequently affected, and also the long bones of arm and leg; the hip joint and the knee joint are also favorite sites for the development of tuberculosis. The lesion starts owing to the lodging in a lymphatic vessel, or more rarely in a blood capillary, of a white blood cell containing tubercle bacilli which may have entered the body in any of the ways described here. Tuberculosis of bones and joints usually runs a much more favorable course in children than in adults, and when death occurs it is generally due to spread of the disease to the lungs or brain. These forms of tuberculosis are considered elsewhere.

PREVENTION OF TUBERCULOSIS

The fight against tuberculosis must consist partly in prophylactic measures to prevent the spread of infection, and partly in curative treatment of the established disease. The object of all the modern methods for the prevention of tuberculosis is the routine avoidance of infection.

The reduction in the mortality rate is undoubtedly due in part to improvement in the conditions of living among the poor, as overcrowding, lack of food, and damp and insanitary dwellings play a large part both in the development of the disease and in the determination of the course that it subsequently runs. The prevention of infection can only be accomplished by removing the sources of infection. These sources are the excretions from human beings and from certain animals suffering from infection with the disease, and also the flesh, skins, and bones of such animals when handled in industry or used as food.

The causative microbes are dispersed about the vicinity of a consumptive patient when he coughs, or may cling to his feeding utensils, and his sputum teems with them. If, therefore, he cannot have a room to himself, and his sputum, personal linen, and utensils are not disinfected efficiently and at once, his disease constitutes a risk for other people, especially for children.

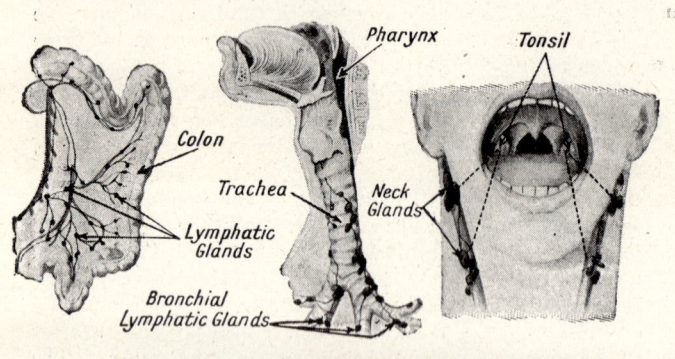

Case finding is perhaps the most important single prophylactic measure. Special instruction is given to doctors, medical students, and other workers for this purpose. Local health agencies are now establishing diagnostic clinics fully equipped with X-ray and fluroscope units. To prevent the further spread of the disease all active cases should be under medical supervision and familiar with the methods by which infection of others is prevented. The unknown case constitutes a major community health problem and every effort should be made toward discovery.

The public-health service, which is also concerned with the reception of reports of cases of tuberculosis, is of value in affording statistical evidence of the incidence of the disease, and also in arranging for the contacts of such cases to receive facilities for examination and observation, in order that any signs of disease may be detected at an early stage. The home conditions under which the tuberculosis has arisen may also be investigated. Because of her many contacts with individuals in the home, school, and industry, the public-health nurse has an ideal opportunity for finding cases in the early stages, before they have had time to progress beyond the hope of cure and before they have developed into sources of infection for other people. Purification of the milk supply, regulations as to the inspection of cows, and the destruction of tuberculous meat are further public health measures which must diminish the incidence of infection by the bovine type of tubercle bacillus.

CHANNELS OF INFECTION OF THE TISSUES

Left: mesenteric glands may become infected with tubercle bacilli coming from the bowel. In a large proportion of this kind of infection in children the microbe is the bovine. Center: infection of bronchial glands from the air passages; the microbes may then pass to lung tissue. Right: infection of neck glands from tonsils.

Public Control. The various state and local health agencies are actively engaged in a campaign to control tuberculosis. The chief aims may be summarized as: (*a*) more adequate treatment of those afflicted with the disease; (*b*) more thoroughgoing efforts to discover minimal cases; (*c*) more general precautions to prevent infection; (*d*) more vigorous building up of individual resistance to the disease; (*e*) more adequate social relief for patients and their dependents; (*f*) the acquisition of new scientific knowledge; (*g*) the better education of the public in the application of knowledge and the use of available facilities; and (*h*) ultimately, provision for sheltered or supervised employment of arrested cases.

TREATMENT OF TUBERCULOSIS

The treatment of tuberculosis has only been placed on a scientific footing since the discovery of the cause of the disease, but no specific remedy has yet been discovered, although it would seem that such an elixir is not very far off. All modern methods of treatment are based on the fact that during the acute stage of the disease rest is the most important curative factor. The influence of food and fresh air is discussed in Chapter 110, where also full details are given of home and sanatorium treatment.

In certain varieties of tuberculosis the use of ultraviolet rays has been attended by excellent results, especially in cases of lupus, glandular infection with abscess, and skin manifestations. The effect of natural and artificial sunlight on tuberculous bones and joints is very marked.

For over fifty years bacteriologists and chemists all over the world have been working to try to produce a specific cure for tuberculosis. Their efforts have thus far failed. Tuberculin no longer enjoys any popularity in this country as a therapeutic agent. The value of B.C.G. vaccine as a prophylactic is still doubtful. Great advances, however, have been made in the surgical measures which can be applied to put a diseased lung at rest.

There is little doubt that although a remedy may be fatal to the tuberculous germs outside the body, and at the same time innocuous to animal tissues, yet such a preparation may be quite unable to heal long-standing tuberculous lesions in the body, or to destroy the germs buried deeply in organs and hedged in by a barrier of scar tissue.

Surgical Tuberculosis. There are many forms of tuberculosis where surgical methods are used for treatment. Acute cases are not suitable, but when the disease takes on a more chronic form it tends to localize, owing to the resistance offered by the tissues, and in many cases it is possible to remove the greater part of the diseased tissue.

Bones and Joints. Tuberculosis of the bones is exceedingly common in children. It frequently affects the end of the shaft where growth is taking place, and where, for this reason, there is increased vascularity. It also frequently affects the epiphyses, and may from them get into the joint. The reaction of bone to the disease is slow, and owing to the fact that pain is at first not great the patient frequently gets about until the disease has progressed considerably. Usually an abscess bursts through the bone and may discharge through the skin. This condition is termed a cold abscess.

The tubercle bacillus may similarly be taken by the blood stream and deposited in the synovial membrane of a joint and gradually lead to serious changes in that joint. Here again the condition is usually painless at first and, unless the bones become involved, may remain painless until great swelling and destruction of the joint result.

The best treatment for both bone and joint tuberculosis is to immobilize completely the affected parts for a prolonged period of time. If abscesses form they can be aspirated. The essential thing is complete rest. Now, it is a very difficult thing to rest any part of the body completely, and surgical ingenuity has been severely taxed to provide splints and appliances which will render completely immobile all the various joints of the body which may be affected by tuberculosis. Special hospitals have been set apart for joint tuberculosis.

Excision. Two or three years is frequently needed in order to allow a bony or arthritic tuberculous focus to subside. From the economic point of view this is a serious matter, for poor parents cannot well provide for their children affected with tuberculosis, and the accommodation in hospitals and sanatoria is not great enough to satisfy the calls upon it. It therefore happens sometimes that the surgeon may think it justifiable to excise a tuberculous joint or bony focus in order to bring about a more speedy cure.

Amputation is very seldom required in children and only in those cases in which serious secondary infection occurs.

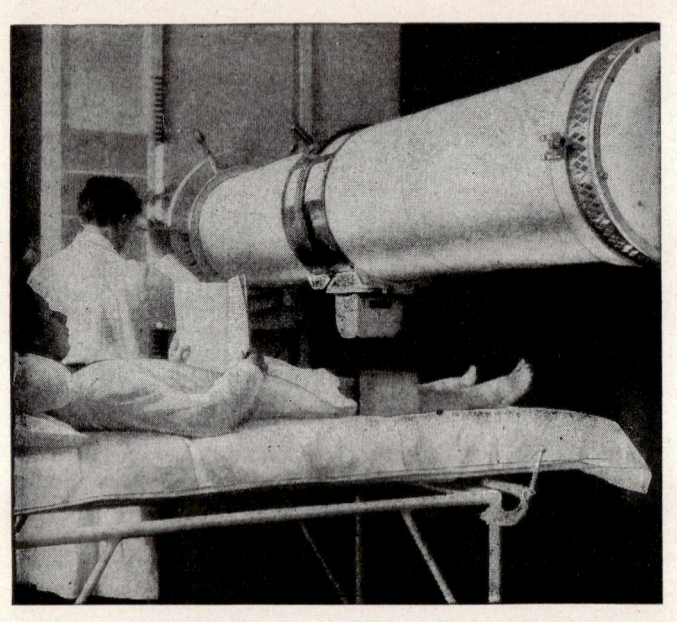

X-RAYS IN THE TREATMENT OF TUBERCULOSIS
The scope of radiotherapy is very wide and now includes the treatment of tuberculosis of the joints by X-rays. Here is seen apparatus used in treating the knee of a patient suffering from this form of the disease.
Wide World Photos

Ankylosis. The common development following tuberculous infection of a joint is ankylosis (see Chapter 166). If this fixation of the joint has occurred in a deformed position, the surgeon may correct it by an osteotomy of the bone some little way from the joint.

Glandular Tuberculosis. The responsibility for treatment of glandular tuberculosis is still disputed between the surgeon and the physician. Scrofulous glands are very common, though less than they were in the time before diseased tonsils were so well treated. Tuberculous mediastinal glands are outside the province of the surgeon, and mesenteric glands affected by tubercles can generally be dealt with satisfactorily by the physician, except when a group of them becomes acutely inflamed and causes peritonitis; but enlargements of glands in the neck, axilla, and groin are usually removable easily, thus leading to a cure of the disease much more quickly than would be possible by other means.

The drawbacks to surgical intervention for cervical glands are that an ugly scar is often left and that occasionally it is very difficult to avoid injury to the spinal accessory nerve, whose section may lead to a slight dropping of the shoulder. In most cases, however, if medical treatment, such as open air, light treatment, cod-liver oil, etc., does not cause great improvement in three months, removal of the glands is a wise procedure.

A tuberculous gland often becomes calcified when the disease has ceased. In the abdomen such a calcified gland is frequently the cause of obstruction of the intestines, owing to a coil of gut becoming adherent and getting kinked. When this condition occurs it requires surgical intervention.

Skin Lesions. Tuberculosis of the skin sometimes needs surgical attention. The verruca necrogenica, or butcher's wart, is a tuberculous lesion and can easily be removed. Lupus, if in a part where no serious deformity would result from its excision, is suitably dealt with by surgery; but if it is in such a region as the face, where mutilation would result from a cutting operation, it is better dealt with by X-ray or radium treatment.

Genitourinary Organs. For early tuberculous disease of one kidney, the removal of it by surgery is the acknowledged best method of treatment; when both kidneys are involved operation is usually inadvisable. Tuberculous inflammation of the bladder is frequently secondary to disease of the kidney, and subsides after the renal disease has been dealt with. If no renal disease exists, the bladder condition is treated by washing out of the bladder or by instillation of antiseptics, and general remedial measures.

Tuberculosis of the testicle is a very common disease, and may occur as a small hard nodule in the epididymis without causing any pain or being noticed by the patient. If the process advances to the stage of abscess, medical measures often suffice, but if the testicle becomes disorganized its removal is indicated. Tuberculosis of the Fallopian tubes is sometimes found in young women, and the best treatment for this is removal of the parts.

VARIETIES OF TUBERCULOSIS

There are many manifestations of tubercular disease, and two of them will be considered in other parts of this work. Tuberculosis of the lungs, or consumption, is dealt with in the section on Respiratory Diseases, Chapters 106-111, while tubercular meningitis, hip-joint disease, etc., are described in the section on Diseases of Children, Chapters 193-199. Other forms of the disease are dealt with below.

Miliary Tuberculosis. By this term is meant an acute form of tuberculosis in which minute nodules are formed in a number of organs of the body, owing to dissemination of the tubercle bacilli by the blood stream. The word miliary, which means resembling a millet seed, is an allusion to their size.

The disease is most frequent and most fatal in early childhood, but is not at all uncommon between the ages of twenty and thirty. It nearly always follows on a chronic tuberculosis of the glands or of bones, but it may be the result of a flare-up following measles, whooping-cough, or typhoid.

There are three main types: acute generalized miliary tuberculosis, the so-called typhoid form; acute pulmonary tuberculosis, in which the nodules are most numerous in the lungs; and acute meningeal tuberculosis. In any one of these types the extent of the miliary involvement will depend upon three things: the number and virulence of the bacilli; the resistance of the patient; and the channels through which the bacilli are mainly distributed.

In the first-mentioned form the tubercles are thickly scattered throughout all the organs of the body. The early symptoms are those of a profound general infection and are due to the toxemia or poisoning caused through the

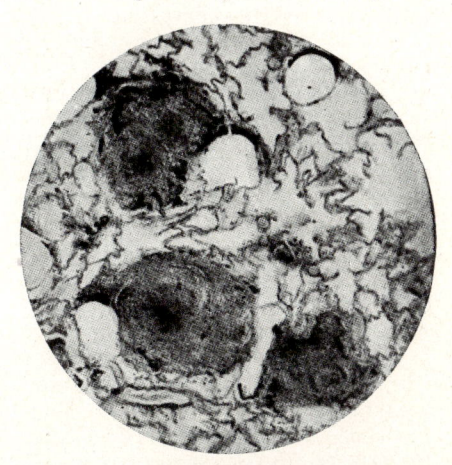

MILITARY TUBERCULOSIS IN THE LUNG
The three dark masses within the circle are the minute nodules known as tubercles, and are composed of large cells formed in response to the activity of tubercle bacilli.

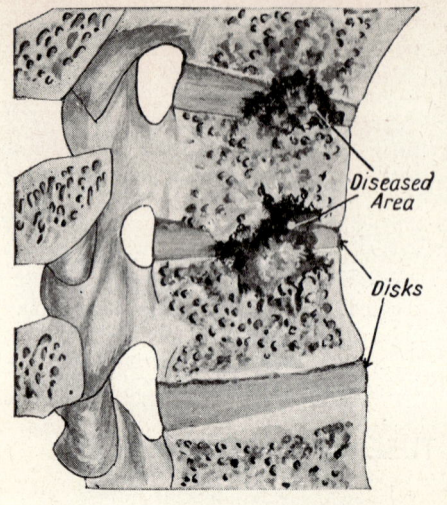

WHY THE SPINAL COLUMN COLLAPSES
The above illustration gives a very clear indication of the manner in which the spine is affected in Pott's disease. The tuberculosis bacilli have attacked adjacent parts of three vertebrae as well as the disks between them.

tubercle bacilli. It begins with weakness, which rapidly increases, and with marked loss of appetite and of weight. Irregular fever is present in children from the first. The pulse is rapid and feeble, the tongue dry, and the cheeks flushed. The spleen is much enlarged, sometimes to five or six times its normal size. Delirium is almost always present, and gradually deepens into a profound stupor. The lung symptoms are those of a slight bronchitis. The sputum is scanty and may contain no tubercle bacilli. The diagnosis from typhoid is often difficult.

In the pulmonary form the onset is usually sudden, but there may have been a previous history of cough. Respiration is rapid and shortness of breath may be distressing. The nose and lips are often blue, the rest of the face being pale. The signs in the lungs are usually those of an acute bronchitis, with patches of bronchopneumonia. The duration of the disease varies from one to several weeks, but it is usually fatal in the end.

The treatment of both these forms is merely that of tuberculosis generally, with special emphasis on proper food, fresh air, and rest. The miliary form of meningeal tuberculosis is really a tubercular meningitis (see Chapter 195).

Lupus. The name lupus is applied to two totally different types of disease of the skin. They are lupus vulgaris and lupus erythematosus, but it is to the former that reference is usually made when a condition is loosely called lupus. It is thought to be caused by the tubercle bacillus.

The distinctive lesion is a soft, "apple jelly" nodule, sometimes the size of a small pea, situated deeply in the true skin, *i.e.* it is subcutaneous, but can be easily seen through the skin.

After a time fresh nodules appear in the neighborhood of the first, and as they increase in size they usually become more or less confluent. By now the patch is slightly raised above the level of the surrounding skin. The process is extremely slow, with the result that the center of the affected area may undergo resolution, with the formation of a scar. This scar is never sound, however, and relapsing nodules can always be found.

In the majority of cases some of the lesions gradually become more and more superficial, until they finally break through the skin, when ulceration is said to have taken place. Infection with the common causative organisms of sepsis now occurs and consequently the surface becomes partially covered with crusts, scabs, and pustules.

Lupus vulgaris is essentially asymmetrical, but as one of the sites of predilection is the nose it may become symmetrical as a result of its spread. On the nose it is almost invariably secondary to disease of the mucous membrane inside that organ. From there it may spread through on to the palate, as well as on to the cheeks. It rarely attacks bone, but the nasal cartilages are all too often destroyed.

As the cause of lupus is—probably—the tubercle bacillus, it is more common

DISEASES CAUSED BY KNOWN GERMS: TUBERCULOSIS

among the poorer classes owing to their mode of living. Where the nose is first affected it is probable that the organism gains an entrance into a small crack after being inhaled with dust, etc. As the disease progresses a nasal discharge appears. This may infect the backs of the hands from rubbing. Occasionally the bacilli may be carried by the blood stream and deposited in many subcutaneous sites simultaneously.

Diagnosis and Treatment. Lupus vulgaris most commonly makes its first appearance during childhood; in consequence it is often regarded as a birthmark. This mistake may have very serious results, for neglect will ultimately end not only in extensive ulceration, but in loss of the nasal cartilages and extreme deformity from scarring. Add to this the facts that the disease is very difficult to deal with and that tuberculosis of other organs may also be present, and it will at once be realized how exceedingly important are early diagnosis and immediate remedial treatment.

Where the patch of lupus is limited in extent and operation can easily be performed, excision should always be carried out. The narrow scar which is left is neat, and there is no chance of local relapse if sufficient of the surrounding healthy tissue has been removed at the same time. Skin grafting may, however, be necessary. When operation is not feasible, certain drugs may be applied in an ointment. Pyrogallol is the best of these and seems to have a selective action in causing necrosis of the diseased tissue.

Ultraviolet-light treatment produces excellent results in selected cases. Well-advanced lesions are often arrested and gradually cleared. The methods in common use are the tungsten arc and carbon arc lamps. Diathermy and ionization are also used. The X-ray treatment has now been forsaken owing to the tendency of cancer to form on surfaces affected by lupus.

It is important to remember that the superficial ulceration and sepsis can be cured with comparative ease by a variety of methods, but this does not mean that the lupus itself is cured. Success is entirely dependent upon early diagnosis followed by immediate and drastic measures.

POTT'S DISEASE
An X-ray of tuberculous disease of the spine. The vertebrae indicated by the arrows are collapsed and misshapen.

Pott's Disease. This disease, named after a distinguished surgeon who was one of the first to describe it adequately consists of tuberculous disease of the spine. Although far commoner in children, onset in adolescent and adult life is not rare. As in tuberculosis elsewhere a slight neglected injury may damage the bones to an extent insufficient in itself to cause serious trouble, but sufficient to furnish a point feeble in resistance to the bacillus of tuberculosis.

Tuberculosis may attack any part of the vertebra, but most commonly it attacks the part which bears the main body weight. The disease eats away the bone, which collapses, thus causing the spine to bend forward at a sharp angle and the spines of the affected vertebra to project backwards. This process is accompanied by stiffness and persistent pain, felt both locally and also in front, to which point it is referred by the nerves which issue from the spine. It may thus be taken for simple stomach ache. Little by little the disease, which

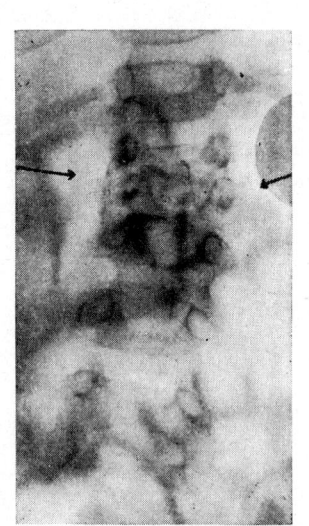

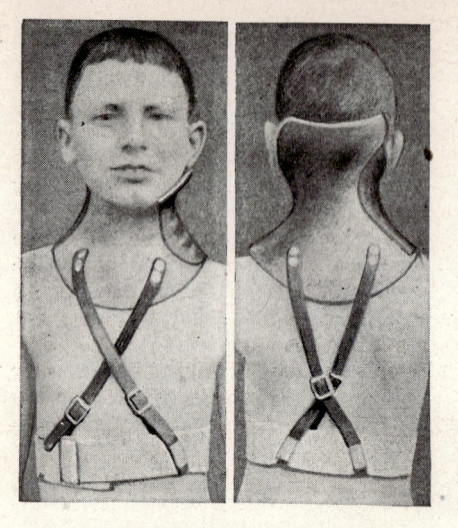

POTT'S DISEASE IN THE NECK
Two views of the application of a celluloid collar to the neck. It supports the chin and the back of the head and, what is quite as important, it prevents all bending movements of the neck, which might be dangerous to life. It lifts the weight of the head off the spine and rests it upon the shoulders.

is at first inside the bone, reaches the outside of the vertebra, and spreads into the surrounding tissues, and a tuberculous abscess forms.

This abscess is very different from the ordinary abscess so long as the ordinary germs of suppuration are excluded. Should they gain access the condition is grave indeed. The spinal cord, the main nerve trunk of the body, passes down the spine in a channel. Distortion of the bony spine by disease may obviously kink this channel to such an extent as to cause pressure on the spinal cord. If this occurs paralysis of all those parts of the body distal to the site of pressure ensues.

Spinal tuberculosis is capable of spontaneous cure, and this is shown by the existence of hunchbacks, in whom resistance to infection has been sufficiently great to enable them to retain their lives while the destroyed bones joined together in a deformed position.

Treatment. No case of tuberculosis of the spine can be adequately treated at home, except at great expense. Institutions exist where such cases can be treated with all the requisite skilled and difficult nursing, while the accommodation is graduated in luxury to suit all purses. In treatment certain things are essential, the first being time. Two years' complete recumbency must be expected in all cases, followed by several more years during which the patient must wear a spinal support and be subject to skilled supervision. Secondly, skilled treatment is essential. All recognized institutions admitting these cases have now an orthopedic surgeon visiting at regular intervals, and resident surgeons who have made a special study of spinal tuberculosis.

If deformity is to be corrected (and it usually is) use must be made of extension. The patient is placed recumbent on a padded metal frame, and by means of pads, or by bending the frame, the spine is gradually bent backwards, or extended.

In the case of cervical (neck) disease it will be necessary to hold the head firmly or even to pull on it in order to prevent the diseased bones from falling together. Various devices are employed for this purpose. Cervical disease is more serious than disease lower down, especially when it is situated in the first vertebra immediately below the skull.

Operations are frequently performed, more especially in the case of adults, to fix the affected vertebrae together and thus shorten the necessary period of treatment. In these cases bone-grafting has been proved very satisfactory.

In Pott's disease heliotherapy (sun treatment) or artificial sunlight is of great benefit, especially in early cases, but this must not be overestimated. Open-air treatment with good food and correct splinting will suffice.

CHAPTER 100

DISEASES CAUSED BY OTHER KNOWN ORGANISMS

Typhus Fever — Trench Fever — Actinomycosis — Diseases Caused by Worms—Distoma—Tapeworm—Hydatid Disease—Roundworm—Ascaris Lumbricoides—Threadworm.

IN this chapter, a study is made first of two diseases which resemble each other in that they are both caused by a type of organism very like the bacterium, and always found in pairs—Rickettsia bodies. These are typhus fever and trench fever. Then follow actinomycosis and worm diseases.

Typhus Fever. The disease which is usually called typhus fever is now very rarely met with in the United States. The name is derived from the Greek word *typhos*, meaning a mist or smoke, owing to the stupor which is a characteristic symptom as well as to the almost perceptible aura associated with the disease.

Typhus is a disease which is begotten of dirt, the infection being spread by lice. It has been called by various names, such as jail fever, camp fever and ship fever; Brill's disease, which was described in New York, and tabardillo, which occurred in Mexico, are also other names for endemic typhus fever. Rocky Mountain spotted fever (see Chapter 98) has been believed to be typhus. Dirt, overcrowding, insanitary towns, prisons, or camps, and cold weather, which militates against personal cleanliness, are potent factors in the origin and spread of the disease.

Typhus fever can be stamped out by the destruction of lice and their breeding grounds. The disappearance of the disease from America has followed in the wake of public-health measures directed to the elimination of slums, improvements in sanitation, and increased facilities for cleanliness. If a case of typhus fever occurs it should be strictly isolated, and all persons who have been in contact with it during its incubation should be kept in quarantine for fifteen days. During this time their temperature should be taken night and morning, and if it rises the case should be transferred to hospital. Further measures include disinfection of clothing, bedding, etc.

The actual cause of typhus fever is the Rickettsia bodies described above, and infection indubitably resides in the blood.

Severe Initial Symptoms. The incubation period of typhus fever is usually twelve days, at the end of which time the disease begins suddenly with headache, giddiness, vomiting, shivering, and rise of temperature. There is great mental prostration and severe pains are complained of in the back and limbs. The appetite is very poor, the bowels are constipated, and the tongue is usually swollen and dry. The face is dusky, somewhat flushed and bloated, and the whites of the eyes are often bloodshot.

As the temperature rises the pulse and respirations also increase in rapidity, and the general condition of the patient becomes that of severe prostration, maniacal symptoms being not unknown. The temperature may reach 103° F. or 104° F. on the first night, and after showing daily remissions for a few days it remains almost continuously at a high level of about 105° F. for nearly a week. At the end of a fortnight from the onset of the disease a fall of temperature by crisis may be expected, and this usually occurs between the thirteenth and seventeenth days.

The Rash. The characteristic rash does not show itself until the fourth or fifth day, and is then first seen under the arms and on the sides of the chest and abdomen. It spreads over the trunk, back, and limbs, but the face is not involved, although it is flushed and congested. The rash consists of three elements: small, raised, round, rose-pink spots or papules in the skin, which later become a dirty brown; similar spots or macules lying beneath the skin and giving rise to a subcuticular mottling; and small petechial hemorrhages, closely resembling fleabites, but having no central puncture. These hemorrhagic spots are usually seen only in severe cases The rash generally begins to fade during the second week.

Course of the Disease. A peculiar smell is associated with typhus, which is described as resembling either the odor of mice or that of rotten straw.

In the second week the general condition of the patient becomes much worse; he is often unconscious and lies with half-closed eyes in a state known as coma-vigil. At the end of the second week he usually takes a turn for the better; the headache is less severe; delirium, if previously present, abates; and with the fall of temperature at the crisis there is a sudden improvement. Refreshing sleep is now obtained, and the patient awakes with his mind considerably clearer, his skin more moist, and with some semblance of a return of normal appetite.

There is always great weakness and prostration, which is slow to disappear during convalescence, and headache, especially after any mental exertion, is present for several months after the recovery.

Very mild forms are occasionally met with, especially among children and in localities where the disease is endemic. Exceptionally severe forms of typhus fever, known as "blasting typhus," are sometimes seen, which prove fatal in two or three days.

Complications. The most frequent complications of typhus are bronchitis,

TYPHUS FEVER — GRAPHIC CHART

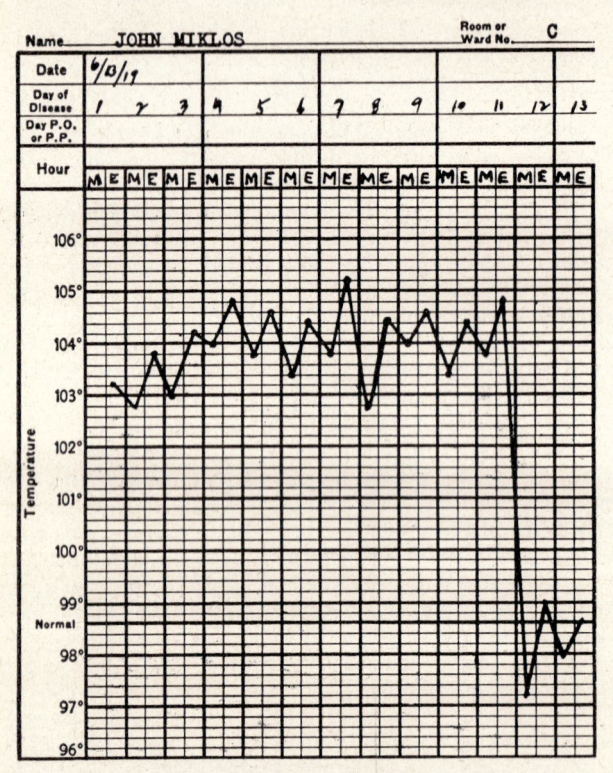

TEMPERATURE CHART IN TYPHUS FEVER

The onset of fever in typhus is sudden. The daily variation, that is, the difference between the temperature readings in the mornings and the evenings, is not very great. After continuing for about twelve days, the temperature suddenly drops and may reach a point below normal.

Courtesy of Physicians' Record Co.

bronchopneumonia, gangrene of the lung, clotting of the blood in a vein of the leg, the formation of an abscess in the parotid gland, and the occurrence of gangrenous bedsores or gangrene of the toes, nose, or hand. Extreme melancholia or even mania sometimes persist after convalescence is established.

Typhus fever is a disease which is progressively more severe as the age of the patient advances. Thus, in children it is seldom fatal, whereas the aged practically never recover. During the middle period of life about 35 per cent of cases die. The mortality of the endemic form is much lower.

Diagnosis. The diagnosis of typhus is not usually difficult during an epidemic. The most characteristic features are the sudden onset with marked prostration, and the bloated, drunken appearance of the face, together with a history of headache, shivering, or rigors and vomiting. The rash is sometimes absent, especially in children, and it may be difficult to see unless the light is subdued when the patient is examined.

It is often difficult to discriminate between typhus and typhoid fever.

Treatment. A patient suffering from typhus should, if possible, be removed to an isolation hospital. All his clothes and bedding and his house should then be thoroughly disinfected in order to destroy lice and their eggs. Fresh air is a very important factor in the recovery of a case of typhus fever. Although the temperature of the room may be as cool as 45° F., a patient suffering from typhus does not complain of the cold and does not catch cold. If his temperature rises above 105° F. it should be lowered a degree or so by tepid sponging. Extra blankets should be used as soon as the crisis occurs.

Skilled nursing is essential in typhus fever, and the mouth must be constantly cleansed. There is often looseness and incontinence of the bowels, and retention of urine may occur, both conditions requiring constant attention. The diet must be restricted to fluids during the acute stages of the illness, and should be administered as for typhoid fever.

After the crisis solid food may be given as the appetite increases and powers of digestion return. Stimulants are usually required at the crisis, and may be given in the form of whisky or brandy. A dessertspoonful every four hours is usually sufficient, unless the patient is a chronic alcoholic.

Sleeplessness is often a very intractable symptom, and hypnotic drugs, such as paraldehyde, should be given early in the disease. The bowels should be kept acting regularly by the aid of enemata, and if diarrhea occurs it must be checked by the use of astringent drugs, such as bismuth, chalk, and opium.

Trench Fever. During the First World War an illness appeared amongst the troops characterized by recurrent attacks of fever, with headache, malaise, and pains in the limbs. It was called trench fever, as it was common among the front-line troops and rare among those stationed at home or at the bases in the rear. This peculiar distribution was found to be due to the fact that the infection is spread by lice. Troops, therefore, who were not able to wash and change their clothes frequently were liable to the disease, and bedding and clothing were the chief means by which trench fever was spread.

It has been conclusively shown that the infection is spread by lice. The causative organism is a form of Rickettsia and the blood of patients suffering from trench fever is capable of giving rise to infection both during the period of fever and for several months after the patient is free of active symptoms.

The incubation period is about seven to nine days. At the end of this time the patient is usually suddenly taken ill with shivering, aching in the limbs, headache, and giddiness; and occasionally nausea, vomiting, and diarrhea may be noticed. The temperature rises rapidly and may reach 103° or 104° F.

The chief symptoms in the disease are headache and pains in the back and limbs, especially in the shinbones. The shin pains are very characteristic, and may be so severe at night as to prevent any possibility of sleep. The spleen is nearly always found to be enlarged. The temperature may pursue a fairly continuously raised course for one or two weeks, and then gradually fall by lysis, or it may be of a typically intermittent character, with sudden rises at intervals, usually of five to seven days. These relapses are very characteristic, the interval between them remaining constant in each case so that their recurrence can be foretold. The temperature at each relapse becomes progressively lower until in a few weeks the fever dies out.

A chronic condition following an attack of trench fever has been noted in many of its victims in which there is debility and disordered action of the heart. Trench fever is never fatal, and as there is no known specific remedy, treatment is directed towards the relief of symptoms and avoidance of infection.

Actinomycosis. This is the name given to any diseased condition resulting from infection by the fungus known as actinomyces or ray fungus. The term actinomyces is now known to include a number of closely allied parasites, the true relations of which have not yet been worked out fully. Speaking generally, the parasite consists of numbers of filaments, each of which is microscopic in size, but which may aggregate together into large masses. These filaments form microscopic spores which have a considerable resistance to heat, but which under suitable conditions are able to sprout and reproduce masses of filaments. In its structural and pathological character this fungus bears a considerable resemblance to the tubercle bacillus, and cases of tuberculosis and actinomycosis have been frequently confounded.

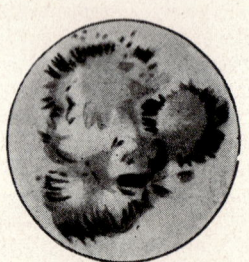

ACTINOMYCES

Microscopic parasite of a fungus disease frequently found in cattle but rarely in man. The disease is stated to be spread by means of infected grain.

Symptoms. Actinomycosis is a disease which is not common in man but occurs with considerable frequency in cattle and less often swine and horses. It most frequently affects the jaw, tongue, throat and face, but may also attack the lungs or the intestines. Lumps or tumors appear. They are hard and may involve bone. Later the lumps may soften, suppurate, and burst, discharging yellow pus.

The malady is rarely communicated to man from animals, though this method of spread occurs in some cases. It is believed to be more usual for the disease to be spread by chewing fresh grains of barley or rye, the surface of which may be infected with the spores of the ray fungus. Such grains have actually been found in the tumor. Carious teeth in some cases are believed to be a path of entrance. The disease has also followed the infliction of a skin wound, but the commonest means of infection are through the mouth, digestive tract, or respiratory system. People who handle raw grain should avoid putting it into their mouths, and should always wash their hands before taking any food.

To protect the public, any parts of an animal found on inspection at the slaughterhouse to be infected by the disease should be condemned as unfit for human food. The whole animal need only be condemned if the disease is widespread throughout the carcass. Milk must be destroyed if the cow is known to be suffering from actinomycosis of the udder.

Treatment. The treatment consists in suitable surgical measures for the opening of the abscesses or even removal of the tumor, and also in giving large doses of iodide of potassium, which drug exercises a great influence in the cure of the disease. Ultraviolet therapy has also been successfully applied.

DISEASES CAUSED BY WORMS

In the following group are included the common worm diseases known in the United States. Those which are found in the tropics (a fair proportion) are discussed later under the heading of tropical diseases, Chapters 152-158.

Distoma. This is the name of a group of worms in the trematode, or fluke, class. Some of the flukes, which are parasitic in man, belong to this group. In most of the species of distomata the sexes are not separate. When laid, the eggs contain a ciliated embryo called a miracidium, which lives for a short time in water, and then enters an intermediary host—usually a fresh-water snail. In the snail it is most frequently found in the liver and digestive organs, where it changes and develops into larval forms called cercariae and radiae. These forms are set free and find their way to the surrounding water, where they live for about forty-eight hours. In some instances they shed their tails and pierce the skin of their definitive hosts, while sometimes they become encysted in another organism. Once inside their definitive host the immature flukes proceed to their selected site. (see Chapters 152-158.)

Tapeworm. Merozoa or cestodes, more commonly known as tapeworms, are distinguished from other internal worms by their segmented bodies and the absence of any digestive system.

They are, with very few exceptions, composed of a head or scolex, by which they attach themselves; and a body of variable length, consisting of segments or proglottides numbering, according to the species, from three to several thousands, which taper off as they near the head, this narrow portion being called the neck. The complete worm is known as a strobilus.

The majority of cestodes occur in vertebrate animals all over the world, and invariably select the small intestine to live in. The four kinds found in man are the Tenia echinococcus, T. saginata, T. solium—dog, beef, and pork tapeworm—and the Bothriocephalus latus, which is more scientifically named the Dibothriocephalus latus.

Anatomy. The scolex or head is usually a blunted cone in shape and bears hooks or suckers or sometimes both, by which the worm attaches itself to the mucous membrane of the bowel.

The variety of form and the complication of structure of the scolex in cestodes are very variable. The suckers may be found in pairs, or fused together, resembling a tube, or they may be provided with stalks, and in one variety they are cup-shaped. The hooks are usually found arranged in a circle.

The segments or proglottides vary considerably in size, number, and shape, but usually are flat, rhomboidal, and hollowed out on the lower surfaces around the insertion of the next segment. Tenia echinococcus has only three segments, whereas over four thousand are found in the fish tapeworm. In all cestodes the segments develop from the scolex, progressing in size and maturity until the complete development of the contained female organs of generation has been attained.

Generally the matured segments become detached in groups at periods of time, but usually after a year or two the remainder of the proglottides may be detached in one chain, leaving only the head behind.

Each segment is encased in a thick, skinlike structure enclosing a plasmic mass called the mesenchyme, embedded in which are the nervous, excretory, muscular, and generative systems. There is no digestive system. The food is obtained by absorption of the chyle from the small intestines of their hosts. Each segment contains male and female reproductive organs.

Life History. The life history of these worms can be divided into larval and adult stages, as these are passed in different hosts. Tenia saginata is found in the ox, T. solium in man, and T. echinococcus develops its adult stage in the dog, though it passes its larval existence in man, and Dibothriocephalus latus in fish; infection can thus be carried by eating uncooked pork and fish or partially cooked animal flesh.

The eggs of the tapeworm, which are oval or spheroidal cells measuring about two one-thousandths of an inch in diameter, develop into embryos with six hooks and may reach their different hosts by a variety of ways. They may hatch out as ciliated organisms, as in the bothriocephalus, having the power to exist in water for a week, where they are swallowed by a fish or mollusc, or they may be passed out through the bowel in a segment or as ova, and eaten by some animal.

Tapeworms in the larval stage were not always recognized as such, but were thought of as other organisms called cysticerci or bladderworms. A cysticercus may be described as the head of a tapeworm growing out of a bladderlike sac or cyst, which becomes filled with a toxic fluid. This larval stage may be passed in the muscle tissue, in which case the entire larva may be surrounded by a cyst. (See Hydatid Disease, below.) The larva in a suitable environment sheds this bladder-tail and begins to grow proglottides from its free end.

A very remarkable phenomenon concerning the cystic development of the larval stage is the formation or budding on the internal surface of the cyst wall of other smaller cysts, containing what are termed daughter scolices or cysts.

Incidence. Tenia solium is most frequently found in Western Europe, especially in countries where uncooked pork is eaten. Dibothriocephalus latus is most prevalent in parts of Russia, more particularly in coastal districts, or in the neighborhood of rivers or lakes, where fish forms the main article of diet. Tenia saginata is widely distributed in Northern India and in parts of the world where cattle are raised under primitive conditions.

Preventive Measures. It is essential that raw beef or pork sausages, raw smoked ham, dishes made from uncooked liver of swine or cattle, also smoked or uncooked fish, should not be eaten. The flesh of the pig in any form should always be carefully inspected for the presence of the condition known as measly pork; curing or smoking is not sufficient to destroy the larvae of these worms. A prolonged temperature of 176° F. will destroy the parasites, but as it takes about eight hours for this temperature to reach the center of a large ham, such a joint should be either cut in half before cooking or boiled for at least that period of time. Freezing will not kill the larvae. Personal cleanliness is most essential in every infected individual if transmission to others is to be avoided.

Treatment. For the successful cure by an anthelmintic it is necessary that the alimentary tract be, as far as possible, empty. It is advisable to prescribe a liquid diet during the previous day and to administer first thing in the morning a saline purgative, followed in two hours' time by the appropriate dose of the drug to be employed.

Some authorities recommend that the doses should be divided, and the second portion given after an interval of two hours; whereas others advise that quarter doses should be administered at intervals of fifteen minutes. If purging has not occurred within four to five hours after the anthelmintic has been taken, another saline purgative should be given. If the drugs administered are male fern or thymol, castor oil must not be given, as the oil dissolves some of their poisonous constituents which may thus be absorbed into the blood.

The resulting bowel movements must be most carefully examined for the minute head of the worm; if this is not found it is probably wise, instead of repeating the treatment, to await repetition of the symptoms, as segments of the worms should be seen within four months.

Suitable Drugs. Of all remedies that have been employed for the cure of tapeworms male fern is the best. The most reliable preparation is the oleoresin of aspidium, U.S.P.; unfortunately it is very nauseous, but this can be overcome by prescribing it in mucilage, or in capsule form.

Some authorities recommend the addition of other anthelmintics such as turpentine, which can be added to male fern in suitable doses. This combination is very useful in dislodging a persistent fixed head, especially that of T. solium. Turpentine is a most valuable drug for this purpose, and when prescribed alone it is usually given in doses of four drachms. In larger doses it is liable to cause poisoning. Thymol is another drug often used successfully in the cure of cestodes. It should never be combined with turpentine or any other oily substance, as the oil acts as a solvent, allowing the thymol to be absorbed.

Hydatid Disease. This disease is caused by the larval form of a small tapeworm, Tenia echinococcus. The adult worm does not infect man, who in this instance acts as an intermediary, while the dog or the wolf acts as the definite host.

When the ova of T. echinococcus reach the stomach of man the little embryos with their six hooks are set free and burrow through the intestinal wall. They reach the liver, lungs, kidneys, peritoneum, or brain, where they develop into hydatid cysts. Sometimes these cysts are found in the long bones, the heart,

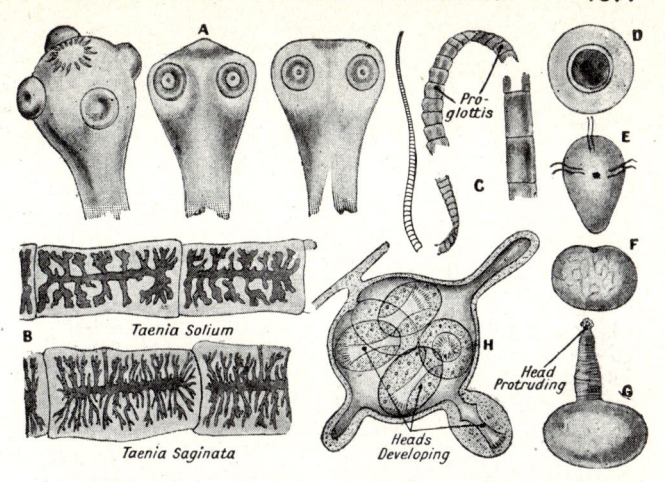

TAPEWORM: DETAILS OF FORM AND DEVELOPMENT
(A) Head of Tenia solium, the pork tapeworm, showing suckers and ring of hooklets. (B) Segments, or proglottides, of T. solium and of T. saginata, the beef tapeworm. (C) Portion of T. solium showing neck and segments. (D) Egg. (E) Embryo. (F) Cyst. (G) Developed cyst of T. solium. In (F) the head is coiled spirally and depressed, while in (G) it is unwound. (H) Brood capsule of T. echinococcus, or hydatid worm.

and the orbital cavity. The cyst or bladder thus produced may attain the size of a human head. Surrounding the cyst there develops a fibrous layer formed from the tissues of the host. From the inner cyst wall outgrowths form which develop into secondary cysts or scolices; these latter are the immature heads of T. echinococcus, which in the intestine of a dog develop into tapeworms.

The contents of these cysts consist of a clear fluid containing no albumin. The cysts may calcify following the death of the parasite, or may rupture and cause suppuration.

Cyst in the Liver. The commonest situation for a hydatid is the liver and when small there are no obvious symptoms, but when large it causes a dragging pain in the abdomen. Rupture of the cyst is spontaneous or the result of strain.

The cyst may rupture into the stomach and intestines, from which there may be a constant discharge for some weeks, resulting in recovery or in death from suppuration. Or it may rupture into the bronchi, and fragments of cysts are coughed up. Death follows from suppuration, hemorrhage, gangrene of the lung, and suffocation. Again, the cyst may rupture into the peritoneum; this usually results in fatal peritonitis. Other directions in which the rupture may take place are the bile ducts, the pericardium, and the vena cava.

Suppuration may take place with or without rupture of the cyst, the symptoms being similar to those of sepsis: chills, sweats, and pyrexia.

Hydatid disease of the liver is diagnosed when there is great and persistent enlargement of the liver associated with good health. Furthermore, the tumor is painless and feels elastic when compressed by the hand.

Cyst in the Lung, etc. The disease is occasionally found in the lung, and the symptoms result from the effect on the lung tissue and pressure on the bronchi. Bronchitis, compression of the lungs, spitting of blood, formation of cavities, and pleurisy are among the usual features.

Hydatid disease of the pleura is less common and resembles ordinary pleural effusion, but the general health remains good until complications arise—such as rupture and suppuration. Hydatid disease of the kidney is not common, but when it does occur it resembles a large hydronephrosis.

The preventive treatment, consisting in precautionary measures against too close association with the definitive host (the sheep dog), should be carefully adhered to. Hydatid disease has been definitely proved in some instances to have been acquired through the disgusting practice of kissing pet dogs, and this dangerous possibility cannot be too widely known.

No medical treatment is of any avail in hydatid disease; the case should be handed over to the surgeon, who will open the cyst and evacuate the contents.

Roundworm. Described by the generic term of roundworms or nematodes, from the Greek word *nema*, a thread, the following worms are found in the human alimentary tract; Ascaris lumbricoides, Oxyuris vermicularis, Ankylostoma duodenale, and Trichocephalus dispar. Filaria bancrofti, which is found in the lymphatic system; F. medinensis, localized in the connective tissue of the lower extremities, and Trichina spiralis, found in the muscles and sometimes in the intestinal canal, are also included among the roundworms.

Ascaris lumbricoides is found in the ox, pig, and man. It is very similar to the ordinary earthworm in appearance, and inhabits the small intestine.

Oxyuris vermicularis, commonly known as the threadworm, is found chiefly in children, its habitat being the large intestine and rectum. Infection takes place through swallowing the ova from contaminated water or food.

Ankylostoma, or *Strongylus duodenalis,* more commonly known as hookworm, produces a very severe anemia, known as ankylostomiasis, hookworm disease, and miner's anemia. This worm is most prevalent in tropical climates, but a good many of the southern states have a high morbidity from this disease. Infection takes place usually through contamination of water or food in districts without drainage; it may also occur through the skin. (See Chapter 156.)

Trichocephalus dispar has a peculiar hairlike anterior extremity and inhabits the cecum.

Filaria bancrofti is found in the lymphatics of the extremities and trunk. This worm is localized to subtropical and tropical climates, and its intermediate host is a mosquito, Culex fatigans. The Filaria medinensis, or Guinea worm, is unknown in Europe, and is chiefly confined to the great portion of Asia, West Africa, and parts of Brazil. (See Chapter 156.)

Trichina spiralis. Found in the voluntary muscles of the body, it gives rise to

DISEASES CAUSED BY OTHER KNOWN ORGANISMS

a disease known as trichinosis. These worms are parasitic to rats and are conveyed by them to the pig.

Ascaris Lumbricoides. Popularly known also as roundworm, this is one of the most common of human parasites, afflicting persons of all ages though most commonly found among children. Usually only one or two are present in an infected person, but sometimes the worms are found in enormous numbers. They are most prevalent in tropical countries, where their existence is favored by the warmth of the climate and by the insanitary habits of the population, but they are not uncommon in various parts of the United States. In appearance the roundworm resembles the common earthworm. The male is from four to six inches long, and the female from ten to twelve inches. They are smooth, cylindrical, and pointed at both ends, and are of a yellow-brown or reddish color. The mode of infection was formerly held to be direct; the eggs of the worm passed by an infected person were believed to gain entrance into another through the medium of drinking water or of dust on food; but experiment has shown that rats or mice may act as the intermediary host, infecting food by their saliva or by their excreta.

The young larva is developed in the egg in a longer or shorter time according to the temperature, and when the egg is swallowed its shell is dissolved in the stomach and the larva is set free and quickly gains maturity.

The adult worm may be ejected from the stomach by vomiting, or it may pass into the small intestine and lower bowel, from which it may be voided. It may crawl up the esophagus and be found

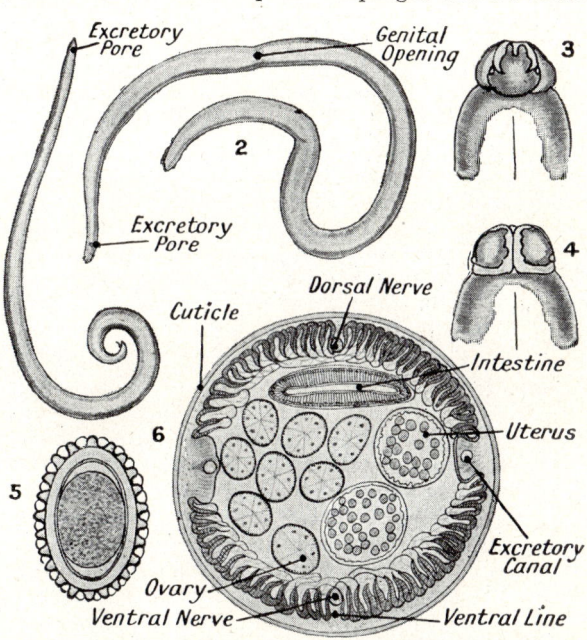

ASCARIS LUMBRICOIDES: TYPE OF ROUNDWORM

The roundworm shown is Ascaris lumbricoides. It inhabits the small intestine and causes varied symptoms. (1) Male; average length four to six inches. (2) Female; average length ten to twelve inches. (3) Head seen from above, and (4) from below. (5) Egg in its shell. (6) Tranverse section of adult female.

at the back of the throat, or it may pass into the windpipe and cause suffocation or even gangrene of the lung tissue. From the intestine it sometimes finds it way into the bile ducts, causing jaundice, or into the appendix, causing appendicitis; if very numerous it may block the bowel.

Symptoms. In many instances the worm gives rise to no noticeable symptoms, but there may be some dyspepsia, nausea, diarrhea, and nervous irritability. In children the symptoms most commonly found are restlessness, foul breath, irritability, picking of the nose, grinding of the teeth, twitching or even convulsions. In some cases there is fever, which may last for a month or more.

Treatment. Treatment is by the drug santonin. This may be given, mixed with sugar, in doses of one-half to one grain for a child, and two or three grains for an adult. It should be given at night, and should be followed by a dose of purgative medicine in the morning. A good plan is to give a dose of santonin on three successive nights, the first and the last dose followed by castor oil in the morning.

Santonin may color the urine a greenish-yellow or saffron tint, and sometimes it causes xanthopsia or yellow vision, when everything that the patient sees looks yellow.

Threadworm. Oxyuris vermicularis is the name given to the thread- or pinworm which frequently infests both children and adults, although the former are much more commonly affected than the latter. The worms breed in the appendix. The male worm measures about a sixteenth of an inch in length. The female is nearly a half inch long. After being fertilized it passes to the rectum, where it lays its eggs or passes out of the anus. Another species of the threadworm is Trichocephalus dispar, popularly known as the whipworm. It is very common in the tropics but not in the United States or Canada. It has a minute head and a long, slender, necklike portion succeeded by a considerably thicker portion, so that the likening of the worm to a whip has some justification. It has an average length of about an inch and a quarter, the female being slightly longer, and the usual place to find it is the cecum, though it may occur in other parts of the alimentary tract.

The eggs are passed in the feces, and must remain for months in water before the embryo is sufficiently developed to hatch out in the stomach of a fresh host. Whipworms may cause appendicitis and also, by piercing the wall of the bowel and allowing escape of its contents, peritonitis. There is no reliable anthelmintic with which to get rid of them. Thymol is said to be sometimes effective. Boiling or filtering water which might be polluted with the eggs is necessary for prevention.

Symptoms. The chief symptoms caused by these worms are irritation in the neighborhood of the anus, frequency of micturition, and sometimes a vaginal discharge in girls. The children often become nervous, thin, and ill, since the presence of the worms usually indicates a catarrhal condition of the large bowel, usually due to a faulty diet. Calomel and santonin in doses of a half grain each may be given to a child of two years on alternate nights for a week, and an enema of quassia or salt and water every evening for eight days. A saline cathartic of magnesium sulphate should be given in the mornings. In addition, a mercury ointment (ten grains to one ounce) should be smeared around the anus, and the child should wear fingerless gloves in bed. Children suffering from worms must sleep in separate beds, and very great care must be taken to prevent their sponges, towels, etc., being used by other people.

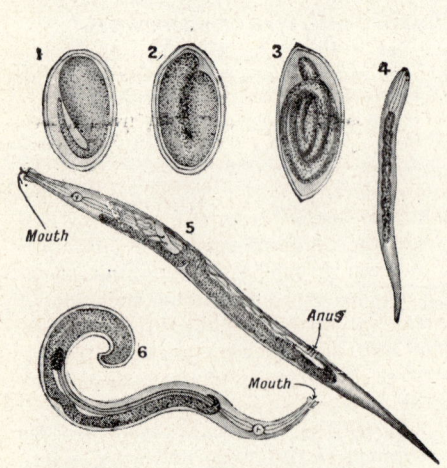

THREADWORM: INTESTINAL PARASITE
The threadworm, Oxyuris vermicularis, inhabits the colon, and in the lower part of the gut gives rise to much irritation. (1-3) Eggs; (4) young worm; (5) adult female; (6) adult male.

CHAPTER 101

VIRUS DISEASES AND RHEUMATIC FEVER

Smallpox — Psittacosis — Mumps — Hydrophobia — Acute Rheumatic Fever.

DESPITE assiduous investigation and modern methods of research, many infectious diseases, some of them of everyday occurrence, still baffle the medical profession as to their causative agents. The ultimate nature of the filtrable virus is still a mystery. In this chapter the commonest of such ailments are described, but, as before, certain types are left out so that they may be included in more appropriate sections.

Smallpox. Smallpox is one of the most severe, although fortunately one of the rarest, of the acute infectious diseases found in the United States today. It is characterized by a rash which commences as a macule, passes through the stages of papule, vesicle, and pustule, and finally dries up to form crusts with marked scarring.

Smallpox is a world-wide disease met with in all climates and affecting all races, but chiefly the colored races and negroes. In places where vaccination is not in vogue children are more often attacked than adults; but infantile vaccination has safeguarded the younger members of a community, so that where it is practised adults are more prone to the disease than children. One attack nearly always renders a person immune for life, but second attacks are not unknown, though they are usually mild.

The infectivity of the disease is very great, as it is spread for a considerable distance through the air; some authorities believe that it can be carried even as far as a mile. The risk of infection at such distances is small, although the disease may readily be contracted by breathing the air of the room occupied by the patient. It is also spread by direct contact with the patient and by using the objects used by him, such as books, clothes, toys, etc. Insects, particularly flies, probably assist in its dissemination.

Early Symptoms. The incubation period is usually twelve days, but may vary from five to fifteen days. The earliest symptoms of illness are headache, marked shivering, severe pains in the back and vomiting. These commence suddenly, with a sharp rise of temperature, sometimes to 103° or 104° F., and all the usual symptoms of fever. On the second day initial or prodromal rashes appear, which are apt to be mistaken at times for those of measles or scarlet fever. These may consist simply of a flushing of the skin or there may be hemorrhages into it, when the prognosis is usually grave.

Rash Distribution. On the third day of illness the temperature generally falls somewhat and the true rash of smallpox appears. It commences on the forehead and wrists as dull red spots or macules, which become raised above the skin, forming papules (see Color plate facing page 1345). The papules spread to the trunk and arms and lastly to the legs, but the rash is almost always densest on the face, forearms, and wrists, showing a tendency to spare the greater part of the trunk and to invade the more exposed parts of the skin. Wherever pressure is applied causing irritation, as by garters, belts, corsets, etc., there the pocks are particularly numerous.

The characteristic distribution of the smallpox rash is important as being a point of great value in differentiating the diagnosis of the disease from that of chicken pox (see Chapter 195). In the latter the rash is situated chiefly on the trunk and face, while it is very scanty on the limbs. In smallpox the mucous membranes are almost always invaded by the rash, which can be seen well developed in the mouth, and which often gives rise to laryngitis.

During the period between the third and the sixth days the rash undergoes a change in character, and the papules become converted into blebs or vesicles which are depressed in the center. At this stage the temperature falls considerably, and in mild cases may become normal, while the patient's general condition is very much improved. On about the eighth day of illness the vesicles become purulent, the clear fluid being converted into pus. Each pustule is surrounded by an inflammatory ring accompanied by much edema. This is particularly marked on the face, which becomes swollen and puffy, and often uniformly covered with the characteristic yellow pustules.

Secondary Fever. Absorption of toxins from these pustules causes a further rise of temperature, which is called the secondary fever, when the patient is extremely uncomfortable with intense irritation wherever the pocks are numerous. The usual signs and symptoms of fever are present, and there is often great stiffness of the hands and fingers. In a severe attack the patient may at this stage pass into the typhoid state, and death frequently ensues. On about the twelfth day of the disease the pustules rupture and blackish crusts form, which separate after a few days, leaving a deep scar. When recovery takes place the temperature falls gradually by lysis (see page 1253), and all the symptoms improve. Some of the crusts are very persistent, and do not separate for a long time. This is particularly the case with those which have formed on the palms of the hands and the soles of the feet.

Variations. The course of the disease just described is that met with in a case of moderate severity. Many other types are seen from time to time, the chief of which are varioloid, discrete or simple, confluent, and hemorrhagic or toxic smallpox. Varioloid cases are those which have been modified by vaccination, and are usually mild, with slight or no secondary fever. Discrete or simple smallpox is the term used to describe mild cases where the pocks are few and symptoms slight.

Confluent smallpox is a very serious condition where the rash is very dense and the pocks are so numerous that they run into one another. The temperature in such cases is very high, and there is much swelling of the skin. Delirium is marked, and death usually occurs at the beginning of the second week.

The most severe type of all is the hemorrhagic or toxic type, which is always fatal. Here the rash is never properly developed, as the patient dies from the toxins absorbed during the first few days of illness. Hemorrhage into the mucous membranes is often seen in these cases, and large quantities of blood are passed in the urine and the stools. Thirst is very marked, and all the initial symptoms of the disease are very severe. Rarely smallpox may be complicated by meningitis. This is also a very rare sequela of vaccination in persons so predisposed. The danger is therefore not removed by abstaining from vaccination.

Complications. The course of smallpox is frequently interrupted by complications, the chief of which affect the larynx, lungs, eyes, and ears.

Laryngitis, when severe, is always of grave significance, but some slight hoarseness or cough is present in a large proportion of cases. Bronchitis and bronchopneumonia are sometimes seen, and occur more frequently in children than in adults.

Inflammatory conditions of all kinds often affect the eyes, simple conjunctivitis being present in a great number of cases, while affections of the deeper structures may also occur.

Infection of the middle ear, which is liable to complicate almost all the infectious diseases, occurs fairly com-

VIRUS DISEASES AND RHEUMATIC FEVER 1405

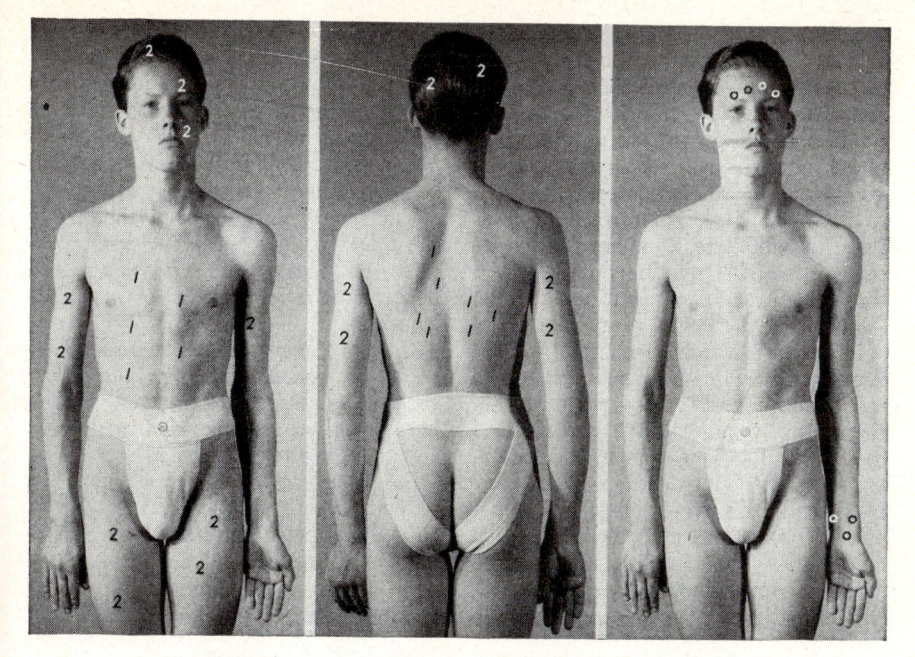

SITUATIONS OF THE RASH IN CHICKENPOX AND SMALLPOX

The vesicles, or little blisters, that constitute the rash of chickenpox appear first on the trunk, back and front, and then on the limbs, face and scalp, as shown in the two left-hand figures. The rash appears in crops. Vesicles may occur in the mouth and throat. The forehead and wrists (right) are usually the first places on which the smallpox rash appears. It occurs as papules, or pimples, later developing into pustules.

monly in smallpox. Other less important complications met with are adenitis, or inflammation of the glands, abscesses, orchitis, and bedsores.

Protective Measures. The treatment of smallpox must be considered both from the point of view of the sick person and from the public-health standpoint. The latter comprises thorough isolation of the patient and the protection of the community in addition to the great prophylactic measure of vaccination.

Smallpox is one of the reportable diseases, and it is the duty of the doctor who diagnoses the condition, as well as the parent or guardian of the patient, to report its occurrence to the proper board of health. The patient may then be isolated in a special contagious-disease hospital. The patient must be strictly isolated until the last crust has fallen off, the skin is thoroughly healed, and all discharges have ceased.

The next important step in stopping the spread of the disease is prompt vaccination of all who have been in contact with the patient. Vaccination is useful in preventing or modifying the disease even when it is delayed some days after the person has been exposed to the infection. Those people who have been in contact with the patient and who are known as "contacts" should be visited daily by an inspector, whose duty it is to report any illness which may arise among them. They can then be isolated immediately the first symptoms become manifest.

The infected house and clothing must be thoroughly disinfected, and schools or institutions visited by inmates of the infected house should be notified.

Epidemics of smallpox should never be allowed to arise, as the disease can be prevented by efficient vaccination and revaccination. In countries where vaccination is compulsory there is no fear of an outbreak, and no provision for smallpox hospitals is necessary. Revaccination should be performed at least twice in a lifetime, at about the age of ten years and again in adult life, and those likely to be exposed to infection should be revaccinated every five years.

Not only is vaccination useful in preventing infection with smallpox, but it will generally prevent its development in those already infected if it is performed during the first few days of incubation.

Treatment. There is no specific remedy for the disease when once it has developed, so efforts must be directed to maintaining the patient's strength, to avoiding septic absorption from the skin with pitting and permanent disfigurement, and to preventing the occurrence of serious complications.

The room in which he is being treated must be airy but not too light, and red curtains and red shades for artificial light are sometimes used to protect the skin from actinic rays and so lessen the irritation on the skin of the face and the subsequent pitting.

In the early stages the diet must be restricted to milk alone, but when the temperature falls in the vesicular stage the food will be increased to build up a reserve of strength to meet the stage of secondary fever, when milk or soft solids are all the foods that can be taken easily.

The skin should receive great attention throughout an attack of smallpox, as one of the worst sequelae of the disease is the pitting of the face. The skin must be sponged daily with tepid water, or warm baths may be used several times a day when the patient can stand them. The face should be covered with a mask of lint kept moist with ice-cold water, or smeared with carbolized vaseline. When the pustules rupture, giving rise to an offensive smell, iodoform may be used with the vaseline. Later, zinc ointment may be applied to the raw areas.

When vomiting is severe in the early stages of the disease, all food must be omitted and only a little ice and champagne given. Pain in the back may often be relieved by phenacetin.

The mouth must be kept thoroughly clean by frequent swabbing with glycerine of borax, while laryngitis and hoarseness are best treated by steam inhalations.

Care of the eyes will reduce the likelihood of serious inflammation; they should be irrigated frequently with boracic lotion and covered with cold compresses to reduce edema.

Sleep must be insured by sponging the patient or by the use of drugs such as chloral or potassium bromide. Stimulants are often required and alcohol may be of great value.

As in all prolonged fevers, skilled nursing is of vast importance; bedsores are particularly liable to develop, and must be avoided by the use of a water bed in severe cases and by constant care of the skin.

Complications such as adenitis, otitis, etc., must be treated as they arise.

Psittacosis. In 1930 Krumwiede demonstrated that the cause of this disease was a filtrable virus. Psittacosis occurs epidemically in parrots and is sometimes transmitted from parrots to humans.

The disease can only be checked by the quarantine of sick birds and restriction of bird importations. Laws along these lines have been adopted in the United States.

Psittacosis is a disease mainly of adults and carries with it a high mortality rate (20 to 40 per cent in epidemics). After an incubation period of about nine days the patient becomes very ill and is soon prostrated. The temperature is high, often rapidly rising to 104° F. The patient complains of chills, headache, nausea and vomiting. After five to six days a gradually developing pneumonia may make the patient critically ill. After a week of high temperature, termination may occur by crisis. Adequate supportive treatment may prevent the occurrence of relapses.

Mumps. Mumps, or, as it is technically called, epidemic parotitis, is an acute infectious disease characterized by swelling of the salivary glands, especially of the parotids. Although the disease is widely distributed throughout the world in temperate, cold, and hot countries, the identity of the virus to which it is due has not yet been discovered with any degree of certainty. It occurs usually in comparatively isolated cases, but epidemics of mumps are not uncommon, especially in schools and other institutions. It is particularly prevalent in winter and in spring, attacking mainly children between the ages of five and fifteen, but adults may be victims of an epidemic and suffer severely. For some reason which is at present obscure boys are much more liable than girls to contract the disease.

Although the virus of mumps is unknown, it is almost certain that infection is conveyed to a healthy person directly from the mouth or throat of the patient, and that fomites (that is, objects contaminated by the patient, such as books, toys, bedding, etc.) do not retain the infection for long. For this reason disinfection after a case of the disease is neither compulsory nor in the least necessary as a rule. The disease is probably contagious for about twenty-four hours before the appearance of the parotid swelling and for at least a week after the swelling has subsided. Isolation for a period of three weeks is usually advisable. The quarantine period for contacts is twenty-six days. One attack generally confers immunity for life, but second or third attacks are not unknown. Relapses are rare.

Symptoms of Infection. The incubation period of mumps is a long one, usually twelve to twenty-six days, during which time there are few if any symptoms. The next stage is one of slight but general discomfort and malaise, with pain in the region of the ear or throat; a slight rise of temperature,

THE CONQUEST OF PESTILENCE IN NEW YORK CITY

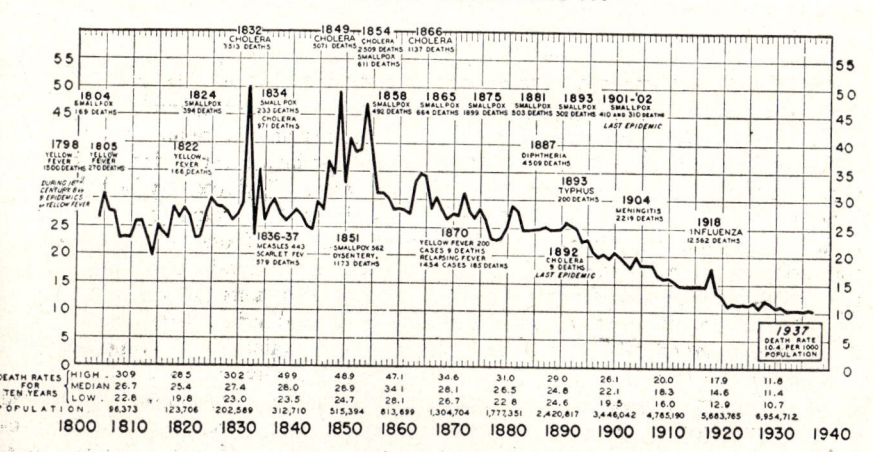

AN ARGUMENT FOR VACCINATION
Note that the last smallpox epidemic in New York City was near the turn of the century; vaccination is compulsory for New York school children.
Bureau of Health Education, Department of Health, New York City; chart by H. M. Cooper

headache, vomiting, nose bleeding, or in the case of a child even convulsions, may also occur. Very often, however, the first sign of the disease is a gradually increasing swelling of the parotid gland in front of and below the ear and along the angle of the lower jaw. Usually, the swelling is at first confined to one side, spreading after a few days to the other side.

In a typical case the swelling and tenderness begin behind the jaw and below the ear, lifting the lobe of the ear; swelling then spreads forward over the jaw and down the neck, and may spread upward to the eyes. The swelling is doughy to the touch. The skin over it is usually unaffected, but may become red and shiny. During this time the temperature is generally rising, and may reach 101° F. to 104° F. Movements of the jaw are painful, the pain varying with the tension present. The secretion of saliva is not usually affected.

It is not uncommon for the other salivary glands to become affected at the same time, especially the glands under the jaw and, less frequently, those under the tongue. The mucous membrane of the mouth and throat may be inflamed; the tear glands at the corner of the eye may also be involved.

An early sign of the disease, often present before any parotid swelling is to be seen, is known as Hathcock's sign, which consists in tenderness on running the finger along the under surface of the lower jaw on the affected side. The spleen is nearly always enlarged, returning to its normal size on recovery.

In the slighter cases there is little more than a mild and temporary local discomfort, but even in the most severe types, with delirium, high fever and great prostration, the course of the disease is nearly always favorable.

Diagnosis and Treatment. The recognition of mumps is usually easy, especially in children. The position of the swelling in front of and below the ear, and the raising of the lobe of the ear on the affected side, will generally be quite enough to fix the diagnosis. It is, however, important to remember that inflammation of the parotid gland does occur from other causes in adults and even, though rarely, in children. Thus, septic parotitis may arise as a sequel to a number of acute infectious diseases, such as typhoid, diphtheria, or scarlet fever, and may also occur with septic conditions of mouth or throat. In these conditions the parotitis is noncontagious, the glands of both sides are affected at the same time, and suppuration is much more common than in mumps. A chronic enlargement of the parotid glands may be a consequence of poisoning by mercury, lead, or iodine; very rarely is it a sequel to mumps.

There is no special treatment for mumps, but the patient should always be kept in bed while the parotid swelling is present. The bowels should be kept freely opened and a light diet given. The mouth must be frequently cleansed with a mild antiseptic solution. Liquid foods are best while the temperature is raised. If there is much pain on moving the jaw, the fluids may be taken through a straw or glass tube. As soon as the swelling lessens and the temperature comes down, the liquids may be thickened; semisolids, such as jellies and custards, or any other bland food requiring little or no mastication may be given. In the milder cases with little constitutional disturbance this diet may be adopted from the beginning.

No medicine is required as a rule, except for high fever or for the relief of pain, when salicylates may be helpful.

Cold or hot compresses, sprinkled with tincture of opium, are sometimes placed on the gland. The dilute methyl salicylate ointment (10 per cent), which is readily absorbed through the skin, is also of value in relieving the pain of mumps. Glycerine of belladonna is another useful application; it is painted over the gland and covered with absorbent cotton. If redness and tenderness become very marked, leeches may be applied or other bloodletting techniques used.

VIRUS DISEASES AND RHEUMATIC FEVER

Very often, however, no local treatment will be necessary except for the use of a simple mouth wash, such as glycothymoline or potassium permanganate, which should always be insisted on in even the mildest cases.

Complications. The possible complications of mumps are numerous, but most of them are not serious. The most important is orchitis, or inflammation of a testis, which, however, many authorities look upon as a symptom of the disease rather than as a complication. Young adults are by far the most frequently affected. The orchitis generally appears about the eighth day, i.e. when the parotid swelling is at its height. One or both of the testicles may be affected, the former being more usual. The inflammation increases for three or four days, and then gradually subsides, as a rule leaving no permanent damage; but in a certain number of cases atrophy or wasting of the organ follows.

The degree of pain which is present in orchitis varies from slight local discomfort, this being aggravated by movement and pressure, to severe stabs of pain radiating down the thigh. In female patients there may be a corresponding inflammation of the ovaries, shown by pain and tenderness in the lower part of the abdomen and by some degree of fever. This, however, seems to be less frequent than is orchitis in the male.

Other complications include inflammation of any of the sexual organs, external or internal, in both sexes. Inflammation of the breasts may also occur, as well as enlargement of the thyroid gland.

Pancreatitis, or inflammation of the pancreas, is not very uncommon. It usually appears within a week of the parotid swelling, and is characterized by more or less severe pain in the upper part of the abdomen, nausea, vomiting and diarrhea.

Suppuration in the parotid gland is occasionally met with, and is always due to other micro-organisms.

Affections of the ear are among the most serious of the complications of mumps, but are comparatively rare. Deafness very often occurs in these cases, and may be permanent. The eyes may also be affected in various ways, but these complications are rare.

Inflammation of the kidneys is much more common, especially in adults suffering from a severe attack of mumps. The urine requires to be periodically examined in these cases, but complete recovery is the rule.

The only remaining group of complications of any importance is that connected with the brain and nervous system. Encephalitis and neuritis are the most serious of these, but fatal cases are extremely rare.

The various complications need special treatment. In orchitis a cathartic should be given at the outset, and the patient kept at rest in bed. The swollen gland must be protected by wrapping in absorbent cotton and supported by means of a bandage. Hot boracic fomentations

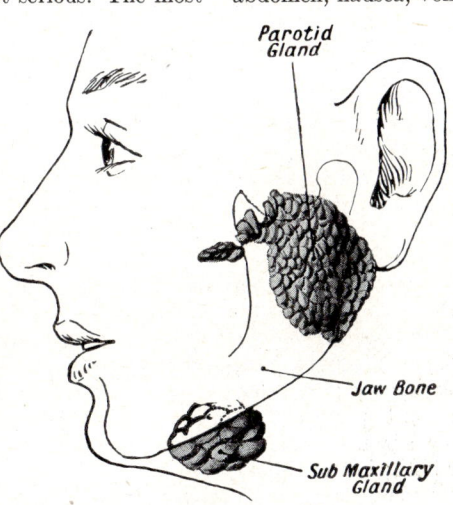

MUMPS: THE GLANDS AFFECTED

The swellings in front of the ears in mumps are due to the inflammation of the parotid glands. Sometimes, however, the submaxillary salivary glands which lie beneath the lower jaw are also swollen and painful.

may be applied, or glycerine of belladonna may be painted on according to the directions already given above. A lead-and-opium lotion is often of service in reducing the swelling and relieving the pain. It is doubtful whether the occurrence of orchitis can be prevented by keeping the patient in bed, but in any case no active exercise should be indulged in for some weeks after recovery. In cases of delirium or symptoms of encephalitis, an ice bag or cap may be applied to the head.

In cases of nephritis, or inflammation of the kidneys, the patient is kept in bed until examination of the urine shows that the condition has cleared up. The diet should be light, and consist principally of milk and milk foods.

Hydrophobia. Hydrophobia is an acute, virulent, infective disease usually resulting from the bite of a rabid dog; but jackals and wolves and, rarely, cats, horses, and even birds may also cause the disease. It is most prevalent in countries where dogs are numerous or poorly controlled or both; in the United States, where it has never secured much of a foothold, it has long since been practically stamped out, thanks to strict muzzling and quarantine regulations. The causative organism, which is a filtrable virus, has been found to be present in the nerve tissues and in the saliva of rabid animals, and it is by means of this saliva, which is carried into the wound by the teeth, that the virus enters the infected person. It immediately attacks the nerve endings, and, entering the nervous system, progresses towards the brain, with fatal results.

The period of incubation, that is, the time that elapses between the injury and the onset of symptoms, is generally found to be between six weeks and three months; but cases have been recorded where it has been as short as two weeks and as long as twenty-seven months. This incubation period depends on two factors: the site and the nature of the wound. The nearer the wound is to the brain, the shorter the distance the virus has to travel. Bites on the face are, accordingly, much more dangerous than bites elsewhere. Large lacerated wounds, by exposing many nerve endings, admit much more of the virus than does a plain bite or a bite through clothing.

A typical case of untreated hydrophobia may be described as follows: The victim, who has been haunted by thoughts of the dread disease throughout the period of incubation, complains of irritation at the site of the wound, with pain in the limb. His fear increases, he becomes depressed and irritable, and seeks solitude. This stage lasts one or two days, when heavy sighs and spasms usher in the second stage. His irritability increases, he becomes terrified, the pains spread to all his limbs and to his body generally. Suddenly the true hydrophobic symptoms are exhibited. He is tormented by thirst, but immediately he attempts to swallow any water he is seized with a suffocating spasm of the larynx which convulses the features. Repeated attempts to drink only result in a repetition of the spasm. Spasms are also brought on by sounds, or by a breath of air on the skin. At first they last but a few minutes; later they last fifteen to twenty minutes. He has frenzies of screaming, throws himself about, beats his hands against the walls and attacks those around him. His eyes roll, his mouth remains open and saliva pours out, since he is unable to swallow it. He develops a hoarse voice, his temperature is raised, his pulse fast and erratic. Sometimes he develops acute mania, but generally he recovers complete consciousness between the attacks. This stage may last two days, until finally consciousness does not return, and collapse ushers in death. Death may result from asphyxia, or from injury caused in his struggles.

Treatment of a Suspected Case. If the virus of hydrophobia reaches the brain the disease is fatal. The sole hope of recovery depends on active measures being taken to arrest and destroy the virus in its course along the nerves.

The police should be immediately notified so that the officer of health for the district may be informed, and the animal seized and handed over to the department of health for examination. The infected person is then advised to place himself at once under medical supervision, or, failing this, he should lose no time in thoroughly disinfecting the wound. It should be freely opened and cauterized either with a piece of red-hot wire or with such powerful agents as fuming nitric acid, undiluted phenol, or silver nitrate pencil. If the latter agents are used, the wound should be finally cleansed with pure water. No effort should be spared to keep up the patient's spirits and to maintain his bodily health. Quiet and absence of excitement are absolutely essential conditions to be maintained.

Pasteur Treatment. Antirabic treatment should be started at once: (1) if the bite or scratches are on the face, head, neck, or hands, or in case of contamination of these parts with saliva; (2) if the bite is a large, lacerating wound on any part of the body; (3) if the biting animal dies within seven days after the biting; (4) if the biting animal cannot be caught; (5) if the biting animal must be killed to effect capture and the head is damaged in the killing; (6) if the laboratory reports that the animal had rabies or that the examination for any reason was unsatisfactory. This treatment consists of subcutaneous inoculations of fixed virus into the skin of the abdomen daily over a period of at least fourteen days. It does not, except in special cases, entail inpatient treatment. This fixed virus is the outcome of Pasteur's great work, and is prepared by dissolving in saline solution the spinal cord of a rabbit which has been infected with the disease. The effect of the inoculations is to develop in the patient an immunity against the virus received by him in the saliva of the rabid animal which has attacked him, the long incubation period enabling immunity to be developed with comparative ease.

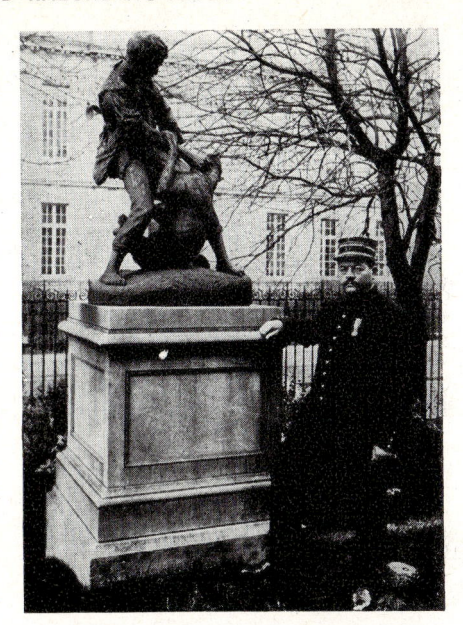

DOCUMENTS IN HEALTH HISTORY

In 1885 a French shepherd boy named Jupille was bitten by a rabid dog; according to medical experience up to that time he faced certain and agonizing death. But Louis Pasteur had been studying the problem of hydrophobia, and inoculated the victim with the weakened hydrophobia virus which he had been testing on animals. Jupille recovered and in this picture stands beside the monument dedicated to Pasteur and commemorating his own experience. Deaths following rabid dog bites were reduced to less than 1 per cent by Pasteur treatment in subsequent years. © *Keystone View Co.*

Symptoms in the Dog. A suspected rabid dog should not be destroyed, but should be isolated. If it can be elicited that it has, in a short time, changed from a docile animal to a snapping, snarling brute, that it has become exceedingly restless and irritable, seeks solitude, staggers in its walk, has difficulty in swallowing, and drips saliva from its mouth, then it is highly suspicious and should be considered rabid. If it dies within ten days, it may certainly be written down as rabid, since it has been definitely proved that a dog cannot be infective for more than ten days before symptoms develop. If on the other hand, it is alive after ten days, then the animal was not rabid, and the person bitten cannot develop hydrophobia. It should be stated that, unlike human victims, the rabid dog shows no aversion to water; rather the opposite.

Acute Rheumatic Fever. The disease called rheumatic fever or acute rheumatism has been known as a scourge of childhood for more than two thousand years, but the exact identity of the agent which causes it is still a matter of dispute. Several varieties of streptococci can give rise to a disease showing similar symptoms in animals. It is probable that in many cases the infection enters the system by way of the tonsils, and that the patient becomes quickly sensitive to one or more of a group of streptococci. Discoveries are being made about rheumatic fever every day, and it is almost certain that within the next ten years the complex problem will be elucidated.

Symptoms. The onset of the disease is commonly rather gradual. For a day or two the patient feels uncomfortable and may complain of a slight soreness in the throat or pains in the limbs.

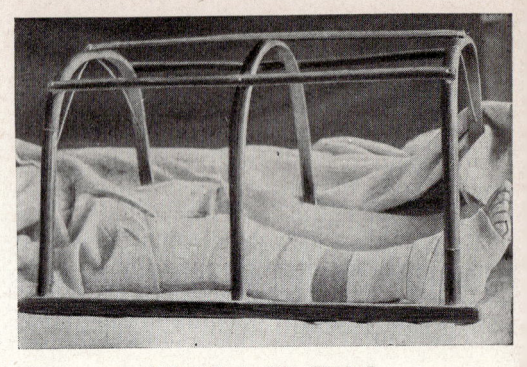

USE OF A BED CRADLE
When joints are acutely tender the presence of bedclothes may become unbearable, and resort should then be had to a bed cradle.

Presently one of the joints, generally a large joint such as the knee, shoulder or ankle, is found to be swollen as well as painful. Within two days the temperature rises to a point between 100° and 104° F. The bowels are constipated, the urine is scanty and high colored, the appetite fails, and the pulse rate is increased. The patient dreads the gentlest touch or the jar of a passing footstep, for the pain in the joints is very severe. The pain is usually worse by night than during the day.

A peculiar feature is the way in which pain and swelling completely disappear from one joint while another becomes involved before the recovery of the first. The swelling takes three or four days to rise and subside. All four limbs usually suffer more or less.

One of the most striking symptoms of rheumatic fever is the sweating. The patient has in a bath of perspiration so profuse as to make even the blankets damp. The sweat has usually a very sour smell. Sometimes an eruption of minute

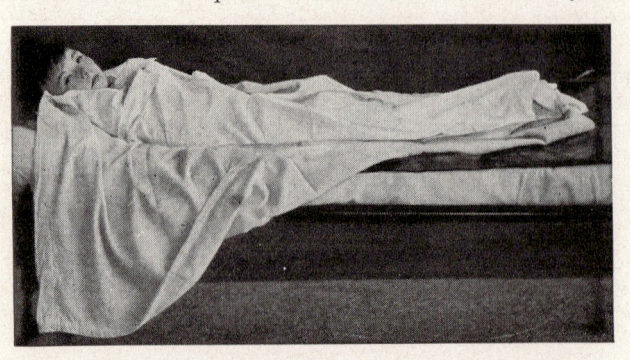

TREATMENT OF HIGH FEVER IN ACUTE RHEUMATISM
A dangerously high temperature may be reduced by wrapping the patient in a sheet wrung out of ice-cold water. This procedure may induce collapse, and should only be used under a doctor's supervision.

VIRUS DISEASES AND RHEUMATIC FEVER

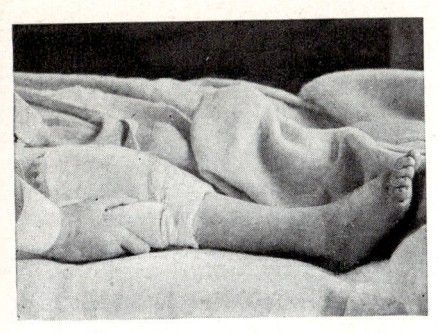

SOOTHING INFLAMED JOINTS
Much comfort may be derived from covering painful joints with hot pads of absorbent cotton, kept in place by a flannel bandage. The joint may be first smeared with a preparation of methyl salicylate, covered with oiled silk.

transparent blisters appears on the skin.

The patient becomes pale and anemic but there is no extreme prostration, no headache and, if uncomplicated, no delirium. The temperature runs an irregular course, with a remission of one or two degrees each morning. Its final decline to normal is gradual. The heart usually becomes slightly enlarged.

Complications. Unfortunately, a large proportion of cases do not run a simple course. By a spread of the infection to the heart and other organs, rheumatic fever often leads to disaster or permanent disablement.

Endocarditis or inflammation of the lining membrane of the heart, and myocarditis or inflammation of the muscular wall, are the most serious and frequent complications occurring in nearly half the cases. In every patient it is necessary for the doctor to watch with the stethoscope for any signs that the valves of the heart have become involved, or for weakness of the muscle. This may happen without giving rise to pain or distress at the time. The younger the patient the greater the liability; if the condition is neglected in early stages permanent heart disease may result.

Hyperpyrexia is a dangerous but rare complication. Its onset is marked by excitement and flushing, accompanied by the sudden disappearance of the rheumatic symptoms. The joints lose their pain and the sweating ceases, but the signs of feverishness increase. Prompt treatment by cool bathing is essential.

Tonsillitis may occur at the commencement or during the course of rheumatic fever. It varies in degree from a mere redness of the throat to a large abscess.

Chorea has a close relationship to acute rheumatic fever. It is most often observed as a late aftereffect, but twitchings may set in during the primary attack.

In many cases the attack of rheumatic fever is so slight that it is overlooked. The boy or girl has a passing chill and seems to recover within a couple of days. There may be soreness of the throat, a trifling rise of temperature, vague muscular pains, and some general discomfort. This is the very important subacute type, which is just as dangerous as the acute type, although it may lack dramatic symptoms. The true nature of the illness becomes apparent only when such complications as heart disease or chorea are found to follow the attack.

Rheumatic fever in young children tends to affect the joints to a less degree than in adults. Skin eruptions and rheu-

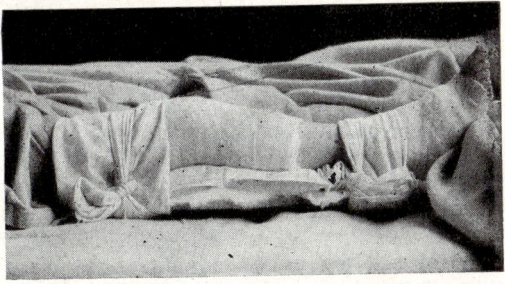

SPLINT FOR A RHEUMATIC KNEE
When a patient is restless it will sometimes be necessary to immobilize a joint by placing the limb on a padded splint. This may procure a sufficient period of uninterrupted sleep. The splint must extend well above and below the joint.

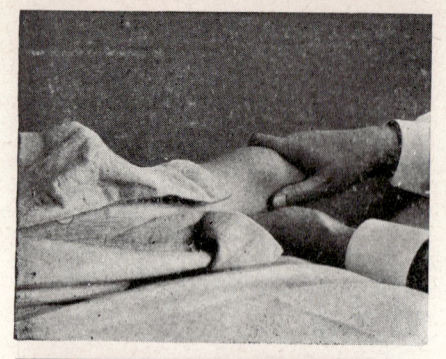

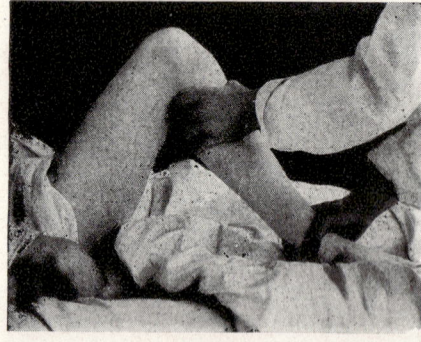

TREATMENT OF JOINTS IN CONVALESCENCE FROM ACUTE RHEUMATIC FEVER

Above, swelling and stiffness of joints may be reduced, when the acute stage has passed, by gentle massage for short periods each day. The muscles of the limbs should also share in the massage. Below, the patient is being encouraged to move his joints for himself. If these exercises are carried out for brief spells several times each day, the patient will find that he has quite a considerable amount of strength when he gets out of bed.

matic nodules (small fibrous thickenings generally on the arms and shoulders) are more common and the disease is often much less acute and therefore more likely to be treated lightly. Heart complications are, however, more likely. The popular expression, "Rheumatic fever in children licks the joints but bites the heart" is all too true. So-called growing pains in a child, with a tendency to excessive sweating, skin rashes, and sore throat, may be the only signs present of a dangerous rheumatic infection.

Liability to Relapse. An attack of rheumatic fever does not confer immunity. On the contrary, it renders the patient more liable to contract the disease again. During convalescence a relapse is not uncommon. The recurrent rheumatism may attain any degree of severity, but it is usually less severe than the original attack. Convalescence is never a rapid process, for the blood is considerably weakened by anemia produced in the body by the rheumatic infection. In children this anemia sometimes fails to respond to treatment, repeated recurrences of joint pains occur, and the general condition may give rise to grave anxiety.

Incidence. Rheumatic fever is pre-eminently a disease of the school age and the young adult. The majority of first

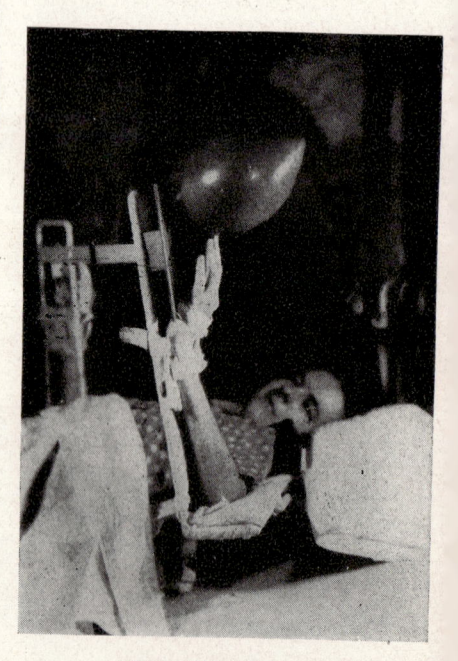

LIGHT EXERCISE IN BED

The care that must be taken not to over-exercise weakened muscles is illustrated here; a child patient at the Riley Hospital, Indianapolis, strengthens her fingers by moving an almost weightless toy balloon.

Courtesy of Mrs. Winifred G. Kahmann

attacks occur in persons between the ages of twelve and twenty-five.

Rheumatic fever is known in most parts of the world, but is especially frequent in the temperate and colder climates. Puerto Rico, Arizona, Florida, and similar regions are relatively free from the disease. In the United States there is some evidence of a seasonal incidence, the late winter and early spring showing the greatest percentage of cases. Apart from this seasonal variation rheumatic fever assumes an epidemic frequency at irregular intervals of three, four, or five years. Large groups of cases then appear within a brief period. Exposure to cold and wet, especially after severe exertion, is often the determining circumstance of an attack. Among certain families extra precautions are necessary because there exists an inherited tendency for its members to contract rheumatic fever.

Treatment. The main principles of treatment are to lessen the inflammation and pain in the joints by rest and soothing applications; to administer the salicylates which appear to have a specific influence on the disease; to protect the heart, so far as possible, from serious and permanent injury by making sure of the needed rest and quiet, and to guard against relapses by careful attention during the prolonged convalescence.

A good strong nurse, a bright airy room, and a proper bed are of the utmost importance. The latter should be firm, stand on a firm floor, and have a soft but firm and flat mattress; a feather mattress is not suitable. The bed must be sufficiently narrow and so placed that the attendant, from either side, can reach any part of the patient's limbs or trunk without interfering with other parts.

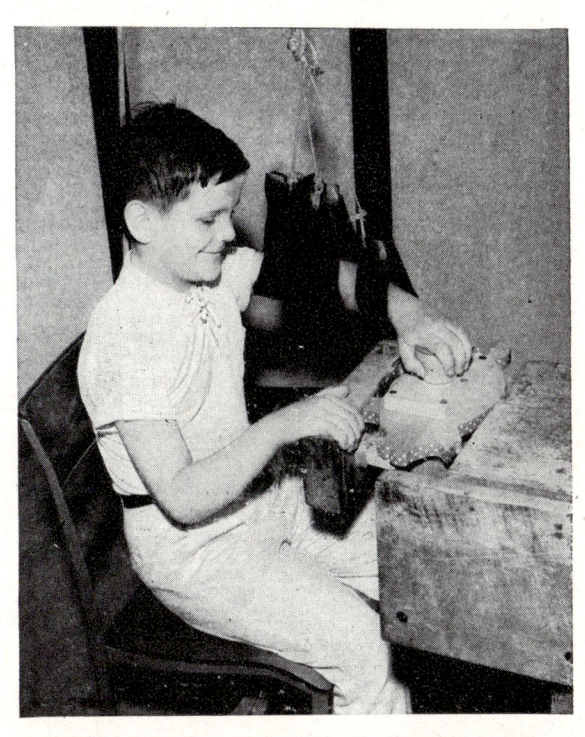

MUSCLE RECOVERY PROMOTED BY ASSISTED WORK
This is an example of the increasingly important curative method called occupational therapy. This boy's arm muscles are too weak for use in ordinary work or exercise, but sound enough to be capable of being strengthened by use. The arm is therefore suspended in a sling and he is enabled to exercise it by work without the strain of supporting it being put upon the weakened muscles. Occupational therapy is administered by trained technicians under prescription from doctors.
Courtesy of The Curative Workshop of Milwaukee

To prevent unpleasantness from the profuse sweating the patient should lie on a soft blanket, and wear a loosely fitting flannel garment, opening down the whole front and freely on the outer sides of the sleeves for easy and frequent changing. He must on no account be allowed to get out of bed to evacuate urine or bowels.

During the feverish stage the diet must be very light, consisting mainly of milk and milk foods, vegetable broths, fruit juices, and occasional lightly boiled eggs. Lemonade or plain water should be taken freely. The inflamed joints should be wrapped in cotton wadding and dressed with methyl salicylate. A bed cradle will keep off the weight of the bedclothes.

The medical treatment consists of the efficient administration of salicylates: ten grains of sodium salicylate every two hours during the day and every four hours at night for an adult, and half these doses for a child, should be given while fever is present. The administration of salicylates should always be in the hands of a physician and the dosage will vary considerably depending on the severity of the case. In most instances the relief of joint pain is very dramatic.

Absolute rest and quiet are essential, and if there has been any suspicion of involvement of the heart this rest and quiet must be prolonged for at least six to eight weeks after the fever. Convalescence must be slow and carefully watched.

Section XIV Blood and Circulatory Diseases

CHAPTER 102

DISEASES OF THE BLOOD AND ASSOCIATED ORGANS

Pallor—General Features of Anemia—Causes of Secondary Anemia — Primary Anemias — General Symptoms — Diagnosis and Treatment — Chlorosis — Pernicious Anemia — Blood Changes — Treatment — Leukemia — Acute Myeloblastic Leukemia — Chronic Myeloid Leukemia — Chronic Lymphatic Leukemia — Hodgkin's Disease — Purpura — Purpura Hemorrhagica — Bleeder's Disease — Plethora — Polycythemia Vera — Splenic Anemia.

SINCE the beginning of the present century much has been done to elucidate many difficult problems of blood disease. Formerly it was considered that certain groups of symptoms were due to defects of the blood alone, but now it is known that all blood diseases involve a study of one or more of the associated organs, particularly the spleen, the liver, the bone marrow and the lymphatic glands. A brief review of the physiology of the blood (Chapter 48) will clearly show why this should be so, and no description of any of the well-established blood diseases is complete without reference to the defects of the above organs.

In some cases, of course, the type of anemia is constitutional, and is quickly remedied when errors of diet or quantitative blood losses are made good. Chlorosis, or the "green sickness," for instance, was one of the products of a misguided policy of the Victorian era which stipulated that young women should be repressed and more or less coddled. The result was chronic constipation and autointoxication which ultimately affected the blood. It is thus evident that the blood is the reflection of the state of the whole body; in almost every case of illness of serious type, the physicians require a complete investigation of the blood to be made at intervals.

The different kinds of blood diseases are dealt with in turn in the following pages; some are the result of abnormalities of the red blood cells, others show defective white cells. In both such conditions there is associated interference with the normal activities of the blood plasma, which conveys the nourishing material to the protoplasmic cells.

The general symptoms of blood disease depend upon the deficiency of the red coloring matter, or, in some cases, the excess of it; weakness, sickness, shortness of breath, general debility; these and many other signs are usually evident.

Pallor. Pallor of increasing character is characteristic of most blood diseases. Permanent pallor is always suggestive of some blood change. In such a case the pallor is shared by the mucous membrane of the lips and the conjunctival lining of the eyelids; unless these are also pale it is improbable that the cause of the pallor is anemia.

Abnormal blood conditions producing pallor may be due to deficiency in the number of red corpuscles, as in the anemia associated with certain infections; or to loss of blood from external injury, internal hemorrhage, or the repeated drain of bleeding piles; or to a deficiency of the iron-containing hemoglobin of the red cells.

THE CONCISE ENCYCLOPEDIA OF HEALTH
GENERAL FEATURES OF ANEMIA

Anemia is the name which is given to any impoverished condition of the blood. From its derivation it means "bloodlessness," and in the widest sense of the term anemia is met with in numberless states of disease. It may be due to impaired formation of any of the constituents of the blood, to any of the causes of pallor mentioned above or to some interference with the activity of the blood-forming tissues themselves.

There are, then, two main groups of anemia: (*a*) Secondary anemia, which is a symptom of some diseased state; (*b*) primary anemia, in which the blood-forming tissues are at fault. To such we may still adhere, although in 1933 it was suggested that properly three groups should be differentiated. So much has been added to the knowledge of the blood since 1920 that nowadays the amount of blood disease seems to be on the increase; actually, however, the investigations are more thorough, and the findings more complete, and therefore blood conditions appear more frequently as features of the clinical picture. Undoubtedly the future will present blood diseases in a much more extended form, and the classification will be more comprehensive and distinct.

Causes of Secondary Anemia. The causes of secondary anemia are:

(1) Hemorrhage. After a large hemorrhage, or as a result of continued loss of small amounts of blood, there is a diminution in the number of the corpuscles of the blood. A large loss of blood will result in the absorption into the blood vessels of water from the tissues, resulting in a diluted blood, which is paler than normal blood and does not carry out its duties satisfactorily. In favorable cases after a hemorrhage the blood becomes normal again in a few weeks.

(2) Acute fever of any kind causes an increased destruction of the blood cells, due to circulation of toxins.

(3) Unhygienic conditions, such as improper food or insufficiency of fresh air and sunlight, result in anemia.

(4) Certain chronic diseases, such as cancer, tuberculosis, kidney disease, syphilis, malaria, chronic suppuration, and chronic infection of the mouth, tonsils, bowel, or other organ may poison the blood and cause anemia.

(5) Some metallic poisons, such as lead and mercury, may cause a degeneration of the bone marrow which produces some of the blood cells.

(6) Among other causes it should be mentioned that some individuals manifest an idiosyncracy to certain drugs and develop a toxic anemia.

Primary Anemias. Among the primary anemias or so-called "blood diseases" the following, fully dealt with under their own headings, are the more important:

(1) Chlorosis, or greensickness, an anemia which affects the female sex almost exclusively between the ages of fifteen and twenty.

(2) Pernicious or Addison's anemia, an anemia of insidious onset which at-

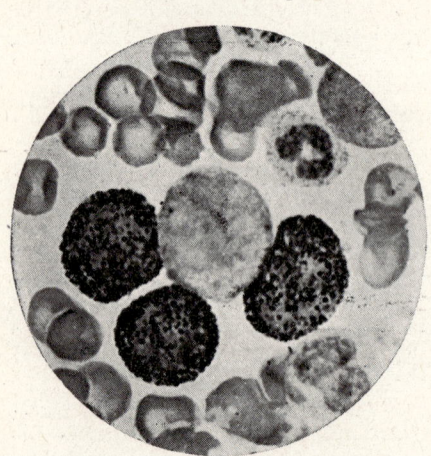

NORMAL AND ABNORMAL CELLS
Bone-marrow cells, knowns as myelocytes, are the precursors of the white cells of the blood and appear in the blood in myeloblastic leukemia. The smaller circles are red blood corpuscles. Magnified 1000 times.

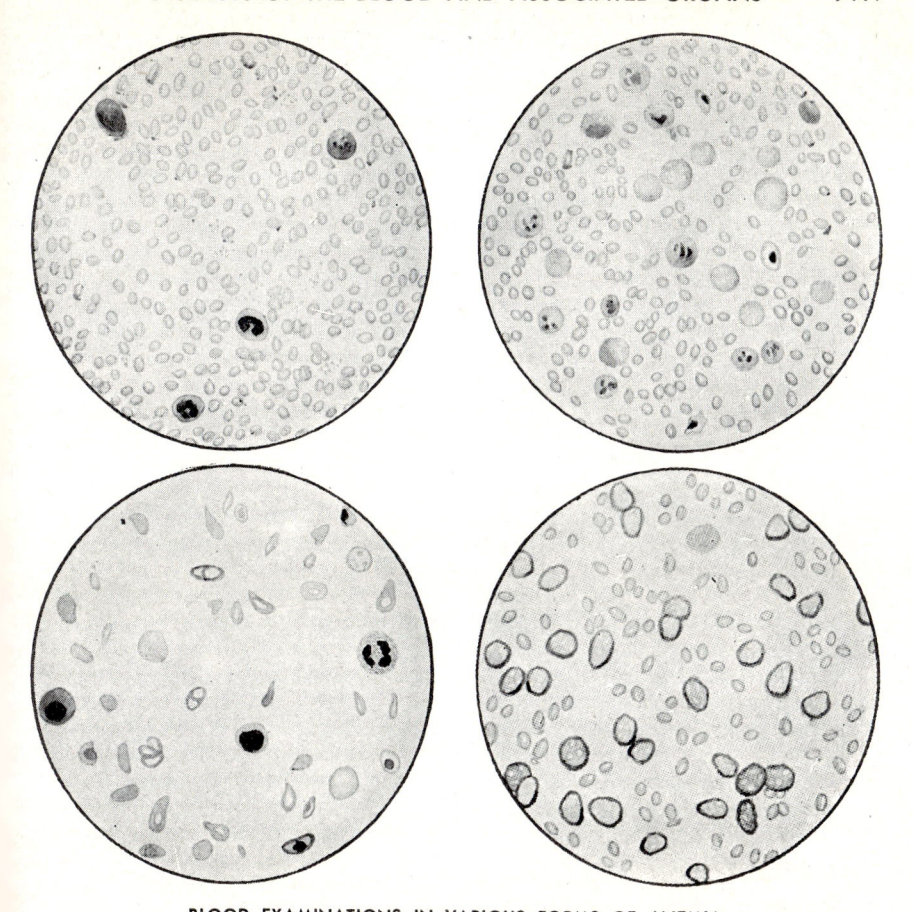

DISEASES OF THE BLOOD AND ASSOCIATED ORGANS 1419

BLOOD EXAMINATIONS IN VARIOUS FORMS OF ANEMIA

Upper left: normal blood showing the usual high proportion of red cells, with occasional white cells and minute blood platelets. Upper right: blood from splenomedullary leukemia: numerous white cells of abnormal type present. Lower left: blood from pernicious anemia: here red cells are scanty, varying in size, and distorted. Lower right: blood from lymphatic leukemia: red cells are diminished, while white cells are more numerous, and of the form known as lymphocytes.

tacks males more often than females, and which can be successfully treated with liver.

(3) Leukemia, a disease of the blood characterized by an increase in the numbers of the white cells beyond the quantity normally present in the blood.

(4) Hodgkin's disease, a disease characterized by enlargement of the spleen, anemia, and progressive enlargement of the lymphatic glands.

(5) Purpura, a condition of the blood which may result in marked anemia. It is characterized by bleeding into the skin, resulting in purple spots.

(6) Hemophilia, or bleeder's disease, a constitutional and hereditary disease which consists in a tendency to bleeding which is difficult to control.

(7) Polycythemia vera, in which the number of red blood cells is too great, and there are plethoric tendencies.

(8) Splenic anemia, a disease of unknown origin associated with enlargement of the spleen.

General Symptoms. In all forms of anemia, whether primary or secondary, the interference with the normal condition of the blood results in definite symptoms. The body is insufficiently aerated and insufficiently supplied with nourishment. The symptoms that result are numerous. There may be at first shortness of breath with general lassitude and weakness, then giddiness, palpitation, headache, and even fainting. Dyspeptic symptoms, with nausea and vomiting, may occur, and diarrhea is frequent.

Diagnosis and Treatment. The diagnosis of a case must rest on a skilled medical examination, and on an examination of the blood itself. Pallor of the skin, while, as already mentioned, a common sign of anemia, is not a sure guide to the diagnosis. It should always be remembered that in certain trades and in certain diseases there may be pallor but no anemia. Pallor may be associated with perfect health, and rosy cheeks may exist in severe anemia.

With regard to the treatment of anemia, the first step is to diagnose with certainty the variety that exists. If it should be a secondary anemia, the treatment must be directed towards removing the cause, when the natural processes of repair will restore the blood to normal. In the primary anemias the diagnosis must be made as accurate as possible by skilled examination. In the graver forms of anemia, the specific treatments are as described later under special headings.

CHLOROSIS

This is a type of anemia which affects the female sex almost exclusively between the ages of about fifteen and twenty, but is becoming much less commonly seen than a few decades ago. Males are rarely affected. It is also called greensickness, as a distinct greenish tint of the face is observed in some severe cases.

Signs. Chlorosis usually begins in females at about the age of puberty and, though no class is immune from attack, it is often associated with unhealthy habits of life. Many authorities make no distinction between this disease and the idiopathic anemia of iron-deficiency which occurs in older women. There is gradually increasing pallor, although at times the disease may be masked by redness of the cheeks. Pallor of the gums and inner aspects of the eyelids often gives a clue to the nature of the disease. In its milder forms chlorosis may give rise to no appreciable symptoms, but if more severe there is general weakness, increasing languor and lassitude, shortness of breath, palpitation, giddiness, fainting attacks, headaches, nausea, specks before the eyes, noises in the ears, constipation, and dyspeptic symptoms.

A frequent symptom which more than all others attracts notice is suppression or diminution of the menstrual flow, though occasionally the flow is excessive. The disease may also cause irritability and a general nervousness. In the graver cases the heart may be seriously weakened and dilatation of the heart result, which may end in permanent damage to the heart muscle. Heart murmurs may be detected by the physician, and may raise the suspicion of valvular heart disease. As a result of chlorosis, clotting of the blood in the veins (thrombosis) may occur, causing swelling of the legs, if it is the leg veins that are involved, but even the veins of the brain have been affected by this process. Affections of the eye occasionally follow chlorosis.

Examination of the blood is the certain means of diagnosing the condition. The red blood cells may be diminished in number, sometimes to about 80 per cent of normal, but the hemoglobin is decreased in a proportionately greater amount, so that each blood corpuscle has

DISEASES OF THE BLOOD AND ASSOCIATED ORGANS

less than its normal amount of hemoglobin. As a rule, however, the characteristic of chlorosis is that the hemoglobin, and not the cells, is reduced. The urine in this variety of anemia is pale in color.

Treatment. The condition is easily curable, but relapses are frequent. Without treatment the disease may last for months or years, but it may end in spontaneous cure.

In marked cases rest in bed for two or three weeks is necessary at the outset to guard against heart strain and fatigue, but plenty of fresh air and simple nourishing food are also necessary. Milk, butter, eggs, meat, and green vegetables, *i.e.* the vitamin foods, are of value. Constipation must be combated by proper habits, suitable food, and exercise, and if necessary with laxatives.

Iron is the drug which yields the best results in treatment. It is often given as an intramuscular injection once or twice a week. The giving of iron by the mouth is still regarded as the best way of treating chlorosis. Iron and ammonium citrates may be given in two-gram doses three times a day or one gram of ferrous sulphate may be taken daily. Blaud's pills, one or more for a dose, are effective. If the stomach is irritable or digestive disturbances result, smaller doses of the iron and ammonium citrates may be given intramuscularly. Laxatives may need to be combined with the medicine to counteract the constipating effect of the iron. Iron medicine should be taken directly after meals and the mouth then washed out, as iron stains the teeth.

As the case improves graduated exercise should be taken in the open air.

Chlorosis has become a relatively un-

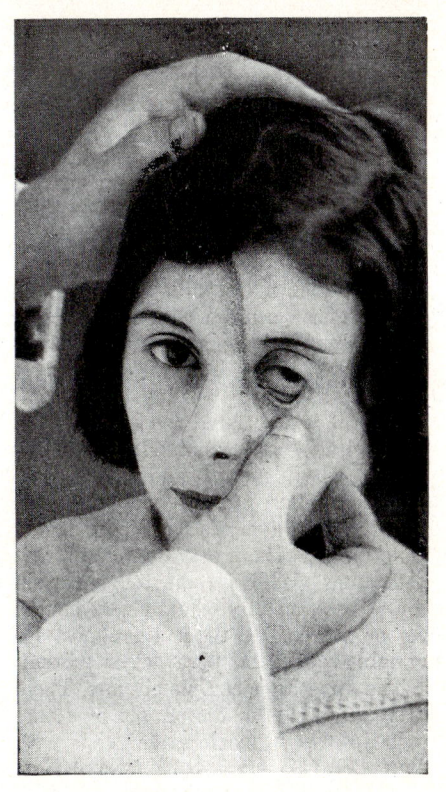

BLOODLESSNESS AND DEBILITY

Impoverishment of the blood may not be manifest on the face, but if the lower eyelid of an anemic person be drawn downwards its lining will be found to be pale.

common disease, and this remarkable diminution has coincided with an increase of open-air sports among girls and improvement in the ventilation of houses and workrooms, and with the greater health-giving influences of the modern girl's costume. In the United States the disease has practically been stamped out.

PERNICIOUS ANEMIA

As its name implies, this is a disease characterized by a very severe anemia. The majority of cases occur about middle life, but no age is exempt. It affects males more frequently than females.

The disease is thought to be due to the deficiency in the body of some substance which controls the proper development of the red blood corpuscles, as they are formed from the erythrocytes in the bone marrow. This substance, known as the P. A. factor, is naturally made in the stomach by the action of a special ferment on the proteins of meat, fish and other animal foods. It is then stored in the liver. Pernicious anemia is thought to be due to defective formation of this P. A. factor.

Signs. The symptoms develop so gradually that the patients cannot say definitely when they began to notice them. The symptom which most commonly leads them to seek advice is muscular weakness. This is invariably present and is nearly always prominent.

With it is associated a marked feeling of lassitude, and any effort speedily causes breathlessness and palpitation. The lips, gums, etc., become very pale and the skin assumes a peculiar lemon yellow color. There may be smooth, reddish areas visible on the tongue or, in some cases, small shallow ulcers on the tip or sides. The teeth are almost invariable septic and pyorrhea is present.

The appetite is completely lost. There may be attacks of discomfort or actual pain in the stomach after food, with nausea and vomiting at times, and diarrhea is not uncommon; but in spite of these symptoms there is no appreciable loss of weight.

An examination of the stomach contents by means of a test meal almost always shows an absence of free hydrochloric acid from the gastric juice. There may be small hemorrhages into the skin and into the back of the eye.

In a few cases, a sensation of numbness and tingling occurs in the legs and feet and, less commonly, in the hands, and this may be followed by a gradual paralysis of the limbs, due to changes in the spinal cord known as subacute combined degeneration. Occasionally this develops before the anemia.

Blood Changes. These are the most important diagnostic signs. The red cells are very greatly reduced in number and may be only between one and two million per cubic millimeter even at the first examination (as opposed to a normal count of about five million per cubic millimeter). Many are altered in shape and no longer have their usual disklike appearance. There are great variations also in size, some being smaller, others much larger than normal, and immature nucleated red cells are present. The most characteristic of these are large red cells about two to four times the normal size, with a large nucleus which fills about half the cell. The amount of hemoglobin is reduced, but not in the same proportion as the number of red cells, so that each of the latter contains rather more hemoglobin than is normally present. The number of leucocytes is also reduced, usually to about 2000 to 4000 per cubic millimeter, that is, there is a leucopenia.

The disease is a very serious one and most of the cases have until more recent times proved fatal within a period of about three years.

Treatment. In 1926, Doctors Minot and Murphy, working in America, discovered that the giving of liver to pernicious anemia patients caused dramatic improvements. In 1929, Isaacs and Sturgis showed that by using portions of the stomach of a pig, these having been dried and cleared of fat, the same effect was obtained. These two discoveries revolutionized the whole outlook of pernicious anemia and altered the prognosis from an almost invariably fatal one to one of considerable hope, so long as the treatment is carried out. Essentially the treatment is palliative and not curative.

With regard to liver and hog-stomach therapy certain principles have been evolved. Every physician is a law unto himself, however, and on various points contradictory reports are made. We may say that the consensus of opinion is as follows:

Taking the fundamental treatment first, liver from the ox, calf, sheep, or lamb may be used, or fish liver as recommended by Davidson; hog's stomach treated as above is available; hydrochloric acid is an adjunct. The liver may be given cooked, raw, or as an extract intravenously or intramuscularly, and it is essential to leave out all the empirical methods and outline those only which have so far proved their worth.

First, there is the Minot-Murphy diet, a system of giving, as a minimum, half a pound of raw calf liver every day. Some patients do well on liver lightly baked, boiled, or stewed. The ideal method is to serve the raw liver in various disguises—as "liver cocktail," by making it into a paste with raw tomatoes and giving it in the form of sandwiches, or by making it up into a salad, along with cheese. Needless to say, in all pernicious anemia states the food should be rich in vitamins and well varied. Cod-liver oil and malt or halibut-liver oil and malt are helpful.

The question of how best to give liver extract is still unanswered. McCrae recommends that intramuscular injections should be given at least every other day, but in the University of Michigan it is held that the number of injections of extract similarly given may be reduced to one per month at least. A routine giving of extract by the veins has been proved of no special advantage except in sudden emergencies, e.g. at the beginning of hospital treatment, when a bad case is seen for the first time. Extracts of liver may be given also by the mouth, sometimes combined with iron, orange juice, tomato juice, etc.

Ventriculin, which is the name given to the extract of hog's stomach which has been deprived of all fat and desiccated before being made into solution, can also be given by the mouth as described above, or by intramuscular or intravenous injection. It is frequently found that pernicious anemia patients suffer from boredom when they have the same type of treatment every day, therefore it is wise occasionally to make some changes.

With regard to acute cases, blood transfusion may be required urgently, after which it may be possible gradually to prescribe intravenous and intramuscular injections, and finally extracts by the mouth or by the most suitable route considering the peculiarities of the case.

Is pernicious anemia a deficiency disease, and so comparable with scurvy and rickets? Dr. D. B. Castle has published results of experiments which appear to show that one of the blood-forming principles is the vitamin known as B_1, of which dried brewer's yeast is a rich source, but which is also present in liver and meat and other foods containing the B_2, vitamin; this affords evidence of the importance of this vitamin element.

All cases when they first come under observation should be kept in bed for some weeks, and, if possible, open-air treatment should be adopted, with due precautions on account of the age of the patient and the poor circulation. The diet should be a mixed one, light and nutritious, of high vitamin value, and must include tender meat.

Septic teeth and pyorrhea must receive proper attention. The bowels must be carefully regulated. Dilute hydrochloric acid and pepsin, which are ingredients of the normal gastric juice, should be given, as they are always much reduced or absent in pernicious anemia. Liver therapy is effective in arresting the further development of central nervous system damage or preventing its occurrence in cases in which it is absent. The aim of treatment, therefore, is not only to bring the blood picture back to normal but also to control the disease of the spinal cord.

LEUKEMIA

Leukemia, from the Greek *leukos*, white, and *haima*, blood, is a disease characterized by a persistent increase in the number of white corpuscles in the blood. There are different varieties of it, which depend upon the type of white cell that shows the greatest increase. When the increase is in the lymphocytes

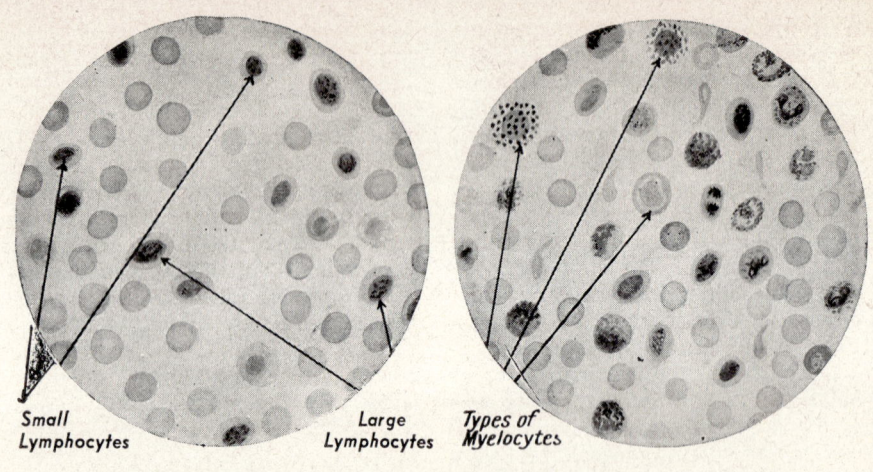

Small Lymphocytes   Large Lymphocytes   Types of Myelocytes

LEUKEMIA: BLOOD DISEASE WITH INCREASED NUMBER OF WHITE CELLS

In leukemia there is a very notable increase in the number of white cells present in the blood, and, as shown in the two specimens of blood exhibited here, there may be a marked difference in the relative proportions of the varieties of white cell. Left: type in which large and small lymphocytes predominate—lymphatic leukemia. Right: myeloblastic leukemia.

the disease is referred to as lymphatic leukemia, which may be acute or chronic. When the increase is in the polymorph leucocytes and these are immature, the condition may again be acute or chronic: the former is called acute myeloblastic leukemia, the latter chronic myeloid leukemia.

The cause of the disease is quite unknown and the definite diagnosis depends upon the microscopic examination of the blood, though there are always symptoms which will lead to a suspicion of the true nature of the condition that has arisen.

Acute Myeloblastic Leukemia. This form of leukemia, with increase of immature leucocytes, has symptoms very similar to those of acute lymphatic leukemia where the increase is in the lymphocytes. Both begin suddenly, the first sign being bleeding from gums, or nose, or into the skin, with feverishness and a rapid development of anemia followed by slight enlargement of lymphatic glands, spleen, and liver. The only difference is that microscopical examination of the blood shows the majority of the white corpuscles (up to 90 per cent in some cases) to be cells called myeloblasts. These are really bone marrow cells which would normally have developed into leucocytes before entering the blood. The disease progresses rapidly to fatal conclusion.

Chronic Myeloid Leukemia. Chronic myeloid leukemia is commonest between twenty-five and forty-five years, and is very rare under twenty years. The onset is very gradual. Often the first sign is abdominal swelling due to a great increase in the size of the spleen.

There is no anemia in the early stages, but this develops later, and the combination of anemia and the pressure of the big spleen leads to weakness and breathlessness. The spleen is always enlarged and sometimes it is enormous. The liver is enlarged, but to a less extent. The glands are seldom swollen. There are usually brief spells of feverishness, but they are slight. Frequently there is edema of the legs.

It is quite common for small hemorrhages to take place into the back of the eyes, which may affect the eyesight, and sometimes bleeding into the internal ear leads to deafness.

The blood, when examined, shows a great increase in the number of white corpuscles, which often reach 200,000 to 300,000 per cubic millimeter, and may be anything up to a million. Where the numbers are very high the blood itself may be of a grayish color instead of the normal crimson. All varieties of white cell are increased.

The disease is invariably fatal, sufferers rarely surviving more than about four years, but temporary remissions in the symptoms are obtained by treatment. The patient should live a healthy outdoor life. Radium or X-ray treatment to the spleen and long bones frequently leads to marked temporary improvement. The drug which is most useful is arsenic, given in the form of Fowler's solution.

Chronic Lymphatic Leukemia. This disease occurs in an older age group and there is usually marked swelling of the lymph glands. The other signs and symptoms are similar to those of chronic myeloid leukemia. Over 90 per cent of the leucocytes are lymphocytes. The spleen is sometimes removed, not as a curative measure, but to alleviate pressure symptoms. X-ray and radium produce remissions in the early stages of the disease.

HODGKIN'S DISEASE

This disease, also known as pseudo-leukemia and lymphadenoma, consists of a progressive enlargement of the lymphatic glands all over the body, and a progressive anemia. It occurs more frequently in males than in females, and it is during young adult life that the majority of cases occur. The name Hodgkin's disease refers to Dr. Thomas Hodgkin (1798-1866), the English physician who first described it.

Signs. In a typical case enlargement of the lymphatic glands is usually one of the first symptoms. Those in the neck are most commonly affected first. Many months may then elapse before the glands in the armpits and groins show any definite increase in size. At this stage the general condition of the patient is quite good. Anemia makes its appearances gradually, however, and is then slowly progressive. General languor, weakness, and loss of weight now become evident. Headaches and constipation may occur.

After some months the patient may complain of a heavy sensation in the "stomach," this being due to the enlargement of the spleen, which usually occurs at this stage of the disease. The spleen itself may be felt as a hard swelling of the upper left quadrant of the abdomen. In time the glands deep in the chest increase in size and, being enclosed in that cavity in close contact with the lungs, heart, and great blood vessels, they press on these important organs. This gradually interferes with their action to the extent of producing cough, breathlessness, pain, and blueness of the face. Intense itching may be experienced all over the body, and the destruction of the blood cells may produce bronzing of the skin. As the disease continues its progress emaciation becomes marked and with it generalized edema makes its appearance. This edema is a waterlogging of the tissues by the blood serum owing to the extreme anemia.

In the earlier stages the blood itself shows very little alteration, but a progressive type of secondary anemia is gradually established. The red cells of the blood become reduced by about half, and their coloring matter (hemoglobin) becomes reduced to about 40 per cent. Occasionally abnormal forms of red cells are seen when the blood film is examined under the microscope. Variations in the number of white cells are not characteristic. The duration of the illness from the time of the first complaint is usually about six months.

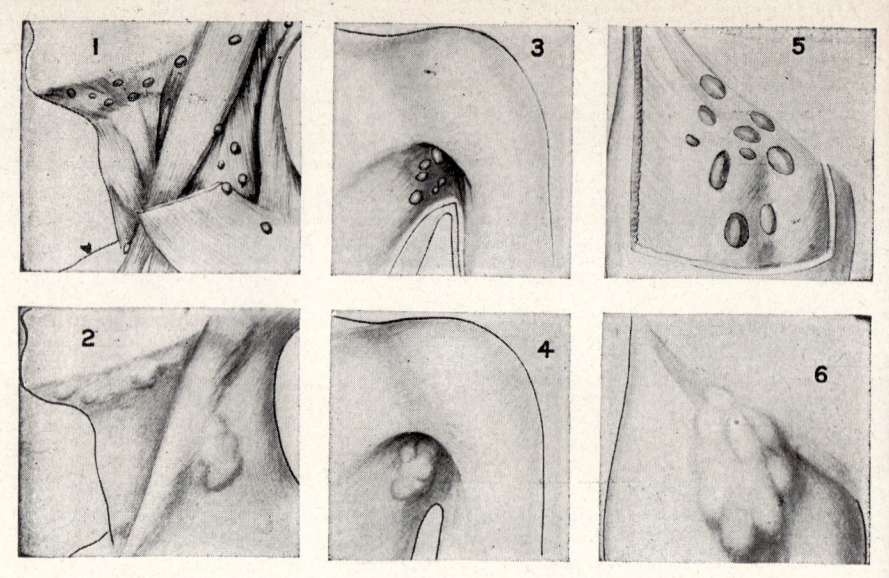

HODGKIN'S DISEASE: SITES OF ENLARGEMENT OF LYMPHATIC GLANDS

In the upper row of figures are exhibited the lymphatic glands in the neck, the armpit, and the groin respectively, and in the lower row swellings caused by the enlargement of the glands in Hodgkin's disease. A general swelling of glands over the body may occur in a number of diseases, but in Hodgkin's disease the enlargements tend to become massive and tumorlike.

Although such is the usual type, there are many other variations which may be assumed by Hodgkin's disease. Of these, the most important is the acute form, in which the whole course is run in the space of a few weeks. In the second category there may be classed those cases in which the glandular enlargement may be localized to certain groups. Should this occur in the glands in the chest or abdomen the increased difficulty in diagnosis is obvious. Yet a third list may be made of those cases in which the fever occurs in waves lasting about ten days, and is followed by a nonfebrile period of similar duration. With the increase in temperature the affected glands swell and become hot and tender, only to quiet down with fall in the fever. These waves may be repeated for many months.

Diagnosis. The diagnosis is often extremely difficult, as the lymphatic glands, being some of the most important defensive organs in the body, may swell for a multitude of reasons. Microscopical examination of a suspected gland will, if other methods fail, reveal to the pathologist the changes characteristic of the disease.

Treatment. Medical treatment up to the present has offered no cure for this disease, and reliance is on surgery, X-ray, and radium. Surgery is first directed at the removal of all foci of infection. The glands, when small and limited, may be excised, but those in the chest and abdomen are not amenable to treatment by this method.

Local application of the X-rays and radium to the enlarged glands and the bone marrow does good by diminishing their size. Radiation therapy in combination with surgical intervention yields the most promise. For the general condition, etc., diet must be supervised, and the distressing symptoms may be dealt with by the use of whatever palliative treatment the physician finds suitable as they arise.

PURPURA

This name is applied to a group of conditions characterized by hemorrhages into the skin and subcutaneous tissues without external injury.

Bleeding into the skin is a symptom sometimes met with in scurvy in the adult, in infantile scurvy, and in hemophilia or bleeder's disease. It also occurs occasionally in infants suffering from congenital syphilis (purpura neonatorum). This form is frequently fatal. It may be met with likewise among the aged.

The cause of purpura is unknown. Probably more than one cause may play a part, *e.g.* allergy and absorption of toxic products from some septic focus in the body. The fatal cases are probably due to micro-organismal infection.

There are several distinct varieties of purpura. Purpura simplex is most common in children, and is usually associated with some feverish disturbance and characterized by the appearance of numerous tiny hemorrhages into the skin, chiefly on the legs. Sometimes the eruption is accompanied by "rheumatic" pains. The spots disappear in the course of a few weeks, leaving no trace.

Purpura rheumatica is known also as peliosis rheumatica. It begins with a short period of irregular temperature, accompanied by pains in the bones, joints, and muscles, by headaches, and by lassitude. Shortly there appears on the legs a crop of macules, varying in size from a millet-seed to a half dollar. These macules are of a dusky red color, and are due to an effusion of blood into the skin. Similar lesions appear later on the chest, the back, the upper limbs, and occasionally on the face. The mucous membranes may also be affected. The hemorrhagic macules come out in successive crops. As a rule the disease runs a favorable course, but occasionally complications may occur in the shape of hemorrhages from the bowels and kidneys, with a return of the fever and vomiting.

Purpura Hemorrhagica. Purpura hemorrhagica is a form of purpura usually met with in young and fragile girls. In this condition the blood platelets are diminished. The condition begins acutely with a sudden rise of temperature, headache, general pains and malaise. The hemorrhagic macules, which occur chiefly in the skin of the legs, though they may be met with all over the skin and even on the face, are irregular in shape, somewhat larger than in the other forms of purpura, and tend to coalesce. The mucous membranes are almost always involved, and there may be bleeding from the nose, the mouth, the throat, the stomach, lungs, bowels, and kidneys, and hemorrhages may occur internally. Similar concealed hemorrhages may occur in the membranous coverings of the brain or the brain itself, causing death.

The disease tends to subside in from six to eight weeks, but in many instances the condition persists for months, and the repeated hemorrhages may deplete the blood so that the sufferer becomes dangerously anemic. Purpura hemorrhagica is occasionally fatal.

There is a special variety of purpura known as Henoch's purpura, which is believed to have an allergic basis. In this all the symptoms of purpura hemorrhagica are greatly intensified. Sudden bleeding occurs from the gastro-intestinal tract. Death may occur within a few days, some cases recover, but relapses are frequent.

Treatment. For all varieties of purpura the treatment is much the same: rest in bed, and light but nourishing diet. The bowels should be kept open regularly; any septic focus should be sought for and dealt with. No local applications are required for the skin. The internal treatment consists in the administration for a prolonged period of iron, quinine, or calcium, and in the acute stages, with pains in the bones and muscles, the salicylates are useful. Transfusion is the most reliable measure in severe cases.

BLEEDER'S DISEASE

Technically known as hemophilia, bleeder's disease is one of the mystery diseases. Everything connected with it is strange and baffling, even its manner of passing from one generation to the next. Thus it is a fact that women very rarely suffer from it; some authorities say never. Yet they act as the medium of its carriage from their fathers to their sons.

For example, neither the sons nor daughters of a bleeder will be bleeders. Nor will his sisters be affected by the disease. But his sisters' sons may be, and his sisters' daughters may transmit the trouble to their sons. Thus, the first question asked when such a case is met with will concern the uncles on the mother's side of the family.

A reference to the chart on page 100 (Volume I) will bear out the general truth just enunciated, and it will be observed that in rare instances a female may show a tendency to bleeding. In the single instance shown in the table the female died of bleeding from a wound which in an ordinary person could quite easily have been stanched. Females belonging to hemophilic families may also suffer from profuse monthly discharges and from dangerous loss of blood after a confinement. It will be further noted that not all males from a hemophilic ancestry are affected with the taint: nor are all the females affected. The proportion of the descendants of a bleeder who inherit the disease will be determined more or less according to the principles of inheritance enunciated by Mendel, explained in Chapter VI. Females in a known bleeder family should not marry.

Ordinary human blood possesses the power, wherever and whenever it leaves the vessels, to coagulate or clot. Consequently injuries are strictly limited in their scope. A blow may cause a certain amount of bleeding under the skin, as in the ordinary case of a black eye, but this is never very great, because clotting at once occurs and plugs up the broken blood vessels.

The bleeder lacks this power of clotting. His blood, on escaping from a vessel, remains fluid, and does not clot. So it goes on flowing freely. Thus, if his nose bleeds he is very likely to suffer a severe blood loss. If he receives a tiny scratch he may lose pints of blood, in spite of every attempt to save him. The consequence is that few bleeders reach manhood and very few live beyond the age of twenty.

Several theories of the origin of this strange affliction are in vogue. One is that an excess of heparin or a related substance exists in the blood and prevents the formation of thrombin from prothrombin, a mechanism which is essential for clotting. Another theory is that the trouble is due to lack of calcium in the blood, and calcium has been given in large doses to correct it.

Treatment. The discovery that snake's venom has the property of clotting the blood with amazing rapidity has led to a series of remarkable experiments which hold out hope of being able to control this once-fatal disease.

The blood from any given sufferer takes thirty-five minutes to clot, but when viper venom, in the dilution of 1 in 10,000, is applied, the blood clots in seventeen seconds.

The viper used in these experiments is Russell's viper, and the venom is extracted by holding the reptile's head in a noose and causing it to bite on a glass covered with a thin sheet of oiled silk. Its fangs pierce this covering and inject the venom into the glass. The venom is dried and then appears in the form of yellow crystals. The poison glands are normally replenished in a week.

Another reptile the venom of which has very powerful coagulating action is the Australian tiger snake. Moreover, it is stated that it possesses certain advantages over viper venom in that it has no tendency to produce acute local hemorrhagic inflammation and that it can be taken orally without danger.

In the absence of viper venom, however, various palliative methods must be tried. Blood transfusion, fresh horse or rabbit serum, local application of adrenalin, the application of fresh tissues in the form of fresh meat of any kind—all these must be given a trial, but no matter how we may look at it, hemophilia is still one of the most dangerous conditions known.

PLETHORA

Derived from a Greek word meaning to become full, the term plethora is applied to an excess of red corpuscles in the blood because of an increase in blood volume.

The plethoric type of individual has a ruddy face, short, thick neck, and general tendency to obesity. While his condition is in some measure the result of hereditary tendencies, it is usually aggravated by indulgence of appetite for food and drink. Although in some cases the subject of plethora in the usually accepted sense—as opposed to the exact scientific sense here discussed—has too much blood, generally such blood excess is absent and the appearance is due to merely local conditions of engorged vessels or to local vascularity such as follows exposure to weather.

Plethoric individuals usually suffer from high blood pressure, and are exposed to the danger of apoplexy or cerebral hemorrhage which accompanies such a condition.

Preventive measures are more useful than curative treatment. Among the former are limitation of intake of food, especially of meat and animal proteins, the insistence upon regular and active exercise, free perspiration, and efficient action of the bowels. When the condition is well established help can still be given by restriction of diet and hygienic measures, and some assistance can be afforded by small doses of potassium iodide, and the use of saline aperients.

Polycythemia Vera. A more serious form of the condition of plethora is met with occasionally, chiefly in men of middle age, in whom, owing to some aberration of the blood-forming organs —the red bone marrow and the spleen— there is a great increase in the number of red blood corpuscles circulating in the blood. At the same time the total volume of the blood is increased so that the vessels are distended with an abnormal amount of blood of an excessively rich cell content. To this condition the names polycythemia vera and erythremia have been given. The exact cause is unknown. In most cases the spleen is enlarged; in some the liver also is swollen.

The complexion may be bright red, or it may be purple. In the latter case there is also swelling and blueness of the ends of the fingers and toes, with curving and thinning of the nails— clubbed fingers. Blood pressure is raised, giving symptoms of headache which may be constant and severe, giddiness, noises in the head, and shortness of breath. There is serious risk of hemorrhage, either from the lung or stomach, or from a cerebral vessel.

The most useful measure of treatment is bleeding. Removal of a pint or more of blood from one of the veins of the arm with replacement by saline solution gives great relief to symptoms, and can be repeated at frequent intervals with renewed benefit.

SPLENIC ANEMIA

This disease is primarily of the spleen and is of unknown origin, for enlargement of that organ gradually comes on without any ascertainable cause. It is an affection of early and middle life. Males are more frequently attacked than are females, while those cases of infantile anemia described by von Jaksch possibly belong to this same group.

Usually the patient first complains of enlargement of the abdomen with a local sensation of weight. This is entirely due to the growth of the spleen, which can then be felt as a smooth and uniform swelling which may occupy the whole of the left side of the abdomen. After a time anemia becomes apparent with a gradual increase in pallor. As this advances the feet begin to swell with edema, and breathlessness on the least exertion causes great distress. In some cases bleeding proves to be a very prominent feature and usually occurs from the esophagus. Occasionally the vomiting of blood may be so severe as to cause suspicion of a gastric ulcer.

Hemorrhage into the intestines may give rise to black feces, while sometimes blood is passed in the urine or is extravasated into the skin and forms purpuric spots. Owing to the extremely chronic nature of the disease any or all of these symptoms may persist for a long time before the terminal signs appear, some ten or twelve years after the first onset of the disease. The anemia becomes chronic and ultimately jaundice and ascites (free fluid in the abdominal cavity) become evident. These features are due to a secondary cirrhosis of the liver, a combination of changes to which the name of Banti's disease is sometimes given.

When examined, the spleen itself is found to be tough and firm, while the blood shows marked diminution in the number of white cells and some loss of red cells. This lack of characteristic changes necessitates great care in the differentiation of the malady from all the diseases in which enlargement of the spleen is evident.

In the early stages treatment of the anemia by the usual means only is indicated. But the ultimate and only radical cure is removal of the spleen itself, and this should be undertaken as early as possible.

CHAPTER 103

COMMON SIGNS OF CIRCULATORY FAILURE

Cyanosis — Anasarca — Edema — Heart and Kidney Edema — Ascites — Syncope — Breathlessness.

APART from pain, abnormalities of the pulse, and the general weakness associated with defects of the heart or of the circulation, there are certain well-marked signs which point to serious interference with the work of the heart, although it is possible that they may also be due to other causes interfering with the circulation.

It must be remembered that the work of the heart is that of a pump which drives the blood through the smallest vessels and so keeps the corpuscles in constant motion and maintains a steady supply of nourishing fluid for the tissues in the form of plasma which oozes out steadily from the capillary walls. It is clear, therefore, that cardiac defects must bring, first, a slowing of the rate at which the red cells travel and consequent lack of fresh oxygen, and, secondly, an increased amount of fluid in the open spaces of the body. Thus we are presented with signs of cyanosis and anasarca respectively. These, as well as the sign of breathlessness, are described in the following pages.

The stoppage of the circulation to the brain may cause a sudden and almost complete loss of consciousness. This generally has origin in some fundamental failure of the regular muscle contraction of the heart and may, indeed, be fatal. Such failures are called syncope.

A great deal depends upon the blood pressure in the smaller arteries. When the peripheral resistance is increased more effort is required to maintain the circulation, therefore the pressure rises, and in the present era of mental and physical stress and strain, raised blood pressure is very common. This matter is dealt with in the chapter on diseases of the blood vessels, but it should be borne in mind that raising or lowering of the blood pressure affects the course of most heart diseases.

Cyanosis. We shall now deal with the causes of the condition called cyanosis. Derived from the Greek word *kyanos*, blue, cyanosis is the name given to a bluish discoloration of the skin due to filling of the capillaries with imperfectly oxygenated blood. It occurs in health as well as in disease, and its importance as a symptom depends entirely upon the circumstances in which it makes its appearance.

The degree of cyanosis depends

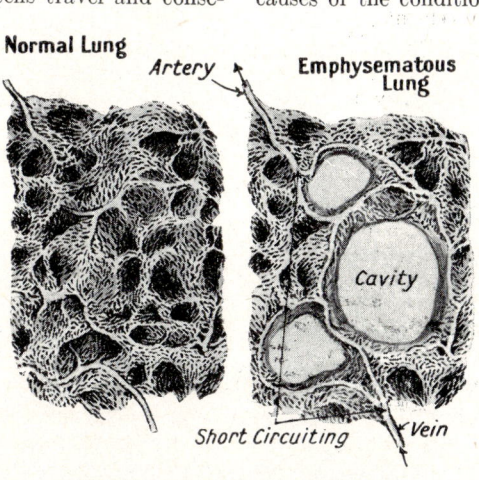

CYANOSIS CAUSED BY EMPHYSEMA
In emphysema of the lungs large numbers of air cells are replaced by large spaces, whereby the aerating surface in the lung is reduced; also impure blood may pass almost directly into the veins by short circuiting.

(1431)

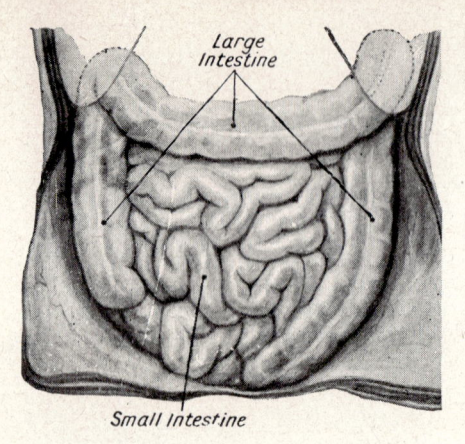

INTESTINAL POISONS AND CYANOSIS

Poisoning by some substances, nitrobenzol, for example, may cause blueness, but this may also result from poisonous substances formed in the intestines themselves—a form which is known as enterogenous cyanosis.

upon the concentration of reduced hemoglobin in the blood. (Reduced hemoglobin is hemoglobin which is not oxygenated.) This may be brought about in a number of different ways—by a weak action of the heart, by shallow action of the lungs which, by their movements, assist the heart's action and charge the blood with oxygen, by anything tending to impede the free flow of blood, or by a shunting of the blood from the right chambers of the heart to the left chambers through unaerated channels.

Many people who are wrongly supposed to suffer from heart weakness are very liable to become blue in the face on slight provocation. There are, indeed, forms of heart disease, such as auricular fibrillation and mitral disease, in which cyanosis is often a prominent feature. On the other hand cyanosis is not an important sign in heart failure, as it rarely occurs early.

A frequent cause of this symptom is a disturbance of the nervous system which controls or regulates the size of the blood vessels in the skin. These blood vessels are so controlled that they open and shut, widen or grow narrow, according to the state of the atmosphere. If, however, the nervous system is irritated by a poison in the blood, very slight degrees of cold will produce very severe results.

Aside from circulatory failure many other conditions make for cyanosis. There may be mechanical interference with the oxygenation of the blood in the lungs, as in severe asthma or tracheal and bronchial stenosis. A toxic basis is postulated for the cyanosis which so frequently accompanies pneumonia. A polycythemia occurs in individuals living in a high altitude. Cyanosis may result in these cases because of the insufficient oxygen supply.

ANASARCA

A general edematous condition of the body is described as anasarca, a term derived from Greek words meaning through and flesh. Fluid may accumulate in the spaces between the cells which compose organs or tissues in and beneath the skin, a condition described as edema; or it may accumulate in serous cavities, the pleural cavity of the chest, for example, and the peritoneal cavity of the abdomen. The latter condition is what is commonly termed dropsy (a popular term which many doctors avoid using), though this term is often applied to the accumulation of fluid in tissues.

The diseases in which anasarca is most commonly seen are Bright's disease and certain forms of heart disease. It may also be found in severe anemia, such as that caused by hookworm disease and in beriberi, etc. Besides treatment directed to the cause of the anasarca, an attempt is made to remove as much fluid as possible from the body by inducing profuse sweating, or by increasing the flow of urine or by mechanical means.

Edema. This is a condition in which fluid passes out from the blood or lymphatic vessels into the tissues, and produces a state of the body analogous to waterlogging. Inasmuch as gravity usually plays an important part in its production the legs are most frequently affected; but the edema may be localized to other parts of the body, such as the face, arms or trunk, according to the various operant causes. In some cases the fluid exudes into the tissues of certain of the internal organs of the body, as the lungs, the larynx, or the uvula.

Edema is shown by the affected part becoming puffy and swollen, and by the possibility of producing pitting. This means that if the tip of a finger be pressed down on the skin a depression or pit is left, which takes some time to fill up. Pressure should be made, if possible, over a bone or tendon, especially when the swelling is very slight, as pitting is more easily brought out there should edema be present. In the leg, the skin over the inner surface of the shin bone, the bony prominences at the sides of the ankle, or the Achilles tendon would suit the purpose.

Edema of the legs may occur in conditions apart from diseases of the heart or kidneys. Thus, in severe cases of varicose veins there is a certain degree of obstruction to the return of blood through the veins, and some swelling of the feet and legs ensues. The blockage of a vein by the formation of a clot of blood, or thrombus, will give rise to swelling of the leg. Pressure of tight garters may also give rise to a mild degree of edema.

In some cases there is an obstruction to the lymphatic circulation of the legs; this may result from the presence of minute worms, such as the Filaria sanguinis hominis, when the legs swell up and elephantiasis results. At times too, after childbirth, the lymphatic vessels are occluded and the leg swells, giving rise to the typical white leg. Pressure of enlarged lymphatic glands and the obstruction of lymphatic vessels due to cancerous growths in the glands will also give rise to an edematous state of the corresponding limb.

There is also a rare condition of edema of the legs which runs in families, in which for no apparent reason the lower limbs become swollen. This is known as Milroy's disease, and once it has appeared it persists for the re-

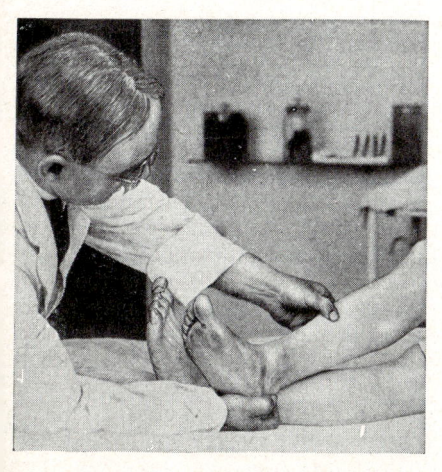

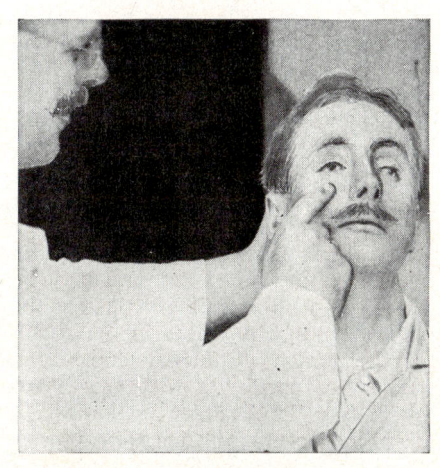

HOW TO TEST FOR THE CONDITION OF ANASARCA
Left: the skin over the inner surface of the shin bone lies almost directly on the bone, and firm pressure will produce pitting should edema be present in the leg. Right: edema of the face, found by pressure on the skin over the bone forming the lower margin of the eye socket, is usually more pronounced after a night's rest in bed.

mainder of the patient's life. Edema of the limbs is one of the characteristic signs of beriberi. In the severe varieties of anemia in adults edema of the ankles is frequently noticed. In anemia the oxygen-carrying power of the blood is impaired and the edema therefore follows the same lines as that seen in heart disease, as explained below.

Obstruction to the main vein returning blood from the head and arms to the heart will give rise to a swelling limited to these parts of the body. Young men especially are at times troubled by the appearance of small areas of swelling of the skin and subcutaneous tissues which are of transient duration. This is known as angioneurotic edema.

Edema of the internal organs is nearly always of grave significance. Acute edema of the lungs is a comparatively infrequent condition associated with rapidly developing heart failure or as a complication of pneumonia. It is at times also met with in pregnancy or in diabetes, and it may occur as a complication of lung surgery. The patient is suddenly seized with great difficulty in breathing, and watery fluid wells up from the lungs in considerable quantities and pours out of the mouth and nose. In chronic edema of the lungs, the lower lobes or bases gradually become waterlogged as the result of failure of the circulation in diseases of the heart and lungs, or as a part of the general edema in kidney diseases.

Edema of the lining membrane of the larynx is a serious condition which may cause death from asphyxia. It results from a variety of causes, and may be associated with chronic affections of the kidney or with abscesses in the region of the throat. In kidney disease the uvula may swell up, with consequent difficulty in breathing or swallowing.

In any acute inflammatory process there is in the early stage an output of fluid from the blood vessels into the connective tissue spaces. Lymph is poured out to dilute the irritant causing inflammation and to repair the damage,

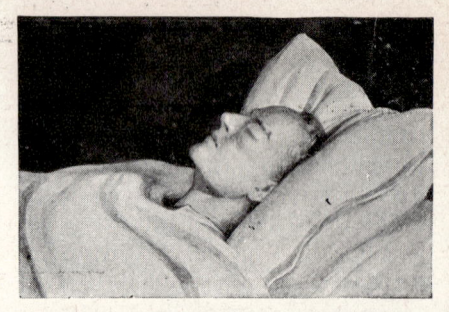

EDEMA: APPEARANCE IN NEPHRITIS

In acute nephritis, or Bright's disease, swelling first appears on the face, and is most marked below the eyes, owing to looseness of the tissue here. The swelling then appears on the legs and may extend further.

but the exact mode of production of the edema of inflammation is unknown. It may give rise to localized swellings of the skin or deeper structures.

When the blood reaches the tissues its current slows down so that the tiny cells to which it is bringing food and oxygen may obtain them. The oxygen which it brings immediately passes through the wall of the blood vessel and is caught up by the cell. The food must flow slowly or percolate through.

The cells take as much of this nourishing fluid as they require; what they leave flows slowly on into tiny vessels called lymphatics. If a lymphatic gets stopped up there will be no escape for the fluid along its normal channels, and the tissues in the neighborhood will swell up with fluid. The larger the lymphatic which is stopped up the larger the area in which edema will occur.

Again, if more fluid leaves the blood vessels than normal, there may not be room in the lymphatic vessels to carry it all away, so swelling will again result.

Thus two causes of edema are some stoppage or obstruction of the lymphatic channels, and too great a flow of fluid out of the blood vessels. Both these causes may contribute to edema. The cause of an increased flow of fluid from the blood vessels may be obstruction of a vein, and edema of the leg from a tight garter may readily occur; or the circulation in the vein may be sluggish as when it is varicose, with the same result.

Treatment. The treatment varies with the cause, and should be directed to the organ or system primarily at fault. Thus, in edema due to heart failure, absolute rest in bed is of the utmost importance. Drugs such as digitalis are of value. At the same time the elimination of fluid which has accumulated in the tissue spaces is helped by increasing the excretion by the kidneys with the aid of diuretic drugs, and by the administration of saline aperients, causing loose, watery evacuations. In very severe cases it may be necessary to allow the fluid to drain from the legs by means of small punctures, made through the skin by Southey's tubes.

The treatment naturally depends on the cause. If the heart or the kidneys are the cause, treatment should be directed to these organs. Like breathlessness, edema is a symptom of many diseases. Nor is there, usually, much doubt as to its origin. Thus, long before it appears in heart cases signs of heart weakness will have been apparent. In any case, however, a doctor should always be consulted.

Heart and Kidney Edema. The edema of heart disease occurs frequently when two of the auricles of the heart have ceased to contract normally. This trouble is called auricular fibrillation because these auricles, instead of beating firmly and strongly, quiver but never contract as a whole.

The cause of the edema in these cases is not very easy to understand. The explanation is that the greatly weakened heart is unable to do its work and so the blood is not pumped properly and tends to accumulate in the veins. This really amounts to a stopping up of the veins, and so of the trunk lymphatic which flows into them.

It is easy to understand why, when the heart begins to beat properly again, the edema at once goes away. Some of the most extreme cases of edema are due to heart disease. Patients may be absolutely waterlogged so that the skin breaks in places and allows the excessive mass of fluid to pour out. This condition is less common than it used to be owing to improved methods of treating heart diseases.

The edema of kidney disease is less severe than that of diseases of the heart and may be confined to the eyelids and face. It is probably due to the action of poisons in the blood which the diseased kidney is failing to get rid of. These poisons make the nerves which control the small blood vessels intensely irritable, with the result that the vessels tend to open wide on the least provocation. The face, being the most exposed part, is most subject to such provocation.

Edema often occurs to a slight extent during attacks of rheumatic fever when the heart irritation is marked.

Ascites. The term ascites, signifies an accumulation of fluid in the peritoneal cavity, and the condition is an important symptom in several diseases. Several gallons of fluid, which is usually of a pale yellowish color, contains albumin, and has a specific gravity of 1.015, may be found. As the fluid in the peritoneal cavity increases, a feeling of weight and discomfort is experienced, and the pa-

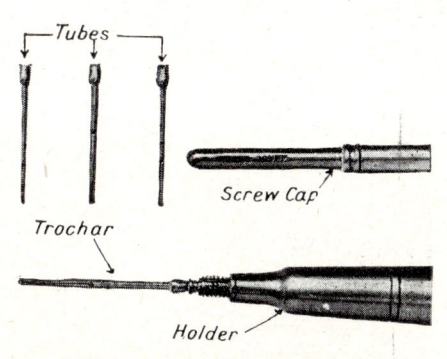

SOUTHEY'S TUBES FOR DRAINAGE
Edema is sometimes treated by inserting several of these little tubes into the subcutaneous tissue. The tubes have lateral openings, and much fluid may be drained off. A sharp trocar is used for inserting.
Courtesy of Arnold & Sons

tient—if still able to walk—walks with head and shoulders thrown back and legs wide apart, thus balancing the load of fluid.

The pressure of the fluid on the great veins passing up from the lower limbs causes the legs to swell, and enlarged veins appear on the surface of the abdomen. The diaphragm is pushed up, displaces the heart and liver, and compresses the base of the lungs.

Ascites may be caused by obstruction of the portal circulation within the liver. Obstruction of the circulation is always followed by edema, and in this case it is fluid in the peritoneal cavity. At times a similar kind of obstruction to the flow of blood through the portal vein may be caused by cancer or by syphilis affecting the liver itself.

Other causes of ascites are obstruction outside the liver, taking place through pressure on the portal vein from cancerous growths and tumors, or by thrombosis (coagulation) of the blood in the portal vein. Or, again, ascites may occur as part of a general edema—as in Bright's disease—in disablement of the right ventricle of the heart through disease of the lungs, and in disease of the left side of the heart.

Much fluid in the peritoneal cavity is recognized by enlargement of the abdomen. The abdomen becomes uniformly enlarged, with a tendency to bulge forward and downward when the patient is erect, but when the patient is recumbent it bulges laterally.

When ascites is a symptom of heart or kidney disease there is no difficulty in diagnosing the cause. When by exclusion of such causes it is evident that the ascites is due to some local abdominal disorder, diagnosis may be very difficult.

Treatment by paracentesis is necessary when the ascites produces great pain and stomach trouble, or through pressure on the diaphragm causes breathlessness and cardiac disturbance. Paracentesis means tapping the peritoneal cavity by means of a trocar and cannula. While the fluid is running out, a binder round the abdomen is tightened at intervals, as the fluid escapes, lest the small abdominal blood vessels should burst on account of being thus suddenly relieved from the pressure of the fluid.

SYNCOPE

This term, derived from the Greek *synkopto*, I strike down, can be best defined as a condition of collapse as a result of insufficient blood supply to the brain. Recovery from a temporary insufficiency can occur and the patient is then said to have a syncopal attack, but should it be of long enough duration death may supervene. Syncope, in its looser meaning refers to any sudden loss of consciousness as in fainting from fright.

The symptoms are those of extreme pallor of the face and mucous membranes, with cold sweats. Dimness of vision, air hunger, restlessness, gasping for breath, and vomiting may precede a passing delirium. There are noises in the ears, and a rapid, feeble, and fluttering pulse. Ultimately unconsciousness appears, but one of the most distressing of all symptoms is the sense of impending death experienced by the victim.

The simplest cause is a deficiency of blood consequent on severe hemorrhage. Such can occur from wounds of important blood vessels, from bursting of aneurysms, and in extreme hemorrhage from lungs or stomach. It is common in certain cardiac affections, and of these aortic regurgitation, heart block, and fatty degeneration are the usual offenders. Frequently it is said that a patient died of shock. In such cases syncope occurs, and examples are readily found in violent emotion, blows on the head or abdomen, and sudden extensive injuries in accidents.

Fatal cases have been known from the drinking of large quantities of cold water by a person hot from exertion. In many minor operations, such as the tapping of ascites and pleural effusions, preparations have to be made in case syncope should suddenly appear, while certain exhausting affections sometimes end in this way.

Various poisons must also be mentioned. Of these digitalis and aconite are pre-eminent, while many people have experienced the effects of too much nicotine and have recovered from the symptoms; but even tobacco has been responsible for attacks of syncope.

BREATHLESSNESS

The scientific term for this condition is dyspnea. Everyone has been breathless at some period of his or her life, which disposes at once of the deeply rooted idea that breathlessness is necessarily a sign of heart disease. It is a sign of distress; and among the causes of distress heart disease is included. But there are many other causes.

Breathlessness is really a sign that the breathless person is making strong efforts to pump blood into his muscles and brain while at the same time he is drawing more and more oxygen into his lungs. The perfectly fit man needs to do very little of this pumping. The unfit man, on the other hand, must make many small, swift efforts, because his heart is flabby and his lungs do not possess good expansion. He therefore breathes with difficulty.

There are diseases which poison the nerves leading from the sensory centers to the organs, and so make them more

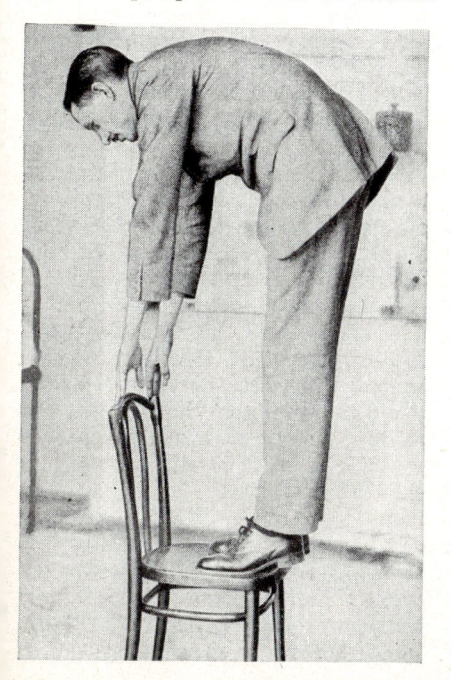

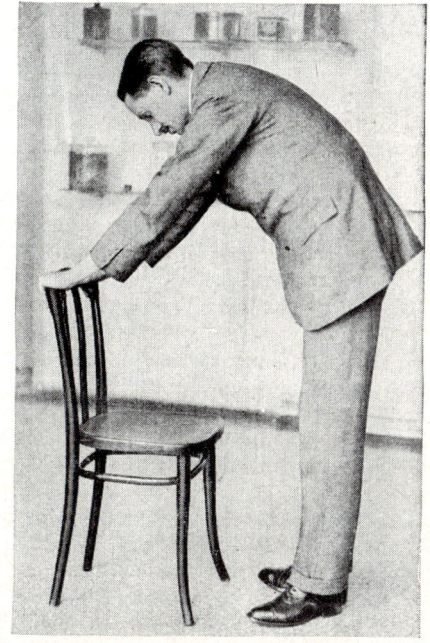

STEPPING UP TESTS FOR BREATHLESSNESS

The man in normal condition ought to be able to carry out this test without becoming seriously breathless, although it is not necessarily a matter for alarm if he does. Step up onto a chair, keeping the body as high as possible. From this position step back off the chair, repeating the motions twenty times in quick succession.

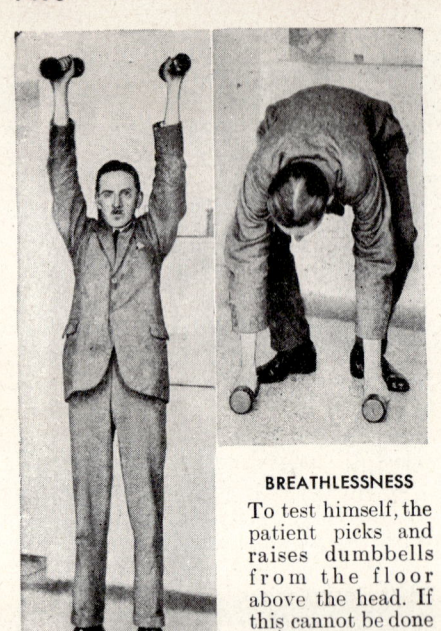

BREATHLESSNESS

To test himself, the patient picks and raises dumbbells from the floor above the head. If this cannot be done fairly rapidly several times without breathlessness, his condition cannot be considered normal.

excitable or irritable than normal. Irritable nerves transform small troubles into great ones.

Finally, breathlessness occurs in people with actual damage to their lungs or heart because these organs are unable to stand any strain. The breathlessness of pulmonary tuberculosis and of heart disease belongs to this class. But it should never be forgotten that this very serious type is comparatively uncommon, accounting for not more than 10 or 15 per cent of all the cases. Breathlessness in such cases must be carefully avoided.

If the heart becomes weakened by prolonged acute fever and infection, breathlessness takes on another and more serious character. In heart disease the breathlessness is not due to poisoning of the nerves, but to actual damage to the heart muscle. In the early stages breathlessness may be caused only by unusual effort. As the heart disease progresses breathlessness ensues more readily on ordinary exertion. Finally, the heart cannot increase its force even by the slightest amount, and so every call upon it to do so results in failure. The patient tries by breathing harder to make up for the heart weakness, substituting lung pumping power for heart pumping power.

Breathlessness cannot be cured, or even properly treated, until its exact cause has been found, and this may be a matter of considerable difficulty. Nevertheless, a few simple rules may be laid down.

1. Anyone who notices that he is becoming breathless when performing work or efforts which did not formerly produce this feeling, should make quite sure that he is breathing properly. Shallow breathing is a common cause of this trouble.

2. Attention should also be given to the bowels, digestion, and diet. Obese individuals get short of breath quickly because of the burden that their circulatory system labors under.

3. The effect of gradually increasing exercise in the open air such as graduated hill climbing can be tried. If this is combined with a change to sea or other bracing air it may effect a cure.

It is wiser, however, to seek medical advice in the early days of the trouble so that the right treatment may be adopted from the start. It is possible that some unsuspected heart or lung condition is the seat of trouble, for example, an undetected rheumatic carditis or a chronic bronchitis.

Even if the heart itself is the cause of the trouble, a great deal can be done to improve matters. Functional weakness can be strengthened and temporary sources of trouble removed. At the worst, the activities of life must be adapted to meet the body's limitations, which in many cases are merely those of advancing years.

CHAPTER 104

DISEASES OF THE HEART

Pericarditis — Acute Fibrinous Pericarditis — Pericarditis with Infusion—Chronic Adhesive Pericarditis—Functional Heart Disease—Disorders of Force and Rhythm—Extrasystoles—Auricular Fibrillation—Auricular Flutter—Heart Block—Use of Electrocardiograph—Diseases of the Heart Muscle — Myocarditis — Hypertrophy — Dilatation — Endocarditis — Valvular Disease of the Heart — Aortic Disease — Mitral Disease — Congenital Heart Disease —Angina Pectoris.

IN dealing with the disease of the heart, it is customary to take first the outer enveloping bag or pericardium, and discuss the common ailments associated with it. Next in order comes the heart muscle itself—the myocardium, and its associated disease myocarditis. Finally, there is the lining membrane, the endocardium, and its diseases are considered under the heading of endocarditis.

Each of these groups has many subdivisions, but despite complexities, cardiologists rarely consider any individual affection of the heart *per se*. The growing custom is to combine the affections of all three regions into the one great disease of carditis, since there is always some pericarditis with myocarditis, and endocarditis is frequently found to affect the myocardium. Thus the situation as a whole must be envisaged, if we are to obtain the correct impressions of the activities of the disease processes in their total.

Owing to improved methods of investigation and to better knowledge of the heart's action, there is a growing tendency to give up the old divisions of organic and functional disease. Certainly there still must be defined a few ailments which affect the work of the heart only, and apparently these have no organic basis so far as the heart itself is concerned, although they may be dependent upon digestive or nervous abnormalities or other conditions. Nor must it be forgotten that organic disease of serious nature may be present with unobtrusive symptoms.

On the whole, however, heart disease, no matter where it may begin, must inevitably in the event of its unhindered progress reach a stage at which, for various fundamental reasons, the pump breaks down. This is called heart failure, and is one of the most dangerous terminal signs of heart disease, giving rise to many of the signs associated with circulatory failure and described in Chapter 103.

With this fact kept steadily in view, a problem otherwise complicated and difficult becomes simple. The presence of an abnormal sound in the heart, for example, is of importance only so far as it is associated with heart failure, *i.e.* failure of the heart to compensate for the mechanical disability. Thus an abnormal sound which has been present for years in a heart which has throughout the period been able to perform vigorous work, and which is continuing so to perform, may be discounted as a sign of danger.

Heart failure may occur without any organic trouble having preceded it; on the other hand, heart failure may never occur though the organ has been quite extensively damaged.

We will now deal in detail with the principal groups of heart diseases.

PERICARDITIS

Inflammation of the bag in which the heart works is called pericarditis. This bag is lubricated inside so that the organ may slip up and down easily with each beat. The first and most obvious effect of pericarditis is failure of lubrication. Friction is set up and the heart rubs on the side of its bag, often causing pain.

It produces, however, such an outflow of fluid that very soon the bag fills up

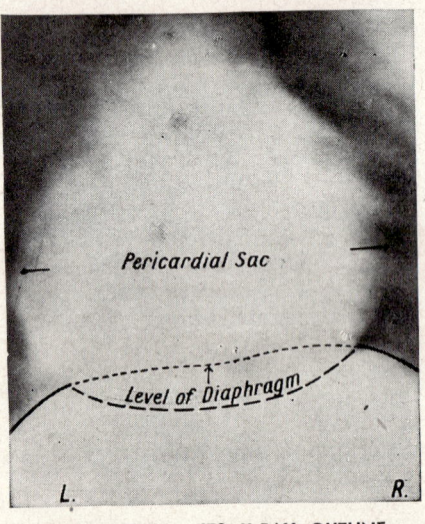

PERICARDIUM: ITS X-RAY OUTLINE
The sac containing the heart is seen to overlap in front the outline of the diaphragm. The heart lies nearer the center of the body than is generally supposed.

and separates the raw surfaces, thus preventing them from rubbing together, and so removing the pain for the time being.

Apart from injury, primary pericarditis is rare. It nearly always occurs as a complication of rheumatic fever, tuberculosis, generalized sepsis, certain fevers (especially scarlet fever), and pneumonia, and it may be the result of spread from pneumonia with pleurisy. All ages and sexes may suffer from pericarditis, but men are more susceptible than women.

Three distinct types may be differentiated, viz., acute fibrinous pericarditis, pericarditis with effusion, and chronic adhesive pericarditis. One type may merge into the other; indeed, it is rare that a case of pericarditis resolves without some adhesions, however small they may be.

Acute Fibrinous Pericarditis. In this condition, there is slight increase of the normal glairy fluid which lubricates the inner lining of the pericardial bag. The fluid tends to clot, and with the constant movements of the beating heart the fibrinous ridges formed resemble the surfaces of the two components of a bread and butter sandwich after they have been separated. Another common name is *cor villosum*—the hairy heart. The outer layers of the myocardium are usually inflamed.

Signs. This is one of the types of heart disease in which there may be few symptoms, although a dangerous state exists. The common complaints are, however, pain over the heart region or at the left shoulder or stomach. Often shortness of breath is a marked feature, together with a short cough. The temperature of the patient may rise to as much as 103° F.

The doctor who auscultates and employs all the other technical methods of diagnosis finds that a definite sensation of rubbing—known as friction—can be experienced by the hand and by the ear. This varies in quality; occasionally it is of a triple character, rather like the cantering of a horse. Often the sound is like the squeak of new leather (the French have styled this *bruit de cuir neuf*).

In a very few cases the exudation is absorbed and leaves no traces. In a great number of cases the exudate behaves like glue and leaves the two layers of the pericardium closely adherent. In the event of much fluid gathering there is great embarrassment of the heart.

Pericarditis with Effusion. The fluid which has collected in the pericardial space may amount to anything from eight to sixty ounces. The pericardial lining is thickened, and the cavity is full of churned-up flakes of fibrin. Sometimes blood or pus is present.

Signs. Again it must be recorded that even with an advanced effusion the complaints may be few. The pain in the chest causes apprehension; it is more of a discomfort than a pain. Shortness of breath and difficulty in swallowing are marked. Restlessness is a trying symptom to deal with, since rest is the very thing the patient requires most. The complexion may be dusky gray. As the disease goes on, sleeplessness and delirium may complicate matters. The patient usually becomes morose. The technical evidences are bulging of the precardial area, obliteration of the beat of the tip of the heart, and imperceptibility of the heart sounds through the stethoscope.

Many effusions come to a head in two days and then clear up. Some, however, go on gradually increasing for weeks, causing great cardiac embarrassment. If the fluid is purulent, the toxemia and local poisoning are severe. In numerous cases the signs are so mild that the diagnosis is not made; this applies especially to the serous effusion, as a rule.

Complete mental and physical rest should be aimed at. An ice-bag over the heart brings great relief. Liquid nourishment should be the rule in the acute stages. In the event of a growing effusion, it is usually necessary to apply some form of counter-irritation to the precardial area. But if there should be the slightest evidence of heart embarrassment beyond tolerable limits, the operation of paracentesis is performed, and the fluid let out. The operation may have to be repeated.

Chronic Adhesive Pericarditis. Assuming that the layers of the pericardium have become thickened and that they are glued together, the danger is not great if the bag of membranes is not weakened and if it is still capable of supporting the heart. If there is severe myocardial involvement, however, the outlook may be bad. With the pericardium often bound down to the inner wall of the chest or to the pleural membranes, there is fundamental disruption of the heart's action, and in addition the heart may enlarge or become dilated. Various signs are known to doctors, one of which, Broadbent's sign, shows a tugging of the points at which the diaphragm muscle is attached to the chest wall; this is the result of internal adhesions.

Treatment is that of the cardiac complications, described later. Sometimes removal of the ribs over the cardiac region frees the heart and gives it less work to do to overcome the restrictive influences of the adhesions.

FUNCTIONAL HEART DISEASE

This is called also disordered action of the heart, nervous heart, and effort syndrome, the latter term meaning a group of symptoms met with in persons who show a diminished power of responding to calls for effort. More recently the terms neurocirculatory asthenia and cardiac neuroses have come into vogue.

Generally speaking, the symptoms complained of are shortness of breath on exertion or excitement, palpitation of the heart or tachycardia, pain over the region of the heart, and giddiness. In addition fainting may occur in some cases, profuse sweating in others, also hot and cold sensations, rheumatic pains, and nervousness. Tremor, blueness of the hands and cheeks (cyanosis), and a tendency to sickness are also symptoms that have been noted.

The name effort syndrome was given to this complaint because of the fact that the symptoms become much more marked during effort or exertion. It has been definitely established that these symptoms do not point to heart disease in the strict sense, for, in all probability, the heart is sound in the great majority of cases.

The cause of functional heart disease is not clearly understood, but people suffering from it tend to show histories of infectious illnesses.

Both environmental and hereditary factors are of importance. Questioning of other members of the family often reveals a familial tendency towards nervous instability. In the patient's history nervousness, fear, and anxiety play significant roles and indeed the patient may have had one or more nervous breakdowns. Slight illness, mental or physical fatigue, excitement are some of the factors which may precipitate a functional heart disorder in these individuals.

It does not appear that "strain," smoking or drinking alcohol exercise any very great effect. It is the mental state which is important and the symptoms can be interpreted as nervous manifestations of a faulty emotional make-up.

Functional heart disease, therefore, is not very widely different from the general picture of ill-health. It is necessary that the patient be examined with minute care, and search made for troubles which, by increasing the irritability of the nervous system, may be maintaining the condition of excitability. Until our knowledge increases, all that we can do is to seek out and treat any focal infection, reassure the patient that his life is in no danger, and enjoin on him habits of restraint and temperance in all things. He should avoid any strenuous living, excess of physical or mental work, and excess of diet. Rest and a change of scene are helpful. Severe cases require skilled phychotherapy.

It is extremely doubtful that neurocirculatory asthenia can lead to organic heart disease.

DISORDERS OF FORCE AND RHYTHM

In Chapter 48 (Volume III) an account is given of the manner in which the beating of the normal healthy heart is regulated. Faults in the regulating mechanism (the sinoauricular node, or pacemaker, which is retarded by the vagus nerve and accelerated by the sympathetic nerve) quickly produce faults in the rhythm of the organ. These faults are of two kinds, temporary and permanent.

The excitability of the pacemaker can be greatly lowered or depressed by vagal influence, *i.e.*, by nervous stimulations reaching the heart along the vagus nerve. Thus, if the vagus nerve is unduly excitable, or if strong stimulations are being applied to it as, for example, by severe stomach derangement, the pacemaker of the heart may practically go out of action for the time being, and one of several possible kinds of disorder will ensue.

The same thing may occur if a poison is circulating in the blood which has a depressing effect on the pacemaker.

When this happens the heart may merely miss a few beats; or the auricles may begin to beat at an exceedingly rapid rate, so fast, indeed, that the ventricles cannot keep pace with them; or the auricles may cease to beat and begin to "fibrillate." These irregularities or arrhythmias cease at once if the pacemaker is released from depressing stimulations or restored from the effects of poisons.

When the pulse rate falls below sixty beats per minute, the condition is often described as bradycardia, or "slow heart." To possess real significance, slow heart must be an exceptional state; that is to say, it must differ from the ordinary pulse rate of the patient. Moreover, in the early stages of many illnesses and during the course of others the pulse is characteristically slow.

The best-known example of this is typhoid fever, in which, though the patient's temperature may be high, a relatively low pulse is the rule. Diges-

DISEASES OF THE HEART

tive and bowel troubles are very often accompanied by a slow pulse. The reason is that the vagus nerve, which acts as the slowing or retarding nerve of the heart, supplies branches to the stomach and bowels. When these latter are upset or diseased this nerve is irritated and impulses are sent to the heart which have the effect of causing it to reduce its rate of beating. A severe shock to the nervous system, a fright, a blow on the abdomen, even a hot room or the sight of blood, may cause this retarding nerve to show great activity.

There is another form of bradycardia which must be included definitely among diseases of the heart. In this form the pulse is usually about thirty-five to forty-five beats per minute. It never varies from this rate, which continues, very often, permanently. This disease is known as heart block (see page 1448), and the cause of the slow rate is a blockage in the path of the nervous influences which, in healthy people, regulate the rate of the heart's action. Neither the quickening nor the retarding nerve can influence it. The sufferer from this condition is naturally very weak.

Strictly speaking, tachycardia means any abnormally rapid action of the heart. Thus, ordinary exertion or excitement produces tachycardia (a pulse rate of perhaps 120 beats per minute), and so also may even a slight attack of fever. But in medical practice the word has come to mean quickness of the heart's rate in the absence of an obvious or ordinary cause.

Of these pathological or abnormal tachycardias two kinds exist: the ordinary variety in which the pulse is merely greatly quickened, and paroxysmal tachycardia, in which bouts of rapid action occur suddenly and, as a rule, pass off suddenly and in which the rate may be as high as 200 or more beats per minute.

In ordinary tachycardia the pulse is more or less permanently increased in rate. In most cases an infective factor is at play. The patient is really suffering from poisoning of his nerves of a degree not severe enough to raise his temperature above normal. The majority of these people have sub-normal temperatures. The irritable, rapid heart is merely one symptom of a general condition of local infection, such as that resulting from septic teeth or tonsils, or from a diseased appendix.

Rheumatic subjects are very apt to suffer from tachycardia, and so are the victims of any chronic disease, because, in all such cases, poisons are present in the circulation during long periods of time. On the other hand, it is a great mistake to regard the rapid heart as a sign of disease in the sense that the patient would be better if his heart were slow. The heart beats quickly because it is irritable, or because its nerves are irritable; the irritability, not the quick beating, is the real fault.

It follows that drugs given to slow down the heart are useless in this complaint. The cause of the irritation must be sought and removed if the fault is to be rectified.

SINOAURICULAR NODE IN THE HEART
This node is sometimes called the pacemaker, because it controls the contractions of the auricles. It is a minute body consisting of a special kind of tissue.

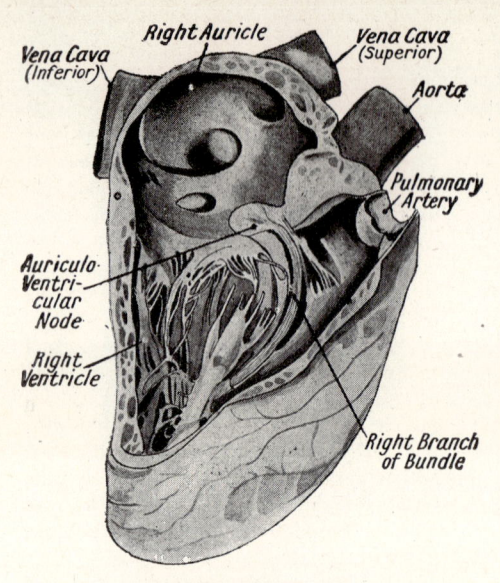

THE BUNDLE OF HIS

Impulses to contraction are carried to the ventricles of the heart by the bundle of His, a band of modified muscle which runs downwards from the auriculoventricular node.

The condition of paroxysmal tachycardia differs fundamentally from the ordinary variety. It points to an abnormality in the nervous control of the heart, and in many cases it is actually auricular flutter (see page 1446). The immediate cause of a paroxysmal tachycardia is the supersession of the normal pacemaker of the heart by some other illegitimate pacemaker. In any case what corresponds to a run of extrasystoles takes place, or, in a case of paroxysmal tachycardia which is really auricular flutter, a fluttering of the auricle. The rate may rise to 220. It is not affected by posture, exertion or excitement. The cause of paroxysmal tachycardia is obscure. In some cases there is organic disease of the heart, but in most the heart is normal in structure to all methods of clinical examination. Liability to the attacks is often associated with neurasthenic conditions. An attack may be brought on by digestive disturbance, excitement, or overexertion, but very often there may be no apparent cause.

But the pacemaker itself may be the seat of disease; in that case it cannot recover, and the disorders following its loss of influence will continue. Again, the auriculoventricular node, which is under the control of the pacemaker, may become the seat of disease; irregularities in the relationship existing between auricles and ventricles will now occur and will be permanent. Finally, the heart nerves, the so-called bundle of His which connects the auriculoventricular node with the two ventricles, may be diseased; in that case both the ventricles, or—if the disease affects only one branch of the heart nerve—one of them, will be cut off from regulating influences.

Thus irregularities of heart rhythm may be due to actual disease or merely to passing influences. In this latter case they cannot properly be classified as organic. In any event, however, they are of four definite types: extrasystoles, auricular fibrillation, auricular flutter, and heart block.

Extrasystoles. As the name implies, an extrasystole is an extra beat of the heart. It is represented in pulse tracings, as a rule, by a small beat which occurs rather before the normal beat should occur. The normal beat is absent and seems to have been "missed." The following beat is always a big one. When these extrasystoles are analyzed it is found that they are either beats of the whole heart (i.e. of auricles and ventricles) or of the ventricles only (so-called auricular extrasystoles and ventricular extrasystoles). The ventricular type is the more common. These extrasystoles are said to occur in every person over forty at some time or other. Unless definite signs of heart failure are present, they mean nothing except that some temporary depressant is acting on the pacemaker. It is a mistake to become alarmed by extrasystoles, but it is well to mention them to a physician.

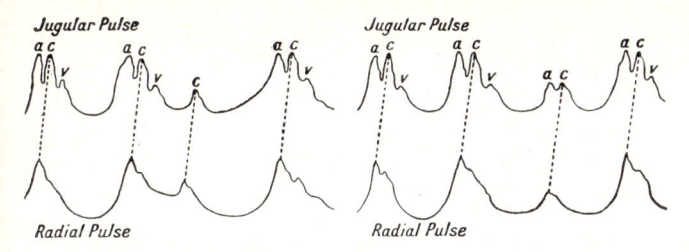

PULSE IRREGULARITY FROM TWO TYPES OF EXTRA SYSTOLE

Left: ventricular extrasystole; the small beat felt at the wrist is shown to be due to the ventricle, because no auricular wave (*a*) precedes it. Right: auricular extrasystole; the small beat at the wrist in this case is shown, by reference to the jugular tracing, to have a different origin; an auricular wave (*a*) is present, so the extra beat is auricular in origin.

The so-called pulsus bigeminus, or twin pulse, consists of extrasystoles occurring after every beat. This form of pulse, which is often a cause of alarm, is not necessarily a sign of serious trouble.

Pulsus alternans, on the other hand, is of an entirely different type. Here a bigger beat is followed by a smaller one, but both are normal. It is a bad sign when other indications are also present.

Sinus arrhythmia, or the "youthful type of irregularity," may be mentioned here, though it is not a sign of ill-health at all, but occurs normally in most young people at some time or other, notably when recovering from illnesses. It is caused by the influence exerted by the breathing on the heart. At each indrawing of air the heart is quickened; at each outgoing of air slowing occurs. Very deep indrawing, on the other hand, tends to slow the heart. The cause of this arrhythmia is the influence exerted by the lungs on the nerves controlling the pacemaker.

In the same way extrasystoles can be abolished almost invariably by slight exertion. It should be noted, however, that the extrasystoles return as soon as the pulse slows down; but this does not matter. What counts is their disappearance.

Auricular Fibrillation. A patient known to be suffering from heart trouble may take a sudden turn for the worse. He may become exceedingly breathless, may find his feet swollen with edema, and may look and feel exceedingly ill. If his pulse is taken it will be found to be extremely irregular, so irregular that the old physicians spoke of this disease as delirium cordis, "heart madness." There will be big beats and small, long beats and short, all wildly jumbled together.

As already stated, the pacemaker controls the auricles. As they beat they send a message to the ventricles, which passes along a peculiar kind of "telegraph wire" hidden within the substance of the heart. The ventricles then beat. This continues, beat after beat, except when the brain interferes and causes the pacemaker either to slow down or to quicken. When that happens the rate of the heart is changed. But the relationship between the chambers is not altered. They go on, as before, beating in pairs, auricles first and then ventricles.

But it happens sometimes that the pacemaker loses control. The result is that the auricle, instead of giving one strong beat, stops beating and quivers or fibrillates—*i.e.* all the cell fibers contract separately and irregularly.

The cause of auricular fibrillation is either weakness of the pacemaker or excessive activity of the fibers themselves. It may happen, for example, that the pacemaker becomes depressed or weak, so that some of the fibers under its control set up what is now called a circus rhythm—a wave of activity flowing round the auricle in a circle. So long as this circus rhythm goes on, regular beating is impossible. But if it can be stopped, the heart at once begins to beat normally again.

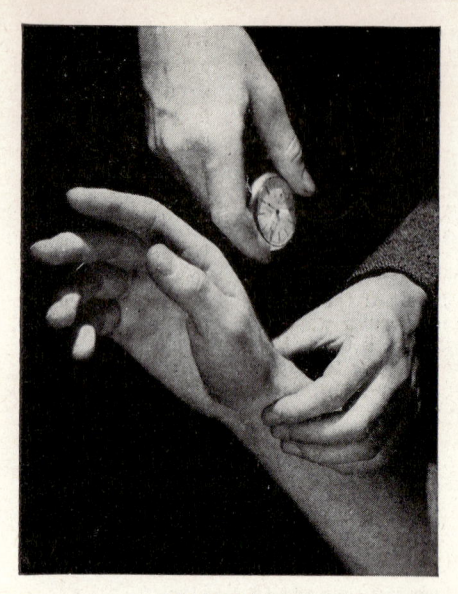

PULSE COUNT

The rapidity of the heartbeat, as perceived at the wrist, is a valuable index to health in many conditions not strictly cardiac. The skilled physician also learns to interpret the character of the pulse—as weak or strong, regular or irregular. Note the position of the examiner's fingers in taking the pulse. It is usual to count beats for twelve or fifteen seconds and then to multiply the result by five or four to express the pulse rate in terms of beats per minute.

© *Ewing Galloway*

Such a recovery is brought about by the use of a drug known as quinidine, which is obtained, like quinine, from cinchona bark. It is, however, a very dangerous drug, only to be used by a specialist. There are cases in which, if it were given, it might do positive harm. The cases in which it succeeds, on the other hand, are made well in a most remarkable fashion.

Apart from quinidine, there is another drug which exercises a wonderful effect on auricular fibrillation. This is digitalis, the extract of the foxglove. Digitalis is safe to use when it is given by an expert. Under its influence the rapid irregular pulse slows down, the edema disappears, and breathlessness is mitigated. The patient who could not leave his bed is often able to get up and go about the world again.

Sometimes, however, auricular fibrillation cures itself. There are forms of this disorder in which it comes and goes. This may be due to a depressing effect on the pacemaker exercised by some of the poisons of disease; for example, the toxic effect of an overactive thyroid. When these toxins begin to appear in the blood the fibers of the auricle are no longer under proper control; when the poisons pass away the control is resumed by the restored pacemaker.

Many people with auricular fibrillation lead more or less active lives as a result of proper treatment. In some cases they seem to suffer but little discomfort; in other cases very great weakness overwhelms them. Auricular fibrillation is most commonly associated with actual disease of the heart—these are the serious cases. But it may occur in hearts which are apparently quite healthy. If it can be stopped in such cases recovery is complete.

Auricular Flutter. Some people complain of what they usually call attacks of "palpitation" of the heart, but when they are questioned it is found that palpitation is not the right word to apply to them. There is no vigorous beating, no "thumping." What the patient experiences is rather a soft, fluttering sensation in the chest. At the same moment he becomes weak and often breathless. He feels very ill.

This is an attack of auricular flutter. What is happening is that the two upper chambers of the heart, the auricles, are beating at double their normal rate, while the two bottom chambers, the ventricles, are trying to keep pace with them. Thus the auricles may be beating at 400 a minute, while the ventricles are doing no more than 180 or 200. All kinds of variations are met with. The flutter begins, as a rule, in an instant; it ends, usually, just as sharply. The patient, from being very ill, becomes suddenly quite well.

DISEASES OF THE HEART

The cause is probably similar to the cause or causes of auricular fibrillation. Many people get small "runs of flutter" at unexpected moments. In some cases they treat these very calmly, knowing that they will soon go away again. In other cases great distress and anxiety are experienced. Some people say that they can stop a flutter by drawing a deep breath. Others declare that a cup of coffee will put an end to the trouble.

INSTRUMENT TO TEST THE HEART

The electrocardiograph automatically makes a diagrammatic record showing the cycle of the heartbeat; this can be filed for comparison with other records made in the same way. By examining two or more of these records (such as that shown on page 1445) a scientific comparison can be made of the action of several hearts or of the same heart at different times. Insurance companies value these records for they remove much uncertainty from diagnosis and health history; nevertheless, the skill of good doctors who have examined hearts by stethoscope has been known to solve diagnostic puzzles that were beyond the help of such technical aids as this.

The condition is only serious when it lasts long, for then the heart becomes exhausted by its enormous rapidity of beating. Modern medicine has various treatments for bringing a flutter to an end when it is thus threatening life. These are of a very specialized kind and

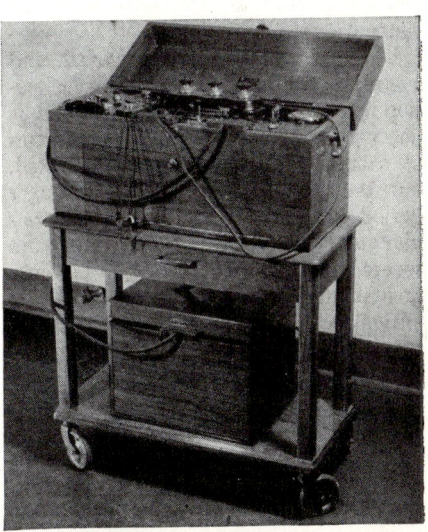

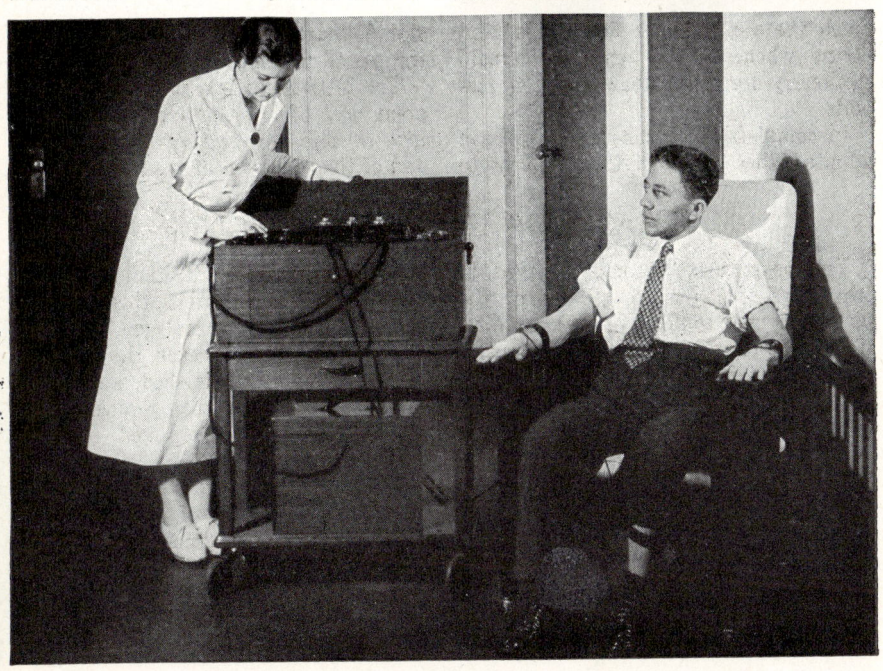

© *Ewing Galloway*

can only be applied by trained consultants who have devoted their lives to this kind of work.

Heart Block. Heart block is the name which Sir James Mackenzie gave to a condition discovered by himself in which a block occurs in the bundle of His, which connects the auricles with the ventricles.

Block is of two kinds, partial and complete. In partial block the connection between auricles and ventricles is not yet entirely severed. In mild cases of partial block the pulse is unaffected, but the jugular pulse shows a longer period than normal between the auricular and ventricular wave. In more severe cases the disparity becomes greater and dropped beats occur—the auricular impulse does not reach the ventricle at all. When this occurs an alarming condition known as the Stokes-Adams syndrome is liable to occur. The patient suddenly falls down and loses consciousness for a short period while muscular spasms occur. The cause is the absence of ventricular beats, no auricular impulse having been able to reach the ventricle. A fit of this kind occurs whenever the ventricles remain stationary for more than eighteen seconds.

In complete block the ventricles have adopted their own rhythm (thirty to forty beats per minute), and no longer depend on the auricles for impulses. The auricles continue to beat at their accustimed rate. There are no fits, but the patient is permanently crippled.

Use of Electrocardiograph. The electrocardiograph is a modification of the Einthoven string galvanometer. This instrument depends for its utility on the fact that when a muscle contracts electrical disturbances are set up. Thus a current passes during the beating of the auricles of the heart, and another current during the beating of the ventricles. These currents cause the "string" of the instrument to oscillate, and the oscillations are photographed through a slit. The plate on which they are photographed moves during the exposure, and thus a tracing is obtained.

Roughly speaking, three waves are recognized in each electrocardiogram. The first, the P wave, is made by the beating of the auricles. It is followed by a sharp upstroke, the R wave, made by the beating of the ventricles. Finally there is the T wave, the significance of which is not agreed on. It is commonly stated that the R-T waves represent the period of ventricular systole.

The instrument is capable of giving a great deal of information about abnormal rhythms or beatings of the heart and of the condition of the heart muscle.

DISEASES OF THE HEART MUSCLE

The heart may become enlarged in two ways, (a) by overgrowth of the muscle (hypertrophy), or (b) by dilation of its chambers. The heart muscle may also be inflamed and associated or not with pericarditis or endocarditis. This condition is called myocarditis.

Myocarditis. The myocardium is liable to various diseases, some of which depend for their origin on infection, while others are caused by lack of a sufficient blood supply. Infections, as a rule, reach the muscle from the inside of the heart, but this is not always the case. The muscle becomes inflamed and then, later, when the infection has passed away, may become fibrous, that is to say, the muscular tissue is replaced by fibrous tissue. When this occurs the strength of the muscle is diminished, and so the force of the heart beat reduced. The term myocarditis is applied to these states.

Myocarditis is more serious the more it weakens the force of the beat. It is seldom an isolated trouble. As a rule other parts of the organ are affected as well as the muscle. By far the most important of these is the bundle of His, to which reference has already been

DISEASES OF THE HEART

made. Inflammation of this heart nerve may result in blocking of the impulses passing along it, *i.e.* in heart block.

The condition is usually associated with rheumatic fever, but it may occur after any acute infection, and in some cases it appears to arise without previous warning of any sort. There is no treatment except rest and care, and the administration of appropriate doses of heart stimulants as the indication arises.

Heart-muscle trouble often arises as a consequence of interference with the blood supply of the organ. The heart is fed by two arteries, the right and left coronaries, and these seem very apt to become the seat of disease changes. When that occurs there is narrowing of the vessels and the amount of blood reaching the heart is reduced. The muscle may become weak and thin, or it may degenerate and become fibrous.

Again, the heart muscle shares in many afflictions which affect other organs of the body. This is specially true of fatty degeneration of the heart. The administration of certain poisons will cause this and so will certain diseases. Droplets of fat appear in the muscle wall. In a few instances the entire wall of the heart becomes fatty and is accordingly so severely weakened that it may then burst and so cause death.

Hypertrophy. In almost every chronic heart affliction, the muscles of the chambers, especially those of the ventricles, become overgrown so that the actual thickness of the chamber wall is increased considerably. This is called hypertrophy. It may arise because of increased work, and is found in the following conditions: all diseases of the heart itself, including valvular defects, pericarditis, etc.; high blood pressure; lung diseases; defects of the aorta. The signs and symptoms are those of myocarditis unless the heart is well compensated, when there may be very few symptoms. The pulsation is usually

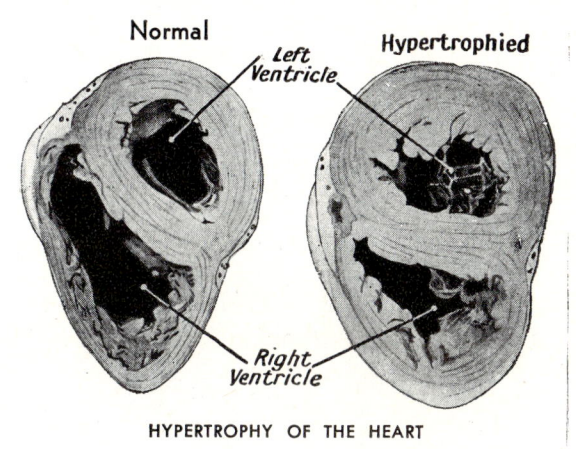

HYPERTROPHY OF THE HEART

Left: normal heart in section. Right: section of hypertrophied heart; the muscular walls of the ventricles are much thickened owing to the development of fresh muscle. The chambers will thus contract more forcibly and maintain the circulation in spite of damaged valves or other obstacles.

more vigorous, and very often the blood pressure is raised.

Dilatation. It cannot be too widely known that dilatation of the heart is not a common complaint, and most so-called cases of it are not cases of dilatation at all, but merely cases in which the heart has been slightly moved over towards the left side by mechanical means.

The heart hangs more or less free in the chest. It can move easily from side to side, after the manner of the pendulum of a clock. This movement alters the position of its left border very considerably and, unless we know exactly where the right border is, we may assume that the organ has swollen out.

Unless the apex or point of the heart is well outside, *i.e.* to the left of, a line drawn vertically through the left nipple, no dilatation need be considered. Normally, the heart lies an inch and a half inside of this line (see color plate facing page 1425) and thus at least two inches

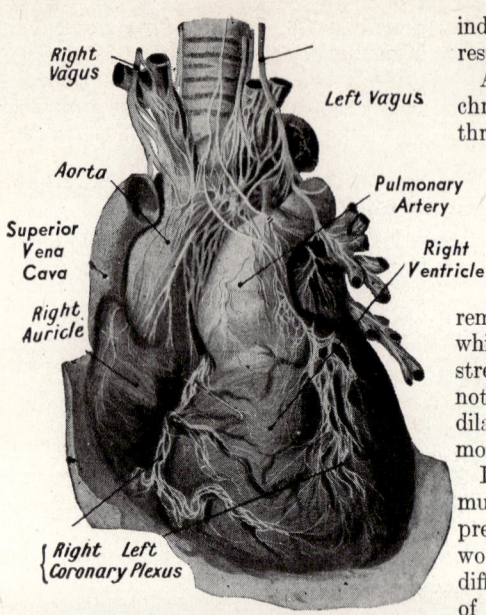

NERVE SUPPLY OF THE HEART

Both the right and left vagus nerves supply branches to the heart. These with branches from the sympathetic nerves form plexuses about the heart. Vagus impulses slow the heart beat; sympathetic impulses quicken and strengthen it.

of change must occur before any anxiety need be felt. Thus the statement often made that a heart is an inch, or two inches, too big simply means nothing at all.

Real dilatation does, however, occur. It is most commonly met with in the course of severe illnesses of the feverish type. In these the heart swells out, becomes extremely weak, and usually also extremely rapid and "soft" in its action. Patients in this condition are very ill indeed, but with recovery the heart resumes its normal size.

A few cases of dilatation exist in the chronic stage. In these the heart is some three or four inches too broad (the left border lying well outside the nipple line). Some of them are cases of real enlargement, as described above and on page 1452 under the heading Aortic Disease, and should not properly be called dilatation. The remainder are actual weak hearts in which the muscle has become wasted and stretched and toneless. Such people cannot stand any exertion; yet unsuspected dilatations are often discovered post mortem in strong, active men.

Dilatation, like other heart symptoms, must never be looked at alone. If it is present in a fit man who goes about his work easily, its significance is obviously different from its significance in a case of extreme weakness.

Nor must it be forgotten that the size of the heart at any given time is under nervous control. The vagus nerve, which slows the organ, also causes it to dilate. Thus, if any poison is acting on the vagus nerve, dilatation is very likely to be met with. This, indeed, occurs in acute and terrible form in a few very severe cases of diphtheria, where the heart expands and never shuts again. It occurs also, to a slighter degree, in other fevers. In these cases the trouble is not in the heart but in the nervous system or blood. When the diphtheria passes off the dilatation goes with it. There are other toxins, e.g. those produced in rheumatic fever, which do not act thus, and with which, as yet, there are no effective means of coping.

ENDOCARDITIS

By this is meant inflammation of the endocardium, the lining membrane of the heart which covers the inner surface of its walls and also the valves. It may be acute and benign or acute and malignant in severity, or may be slow and prolonged in its course.

Rheumatic infection is the commonest cause of acute endocarditis, but scarlet fever, septic infection, pneumonia, tonsillitis, and other acute infections may give rise to it. Inflammation set up in the valves of the heart is the important feature. This may be of a very severe and rapidly destructive nature, or slow and steady in its action. Mild inflammation may allow of complete recovery of the valve structure, but in most cases the inflammation, if the patient recovers from the acute attack, leads to much damage. In the process of healing the valve becomes shrunken and deformed from formation of scar tissue, with the result that it can no longer function efficiently in closing the opening at which it is situated. Thus results valvular disease of the heart, also termed chronic endocarditis; or it may be referred to, in terms of the valve affected, as mitral or aortic disease.

Acute benign endocarditis occurs oftenest in children and young adults suffering from acute rheumatic fever. As a rule one set of valves only is affected. What are known as "vegetations" —small tags or cauliflowerlike excrescences made up of inflammatory products—form on the surface of the valve or heart wall. These may become detached and form emboli (see page 1461), and may then give rise to certain special symptoms.

The disease itself may give rise to no marked symptoms when it is of a mild and slow-acting character. It may give rise to fever, but this will often be regarded as due to the infective disease responsible for the heart trouble. In other cases there are more or less severe symptoms pointing to the heart being involved. These may consist of discomfort or pain in the chest, palpitation, shortness of breath, rapid irregular pulse, faintness, or even of heart failure when the heart muscle becomes involved in the inflammation. The doctor may or may not find a murmur developing due to the roughening or incompetence of the affected valve. The diagnosis of early endocarditis often presents great difficulty unless heart symptoms are markedly present.

The course of the disease in such cases is very variable. It may progress in severity and develop into the malignant type, or after an apparent recovery reappear as soon as the patient gets about again. The resultant crippling of the valve may not produce any obvious symptoms for some time, but sooner or later gives evidence that it has occurred. It may only be discovered accidentally at a later date in the course of a medical examination.

The malignant type, which is most often associated with rheumatic or syphilitic heart conditions, is a very fatal disease. It is also known as bacterial or ulcerative endocarditis. The inflammatory process is very severe and associated with high fever, generally of an intermittent type, anemia, marked heart symptoms, great prostration, great liability to highly infective emboli (py-

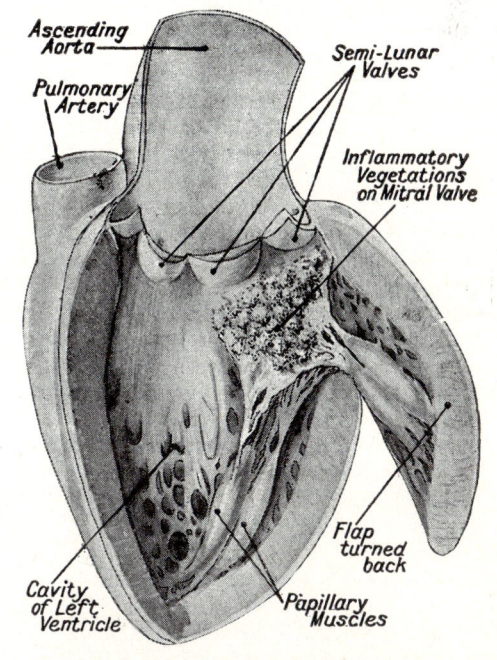

INFLAMMATION OF THE HEART LINING

Left ventricle, subject to endocarditis, one result being that the mitral valve is covered with granular masses, or vegetations. These are dangerous because one of them may be detached and carried off by the blood stream perhaps to the brain, and produce embolism.

emia) and all signs of very severe illness.

Chronic endocarditis is nearly always secondary to the acute benign variety. More rarely it may be primary and due to prolonged strain of the heart, local septic conditions elsewhere in the body, chronic rheumatic fever, and various conditions leading to prolonged poisoning of the blood.

The prevention of endocarditis or of its after-results lies in the prevention of acute rheumatic fever in children and young adults and in the proper treatment of even the slightest symptoms of rheumatic infection. "Growing pains" (see Chapter 199), which were at one time regarded as signs of commencing rheumatic trouble, have recently been found to be nothing like so serious. Definite attacks of rheumatic fever or acute rheumatism in children and young adults must be regarded very seriously and the patient must be kept at absolute rest in bed for many weeks.

If endocarditis ensues, absolute rest must be insisted on for at least three months or longer, and the child watched during apparent convalescence for any relapse. Activity must be resumed very gradually and its effects noted as to shortness of breath, fatigue, heart discomfort, or undue rapidity of pulse.

VALVULAR DISEASE OF THE HEART

Any of the four valves of the heart may be damaged by disease, but those which most commonly suffer are the mitral and the aortic, hence the terms mitral disease and aortic disease. These diseases are really forms of endocarditis, for the lining membrane of the heart is spread over every structure in it, including the cusps of the valves.

Aortic Disease. Aortic disease is disease of the valves in the main blood vessel leading out of the heart, the aorta. Obviously, such disease, if it injures the valve at all seriously, will allow the blood to flow backwards into the heart when that organ is resting between its beats. It will allow, that is to say, a return into the heart of the blood already pumped out of it. The heart is doing all its work twice and thrice over. In order to keep up any sort of a circulation it has to work very much harder than normal and rest very much less. And, even so, the force of the circulation is always greatly diminished, so that the victim of this grave disease soon shows signs of a want of blood supply.

He becomes, in fact, afflicted with blood starvation. The thousands of millions of tiny cells in the body carrying on digestion, muscular movement, nerve activity, and many other forms of work depend absolutely on the blood to bring their food to them. In other words, they depend on the force of the circulation. If that becomes irregular, food does not arrive in sufficient quantity to keep them in full health. Thus a backflow of blood, or regurgitation, means weakness of every cell in the body. A man with aortic disease is an easy prey of a multitude of ailments, and, in fact, often dies of one or other of these before his heart disease has advanced far enough to end his life.

But nature always tries hard to make up for a loss in one direction by greater strength in another. This tendency is specially well seen in aortic disease, the sufferers from which have, as a rule, enormously enlarged hearts. Indeed, their hearts seem actually to grow bigger in proportion to the amount of extra work they are called on to perform. The walls of these hearts are greatly thickened and very powerful. Thus, what is lost in backflow of blood is made up for, or compensated, by extra force in the heartbeat. It happens in a good many cases that the damage to the valves is not very extensive, and that the disease causing the damage heals, so that the trouble gets no worse. The enlargement of the heart may then be enough to keep the circulation going fairly effectively. A patient in that condition may get

DISEASES OF THE HEART

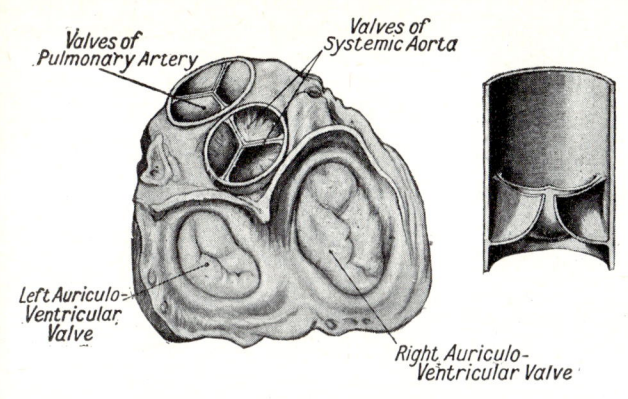

POSITION OF IMPORTANT HEART VALVES
The aorta rises from the left ventricle of the heart. The diagrams show, left, heart valves viewed from above, after removal of auricles and greater part of aorta; right, section of wall of systemic aorta, showing arrangement of valves.

along pretty well, and may even live out his full term of life.

In other cases, however, the disease of the valves goes on unchecked until these are more or less completely damaged. When that occurs even the enlarged heart is not strong enough to do the work required of it, and gradually—or suddenly—the end is reached. It is important in this connection to remember that hypertrophy as seen in aortic disease is a benefit and not a misfortune. It is quite different from the dilated heart which occurs in other conditions, and which is a sign of weakness or sometimes of damage.

Aortic disease, like other diseases of the heart, is specially liable to follow rheumatic fever and syphilis, and it has been found that the more serious types of aortic disease are of syphilitic origin. It must also be allowed that cases arise without any previous history of any disease at all. Most often the pathology in these cases is rheumatic in type.

Signs. The disease begins, as a rule, very quietly and insidiously, and may be present for a long time before its victim is aware of his disability. Frequently it is discovered by accident during an examination for life insurance or during the course of some apparently trifling illness. There must be a considerable number of cases of aortic disease which are never discovered at all—those cases in which a slight damage to the valves is compensated by enlargement of the heart and in which the original trouble heals and does not progress. There are other cases in which the damage is so slight that very little disability occurs.

But these, unfortunately, are the exception rather than the rule. There is little room for doubt that the tendency in damage of the aortic valves is downwards. The disease of the valves, under the severe stress of the working conditions imposed, too often continues; the "leak" or hole in the valves, when closed, becomes more extensive, and so the

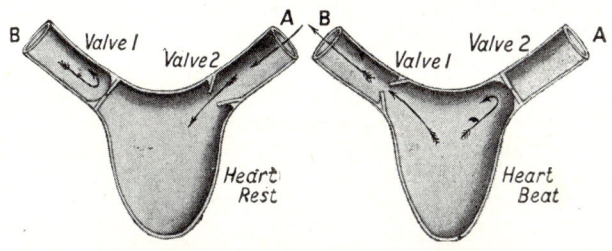

AORTIC DISEASE: MECHANISM OF HEART VALVES
Left: heart in rest. The blood is flowing into the heart at A through the open inlet Valve 2. The blood in the outer vessel, the aorta, cannot flow back into the heart from B because Valve 1 is shut. Right: heartbeat. The blood is flowing out at B, driven by the beat of the heart. Valve 1 in the outlet vessel is open, while Valve 2 in the inlet vessel is shut, to prevent the blood flowing back towards A.

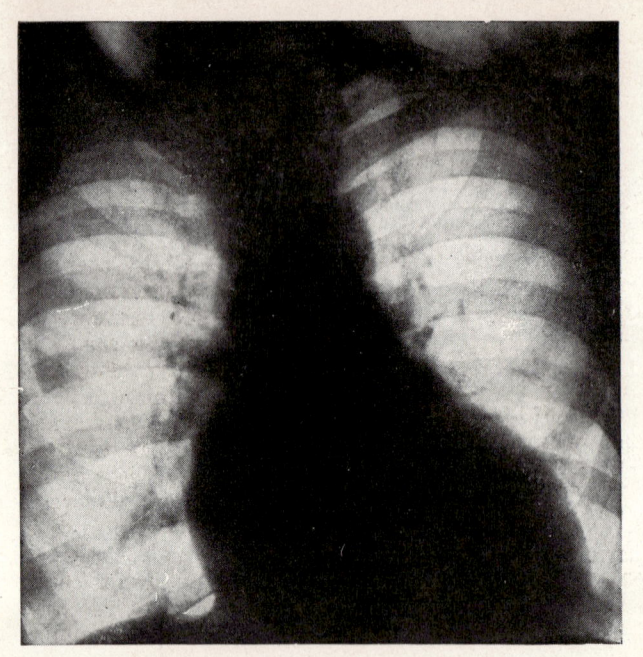

ENLARGED HEART IN AORTIC DISEASE

This X-ray photograph of a heart enlarged by aortic disease shows how considerably the left border of the organ may be extended beyond the line within which it is normally confined, as explained in the diagram on page 1455. The enlargement has compensating advantages in this disease.

burden thrown on the heart increases steadily. Moreover, the original disease, from which the aortic disease took its origin in the first instance, tends to increase in strength.

The patient becomes weaker, more anemic, more apt to suffer from breathlessness, pain over the heart, and fainting attacks. He may drop down dead—this termination is common in aortic cases of syphilitic origin—or he may gradually become a cripple and finally remain confined to bed.

The disease cannot be recognized by anyone who lacks professional training, and frequently reference has to be made to a heart specialist before a final decision can be arrived at. This decision depends on several signs, which are often difficult to interpret. In the first place there is the so-called aortic murmur, or bruit. This is heard by the stethoscope. It is a soft, blowing sound which replaces the second sound made by the heart.

The second sign which is always looked for is enlargement of the heart. The doctor taps, or percusses, from the clear, air-filled lung to the dull, solid heart. He does this with special care on the left side, since it is difficult to tap the right side of the heart on account of the fact that it lies under, or nearly under, the breast bone. The left border of a normal, unenlarged heart lies about three-quarters of an inch inside a line drawn vertically through the nipple. In case of aortic disease the left border may lie as far as three or even four inches outside of the nipple line. When such enlargement is found together with the murmur, there is little doubt as to the nature of the case.

A third sign, to which importance is always attached, is the so-called water-hammer pulse. On feeling the pulse, the doctor is aware of a thumping against his finger which the pulse of a healthy person does not give. This thump is followed by a swift emptying of the vessel, so that the pulse falls away under the finger.

The reason for this is obvious when we remember the nature of the disease. The enlarged and powerful heart gives a strong beat—the thump—but when the beat is over the blood in the artery runs back again through the hole in the damaged valve. Thus the vessel is swiftly emptied backwards. This pulse is also called Corrigan's pulse, from the name of its discoverer. It must be added that no one except a trained physician can properly detect its presence. People who commit the folly of feeling their own pulses are simply deluding themselves, since years of special study are necessary to enable anyone to obtain information from this source. There is nothing easier than to imagine that one has a water-hammer pulse.

Treatment. The treatment of aortic disease depends first of all on its cause. If this is rheumatic fever, everything possible must be done to check the spread of that affliction. If at all possible, the patient should live in a dry, sunny climate, for this may cure him, or at least put a stop to his heart disease. Where life must be spent in less satisfactory climatic conditions, chills and damp should be avoided, and the clothing so adapted that it will tend to keep the body at or about the same temperature in all weathers. The patient should eat frugally and make sure that his diet contains the essential elements of health, the vitamins which are found in animal fat (butter, milk, etc.), in whole-wheat bread, and in fresh fruit and green vegetables.

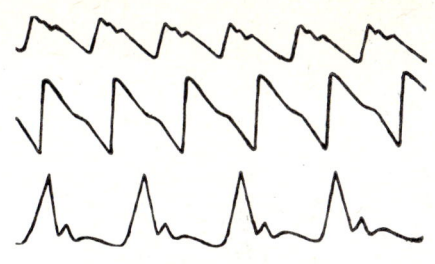

CORRIGAN'S PULSE: A TRACING

The lowest of the tracings given above, which are graphic records of what takes place during the beats of the pulse, shows the Corrigan pulse, sometimes called the water-hammer pulse. Pressure is not sustained as in the other two, which are normal.

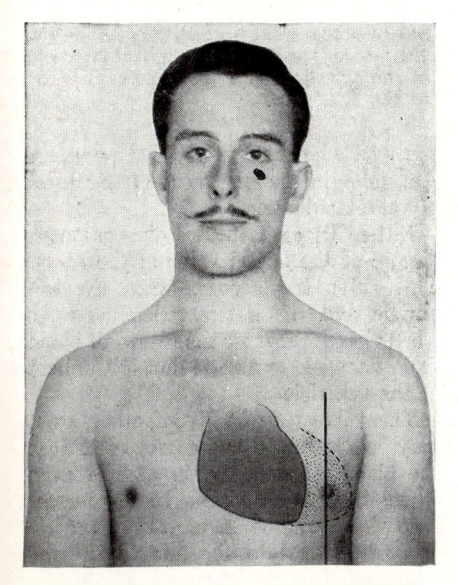

POSSIBLE EFFECT OF AORTIC DISEASE

The normal heart has its left margin well inside a line drawn vertically through the left nipple. The dotted outline shows how far beyond this it may be enlarged by aortic disease.

Where syphilis is the basal cause, antisyphilitic treatment is given with hope that it will bring about a certain measure of improvement. In cases thus treated the disease of the valves is frequently checked. The difficulty is that by the time syphilis of the aorta manifests itself clinically it has usually progressed so far that the prognosis is not very good. Another difficulty is that antisyphilitic treatment in these cases sometimes causes a rapid progression of the disease.

The treatment of the disease itself is still very unsatisfactory. The patient must be made to realize that he is living under severe handicap, and that in consequence all sudden shocks and all heavy exertions are dangerous to him. He must lead a quiet, sheltered life, in as equable a climate as possible, and must avoid all strenuous pursuits. This, however, does not mean that he must spend his life in bed. His doctor will guide him as to what he may and what he may not do, and this advice is likely to vary considerably in different cases and in different circum-

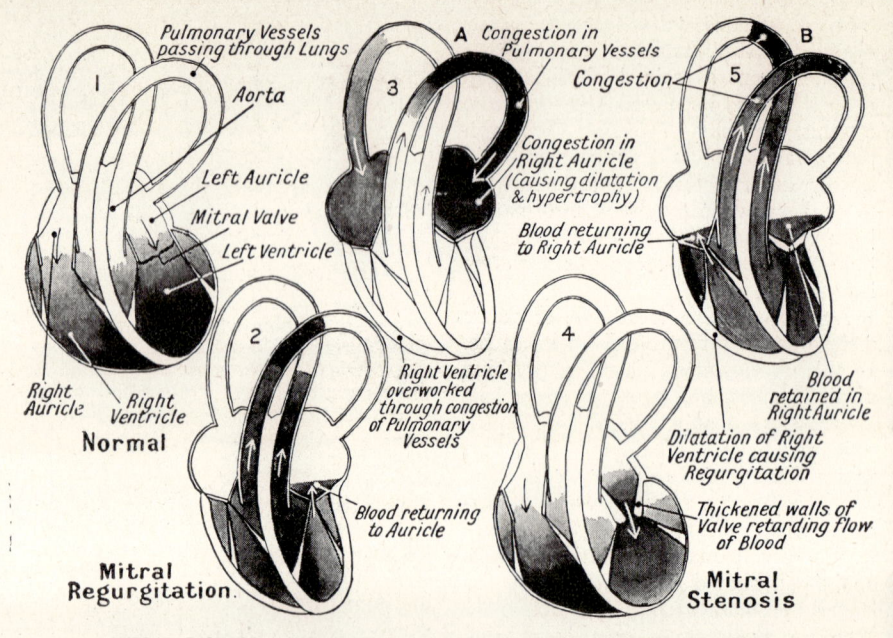

MITRAL DISEASE: DISORDERED HEART VALVE AND ITS CONSEQUENCES

(1) In the normal heart action, the auricles empty themselves into the ventricles, and when the latter contract all the blood is pumped into the great vessels. (2) In mitral regurgitation, part of the blood flows back into the left auricle and (4) in mitral stenosis, part may be left in the auricle; (3) overfilling of the auricle ensues and engorgement of the lungs and then (5) of the right heart.

stances. Shortness of breath or discomfort in the region of the heart indicates that physical effort is excessive or is being made too quickly. Thus, if the disease of the valves has healed and the patient is well except for some small remaining damage, considerable activity is permissible. If the damage is greater, but the progress of disease has been stayed, less exercise will be possible, and so on.

Indigestion is very apt to bring on heart attacks in such people, owing to the nervous connection existing between the stomach and the heart, and sudden death is comparatively frequent as a termination of aortic disease.

Many drugs have been given from time to time. Some of these are simply remedies for chronic syphilis; others belong to the group used in angina pectoris (amylnitrite and nitroglycerine). It is doubtful whether any of them possesses real value in the treatment of this form of valvular disease.

Mitral Disease. Mitral disease means disease of the mitral valve of the heart. This valve is placed between the left auricle and the left ventricle, and so, when closed, prevents the return of blood from ventricle to auricle during the beat of the ventricle.

The valve may be incompetent, or it may be contracted and narrowed so that the blood his difficulty in passing even when the valve is open. In the former case there will be regurgitation, or reflux of blood into the auricle; in the latter the ventricle will be inadequately filled at each diastole, *i.e.*, each rest period. Both these troubles may occur in the same valve at the same time, because a diseased valve may act as an obstruction to the flow of blood when

DISEASES OF THE HEART

open and yet be unable to prevent the back flow of blood when closed.

In mitral incompetence the valve, owing to injury to its form, does not close completely. Blood then flows back into the left auricle, the cavity of which, having to accommodate this blood in addition to that which it receives from the great veins, becomes dilated. Increased back pressure towards the lungs is set up, and so a serious disorganization of the circulation. The signs of mitral regurgitation are those of embarrassment of the heart. There is usually breathlessness on exertion. There is also, commonly, blueness or cyanosis. The left ventricle becomes dilated and enlarged so as to be able to propel a larger quantity of blood, and there is always a murmur which replaces the first heart sound and which is caused by the reflux of blood through the incompetent valve. The outlook is not necessarily bad, and many cases of simple mitral regurgitation live long.

In mitral stenosis there is narrowing of the opening, or orifice, between the left auricle and left ventricle. The narrowing is usually a consequence of valvular disease, and as a rule it tends to progress. Its effect is to interpose a barrier into the circulation. The left heart receives less blood than normal and there is a damming up of blood on the right side, i.e. in the lungs and veins. Thus the patient is cyanotic in severe cases, and is, as a rule, manifestly short of breath and palpably embarrassed in physical activity.

The heart is not usually enlarged, though the left auricle may become hypertrophied and later the right ventricle also, owing to the increased work necessitated by the obstruction. But a rough murmur, the so-called presystolic murmur, precedes the first cardiac sound, and a thrill can be felt in the chest wall over the heart. The murmur and thrill are caused by the blood rushing through the narrow mitral orifice on its way from the auricle to the ventricle.

The outlook in mitral stenosis is not good and patients with this disease have to lead careful lives. It occurs as a sequel to rheumatic fever. Treatment in general is on the same lines as that of aortic disease.

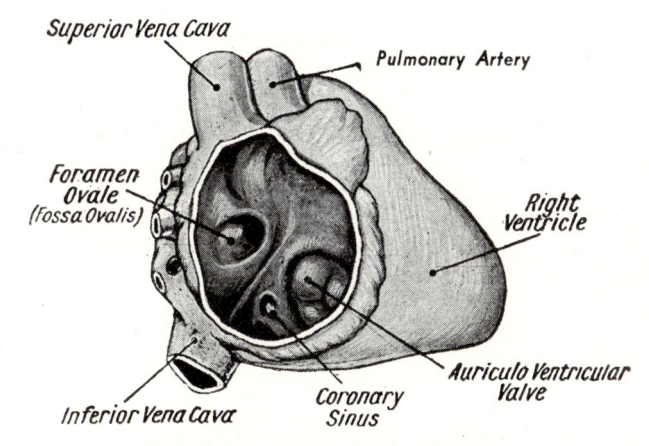

CONGENITAL CIRCULATION DEFECT

The foramen ovale, the opening connecting the right and left auricles, should close before birth. Failure to do so, as seen here, causes an admixture of pure and impure blood, resulting perhaps in general cyanosis or marked blueness of the skin.

CONGENITAL HEART DISEASE

Congenital malformation of the heart is often termed "blue disease," because of the dark discoloration of the skin that forms a striking feature in most cases of this disorder. There are many cases which never manifest any cyanosis and there is a group in which cyanosis is present only at times when the heart is called upon to do an unusual amount of work.

In most instances the condition is due to failure of the embryo heart to complete the series of changes which mark the nine months of intrauterine existence. At an early period the heart consists of only two cavities—the auricle and the ventricle—without any wall to make a right and left division. The distribution of blood through the heart of the unborn child is necessarily very different from that which occurs after birth, for the embryo receives its nutriment from the mother by way of the umbilical cord, and it cannot use its lungs. The partition between the right and left auricles does not become complete until after birth. Blood from the placenta, passing to the fetus by the umbilical vein, ultimately reaches the right auricle. Most of it then goes through the gap called the foramen ovale into the left auricle, then to the left ventricle, and so to the body through the aorta.

Since development may become arrested at any stage, it will be readily understood that the variety among abnormalities occurring in the heart before birth is very great. As a rule several varieties of deformity exist; single defects are rare. The commonest form is an undue narrowing of the pulmonary artery at its origin from the right ventricle.

Signs. Subjects of blue disease are usually weak and sickly from birth, and many of the graver type suffer from convulsions, which may prove fatal. The usual symptoms comprise shortness of breath, blueness of the skin, and swelling of the ankles. In the later stages the swelling may affect the whole body, and all the signs of gradual heart failure follow.

The growth of the patient, both mental and physical, is retarded. A chronic enlargement of the last joint of each finger, known as clubbing of the fingers, is common. Fainting attacks may occur. These patients usually complain of feeling cold, and they are very liable to contract bronchitis. Tuberculosis of the lungs is a frequent complication. The peculiar loud and long murmurs which can be heard by listening over the cardiac region with a stethoscope are of great assistance in diagnosis, while other signs are that the pulse is usually quickened and the heart somewhat enlarged.

The blueness, which is a more conspicuous feature of this disease than of any other, becomes more evident on exertion or on crying. It is most marked in the fingernails, the lips, the tip of the nose, and the ears.

Treatment. Preventive treatment is at present impossible, since the condition cannot be diagnosed before birth. These patients are more prone to develop a bacterial endocarditis than are individuals with normal hearts. It is for this reason that they must be carefully protected from infections of all kinds.

The infants should be wrapped in cotton and kept in an equable temperature. Later, flannel clothing should always be worn. These patients must be shielded from inclement weather, and all exertion should be carefully restricted. Abundant fresh air and sunlight, with simple nourishing food, will help.

Digitalis is a useful drug when signs of heart failure become manifest. The general treatment applicable to ordinary acquired heart disease will also be employed in this condition.

ANGINA PECTORIS

The distressing malady termed angina pectoris has been the subject of research and study for hundreds of years. No disease has so baffled physicians.

The ailment in its severest form is characterized by a violent and terrible pain in the chest. This may come on with extreme suddenness so that the victim appears to be gripped in a vise. His face grows deathly pale, perspiration breaks out on his brow, his breathing is "strangled" and frequently he has the sensation of approaching death. Happily, that extreme form of heart pain is rare. Much more common is the milder condition, rarely fatal, in which attacks of a less severe form occur on exertion or during excitement.

That, until the year 1914, was the whole story of angina pectoris, though it was usually believed that, whereas male victims of the disease commonly died of it sooner or later, women victims were unlikely to die. The condition, however, is equally fatal for both sexes, but a higher incidence occurs among males.

Today we know that heart pain is not due to one disease but to many, and that most of the pains felt in the chest are not angina pectoris at all.

The beginning of this new knowledge occurred during the First World War, when it was found that a large number of young soldiers complained of pain over the heart when they exerted themselves. At first doctors suspected angina pectoris. Presently, however, the term "soldier's heart" began to be used.

From this starting point the new study of pains in the chest advanced rapidly. It was found that the same kind of pain might arise from a variety of causes, some of them dangerous, others comparatively harmless. For example, many victims of nervousness suffer from heart pain; so do many young people with rheumatic fever. In all these cases the pain, though it may be very severe, is not dangerous to life. There is thus a whole world of difference between true angina pectoris—a disease now believed attributable to a deficient blood supply to the myocardium as a result of arteriosclerotic changes in the coronary vessels—and false angina pectoris, which is very common.

It is by no means easy in all cases to make a distinction. Yet there are facts which enable one to arrive at a conclusion in most instances. It is necessary to remember that the heart is perhaps the most sensitive and responsive organ in the body. When the nerves connect-

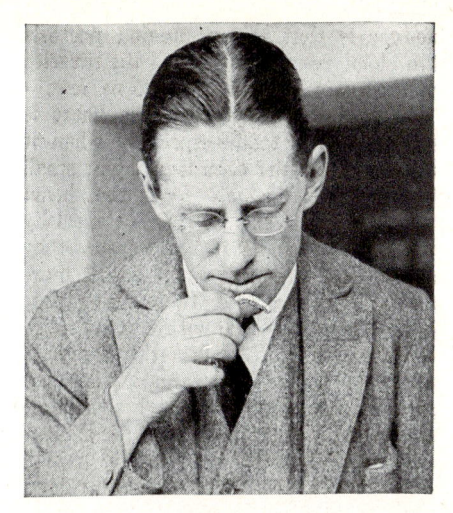

ANGINA PECTORIS: EASING AN ATTACK
Inhalation of amyl nitrite will ease the pain of an attack of angina pectoris almost instantly by its capacity to relieve the strain on the heart.

ing the heart with the senses are poisoned and so made irritable, the very smallest events in the outside world become magnified into great and terrible calls for effort. And so the heart which is "controlled" by these nerves is always beating at its fullest strength; that is to say, it is always tired.

The owner of that heart will complain of severe pain in the chest—pain which may easily be mistaken for angina pectoris. But the real cause of the pain will not be the heart but the toxin which is acting on the nerves. If that toxin can be removed the pain will soon disappear.

Anginal pain may occur with the tachycardia of hyperthyroidism. Many cases of false angina pectoris are due to overeating, oversmoking, or overindulgence. Anything, in fact, which poisons the nerves may give rise to pain in the chest. There are thousands of these cases. They can all be cured, if the real cause is discovered and treated.

What, then, is the difference between pain due to exertion or of nervous origin, on the one hand, and pain due to the heart itself, on the other hand? The answer is that in real angina pectoris the blood vessels which feed the muscles of the heart have become too narrow.

In real angina pectoris the heart is starved of its food—especially when it is working harder than usual. The small blood vessels which feed the heart muscles are very elastic in healthy people. As the heart beats faster they stretch and widen so as to give it more and still more blood. If, however, they have become diseased with what is called arteriosclerosis, they lose this elasticity and grow hard. They cannot widen and so cannot supply more blood when more is needed. And so the starved heart becomes exhausted and terrible pain is felt over the chest and sometimes down the left arm. The heart may stop, or it may go on with difficulty. In any case, the patient will suffer great agony and experience great fear. He must carefully avoid exertion or excitement and must lead a very quiet life. By doing this he may manage, for a time at any rate, to avoid the attacks.

In all cases of pain in the chest it is the condition of the arteries that counts. If these, so far as they can be felt, seem to be soft and healthy, if the patient is a female, or a youngish man, if the attacks are of moderate severity and are not always brought on by exertion, and yield to treatment of the underlying condition, the patient is probably suffering from false angina pectoris; if, on the contrary, the arteries are hard and inelastic, and if the patient is a man past middle age, the attacks definitely induced by exertion or excitement and accompanied by a sense of impending death, true angina pectoris is present.

Electrocardiographic evidence of heart damage aids in the differentiation.

Treatment. Obviously the treatment must be suited to the nature of the complaint. Thus, if a boy who is playing strenuous games complains of pains in his chest, the treatment will be to give him a rest and let him recover his strength. Again, if the pain occurs in people who show other signs of a toxic condition, e.g. Grave's disease, the treatment must be directed to eradicating the underlying cause.

The treatment of true angina pectoris is quite different. Here the worn-out blood vessels are full of lime—hard and fragile; it is scarcely possible to cure them. All that can be done is to ease the strain on them so far as possible, and at the same time supply the patient with some means of helping himself.

The best way of achieving this latter object is to give the drug known as amyl nitrite. This remarkable substance has the power of causing the skin all over the body to flush. Flushing, of course, means that the skin has filled full of blood, and this again means that, for the moment, the pressure in the blood vessels has grown less. The blood pressure in the larger arteries, as well as in the smaller, is lowered and the work of the heart is lightened thereby. This brings the desired relief. The amyl nitrite is supplied in little glass bulbs covered with a thin layer of silk. The bulbs are broken between the finger and thumb, and the silk bag containing them can then be raised to the nose and the amyl nitrite inhaled. Even one or two sniffs of it are usually sufficient to ease the pain and bring the attack of angina pectoris to an end. After the attack small doses of other preparations of the nitrites are often given.

These drugs are dangerous and should never, in any circumstances, be used without medical authority. It is quite common to find people who are not suffering from angina pectoris at all sniffing amyl nitrite because of some chest pain.

The sufferer from true angina pectoris must live within the limits of his heart's strength. The diet in these cases should be frugal. Alcohol should not be taken and smoking must be cut down. Otherwise, any foods that are fancied and which prove to be within the patient's digestive powers may be given. The clothing should be warm and light, and strains, chills, excitement and worries should be avoided as far as possible.

CHAPTER 105

DISORDERS OF THE BLOOD VESSELS

Embolism — Thrombosis — Arteriosclerosis — Causes — Nature of the Condition—Treatment—Diet—Aneurysm— Diseases of the Veins — Phlebitis — Varicose Veins — Varicocele and Hemorrhoids—Raynaud's Disease.

THE blood vessels of the body, which have been described in Chapter 48, are of three main kinds—arteries, veins, and capillaries—and are the passages by which the blood is conveyed to the various parts of the body. The blood vessels are subject to a number of disorders, and we shall deal first with those arising from some obstruction in the vessel.

Embolism. As blood escapes from the vessels it clots. If this did not occur, anyone who cut his finger would bleed to death rapidly or slowly depending on the rate of blood flow. Normally, clotting does not take place within the blood vessels so long as the lining cells of these are healthy. If, however, this delicate lining gets broken, a clot will usually form at the place where the break has occurred.

Causes. A common cause of such damage is a varicose vein (see page 1475). A varicose vein is always a damaged vein. Very often it becomes inflamed, and may then contain small blood clots adhering to its damaged walls. If they get loose and flow into any small blood vessel they will probably plug it up, a process termed embolism.

Embolisms may occur anywhere in the body, but the commonest places for them to occur are the tiny vessels of the lungs. This is known as a pulmonary embolism. The effect is to cut off the blood from a portion of the lung, and since the larger the vessel which is plugged the larger will be the portion of lung deprived of blood, the severity of the symptoms will depend on the size of the vessel affected.

These symptoms usually, but not invariably, include a sharp stabbing pain in the chest. At the same moment the patient becomes very breathless and may become quite collapsed. Spitting of blood almost always occurs. The patient is gravely ill, and should be put to bed without delay, and medical help summoned. If the lung "dies" an abscess may form, or the dead portion may simply shrivel up. Recovery is common enough but depends on the size of the plugged vessel and on the patient's recuperative power.

Embolism may also occur in the liver. Clots coming to the liver arise in the

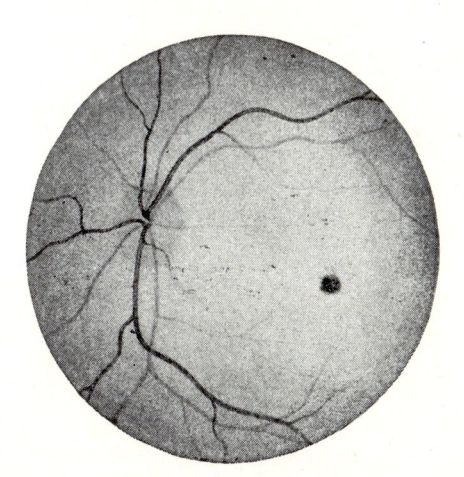

EMBOLISM IN THE EYE
The effect of plugging an end artery is shown in this picture of embolism in a retinal artery. The black spot indicates site of the fovea centralis; the pale area is bloodless. Compare the normal eye in the color plate facing page 152.
Courtesy of Theodore Hamblin, Ltd.

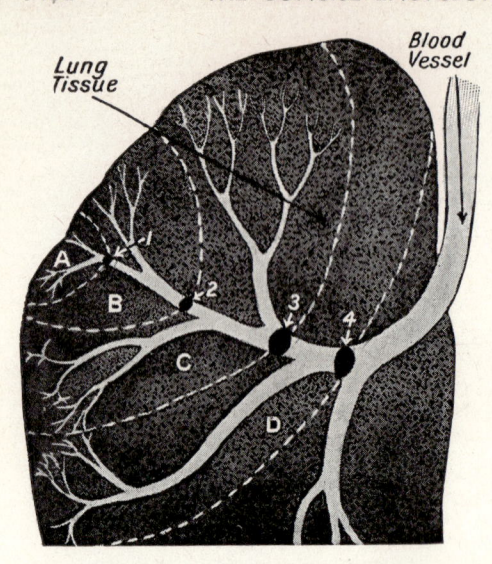

EMBOLISM: PLUG IN BLOOD VESSEL

At 1, 2, 3, 4, are plugs in blood vessels, and A, B, C, D indicate areas of lung supplied by the corresponding vessels. The farther back in the arterial supply the embolism is located, the larger the area of lung which is involved.

veins of the bowels because the blood from the bowels flows directly through this organ. A sharp pain is felt in the right side, as a rule, and signs of collapse may show themselves. On the other hand these symptoms may be absent. Usually the condition is not so severe as embolism of the lungs. The patient should be put to bed immediately, nevertheless, and a doctor should be called.

Clots in the veins seldom plug any vessels except those of the lungs and liver, for the good reason that these organs act as filters and prevent them going any further. They cannot pass through the tiny vessels which they would require to pass in order to reach the arteries. Nevertheless, the danger is great enough and people with varicose veins should realize it. To pinch or slap a varicose vein in which a clot is lodging or handle the vein roughly is very dangerous, since it may set a large clot adrift with serious, or even fatal, results.

Another frequent cause of embolism is inflammation of veins elsewhere in the body, giving rise to clotting. Clotting may occur in the veins of the uterus after childbirth, and in the veins of the abdomen or elsewhere after a surgical operation. The latter is a frequent cause of sudden death during convalescence after operations.

But these clots are not the only or even the most serious cause of embolism. Another cause is inflammation of the lining of the heart, or endocarditis, which was dealt with in Chapter 104, or of the arteries, as described below. Such inflammation may be slight or it may be severe and widespread, so that the blood is poisoned and is full of living germs. In any case, plugs get formed, consisting either of "vegetations," little hard growths, or actual masses of germs mixed up with shreds of material from the inflamed blood vessels. These small poisoned clots or clumps of germs may get adrift in the blood stream. If they do they may be carried to the most vital organs of the body. The blood in the arteries flows directly to the brain, and it also feeds the whole body, including the liver, kidneys, stomach, and heart.

Thus, a plug arising in the heart lining may instantly pass into the small vessels which feed the heart muscle, the vessels that are the very first branches to be given off from the main arterial trunk. When this occurs sudden death is always the result. The heart loses its blood supply and immediately stops. Such cases occur, as a rule, in patients suffering from severe forms of heart disease, but it is possible that they may occur in quite mild conditions of the same kind. The heart's own blood vessels are called coronary arteries, and so this plugging of the heart's blood vessels is usually spoken of as coronary embolism.

In cerebral embolism the brain is the seat of plugging. The patient shows symptoms of severe brain trouble in an instant. Thus, he may become paralyzed down one or both sides of his body, or in one or all limbs; he may go blind or deaf; he may lose his speech; or he may die on the spot. It depends entirely upon what part of the brain the plug happens to lodge in.

Other forms of plugging of this kind are found in the liver (hepatic infarction), kidney, spleen, and even in the eyes and ears and skin —anywhere, in fact, where there are small blood vessels. The word infarct is used to describe the portion of flesh or organ which loses its blood supply and so may die. Naturally such a starved portion is apt to be attacked by germs, because until it gets blood again it is too weak to defend itself. Thus, an embolism is often followed by an abscess or an inflammation. In cases in which the inflammation in the heart and blood vessels is extensive, hundreds of small, or multiple, embolisms may be found all over the body after death. These show that the blood was tending to clot even in the vessels.

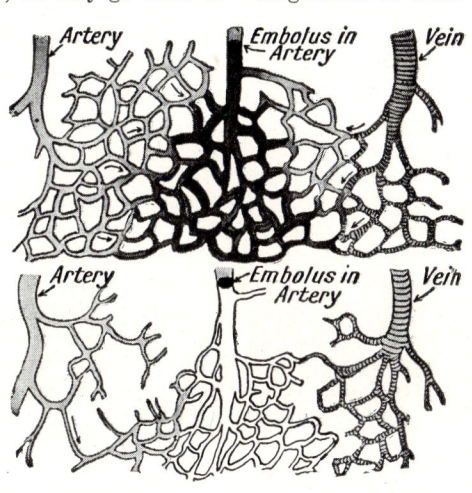

Additional Causes. Two other causes of embolism remain to be described— air and fat. When a man cuts his throat, air is often sucked into the severed ends of the veins. If this air should reach the heart instant death will usually occur, for the air forms bubbles in the blood and stops the circulation. Air sometimes enters the blood also through wounds in the lungs. Fat embolism occurs following trauma to fatty tissue.

INFARCTION BY PLUG IN AN ARTERY
Above, an embolus plugs an artery: blood passes into the empty vessels from the veins and possibly adjoining arteries and engorges them; but if not, the affected area forms a white infarction, as below.

Thrombosis. The word thrombosis is derived from the Greek term *thrombos*, meaning a clot, and refers to abnormal coagulation of blood within the heart or blood vessels during life. This may occur in any part of the body, and its effects are widely different according to the part involved. In the main, the symptoms of such a condition are due to the blockage of blood supply.

In certain cases thrombosis is a beneficial happening. In accidents a large blood vessel may be partly or completely severed. If no surgical attendance is at hand, the sufferer might bleed to death if it were not for thrombosis arising in the damaged vessel. In some cases of aneurysm, also, benefit may occur as the result of thrombosis, for clots may be deposited on the wall of the aneurysm which serve to thicken and strengthen it. In general, however, the results of thrombosis are harmful. In the leg, pain, swelling, and disablement arise. In the brain, some degree of paralysis may result. In the heart, the issue may be sudden death.

Causes. When healthy blood is circulating naturally in healthy blood vessels, thrombosis never occurs. The conditions favorable to it are alterations in the blood current, changes in the vessel walls, and alterations in condition and constitution of the blood itself.

Anything which slows the blood current favors thrombosis. The factor may be narrowing of the blood vessels, weakness of the heart, or pressure upon the veins. Cases due to slowing of the blood current are frequently seen in the course of prolonged fevers or other exhausting conditions, such as the marasmus of babies. In extreme old age, also, this type of thrombosis is common. The parts usually affected include the heart, the large vessels of the legs, and the venous sinuses that course through the brain.

Changes in the vessel walls play an important part in thrombosis. Any roughening or injury of the membrane lining a blood vessel attracts the minute blood platelets. These adhere to the part and a blood clot gradually forms upon them. Atheroma (see page 1467), degenerative changes of the arteries, injury, and endocarditis are all examples of conditions which lead to thrombosis.

Some bacteria—for example, staphylococci—are specially liable to induce clotting of the blood; hence the tendency to thrombosis which so often complicates typhoid fever and septic blood poisoning.

When thrombosis has once begun, the clot itself disturbs the blood stream and further blood clots are added to it. It often extends as far as the place where the blocked vessel joins a larger trunk. The speed of the blood current in the larger vessel may prevent further spread of the clot, but there is a risk that a small piece may be washed off and block a small artery.

Sites of Clotting. Although thrombosis may occur in any part of the circulatory system it is found to be much commoner in vessels of medium size. Great arteries like the aorta and very small vessels commonly escape. Veins are much more often affected than are arteries. The reason for this is apparent, for the blood stream moves more slowly in veins and the blood itself contains a higher proportion of carbon dioxide gas.

The lower limb is the part most frequently affected. In the arteries, thrombosis may occur in the substance of the heart or in the brain. In such cases it is generally the result of arterial disease or of embolism.

Effects of Thrombosis. The effects vary with the part concerned. Frequently the surrounding blood vessels enlarge so promptly that no untoward results are seen. There is always a tendency for other branches to take over the duties of the vessel which has become blocked. When a large vein is attacked, venous congestion and edema

THROMBOSIS: CLOTTING IN BLOOD VESSEL
Left: thrombosis has taken place in the long saphenous vein in the left leg; a portion of the thrombus has become detached and has been carried to the right lung, where it has caused embolism. Right: a thrombus in the right femoral vein has been converted into fibrous tissue, blocking the circulation.

may follow. Thrombosis of an artery causes local anemia and, if the surrounding vessels do not quickly respond to the situation, decay and death of the tissues follow.

If the thrombosis is associated with a general infection it is usual for germs to settle at the spot. A septic softening with the formation of matter ensues, and fragments of inflammatory material may be carried to distant parts of the body. In such cases each portion of the decomposing thrombus is liable to start a fresh spot of infection and another abscess may result. In any case the tissues supplied by the thrombosed artery suffer, but they may recover if the part can receive blood from neighboring vessels.

Symptoms and Treatment. The symptoms affecting a large vein may be exemplified by a brief account of a case involving the great veins of the thigh. This condition sometimes arises after childbirth or after operations on the pelvic organs. At the onset there is often a chill and a general feeling of weakness and illness. There is some pain, which may be of a dull, aching character or sharp and shooting. Examination shows a firm, rounded, tender cord if the affected vein is near the surface. The ankle and leg become edematous, being cold, swollen and weak.

The main treatment is twofold. In the first place, appropriate measures must be taken for the relief of any disease which underlies the thrombosis. Syphilis, anemia, or arteriosclerosis may be found. In the second place, it is necessary to encourage the absorption of the thrombus and to obviate the risk of an embolism due to the separation of a portion of it.

The treatment of thrombosis must include absolute rest. In the common type of thrombosis affecting the leg, the patient is kept in bed and the limb elevated on pillows or a special wooden cradle. The support must be well padded, and especially must the heel be protected from pressure. The patient must never be allowed to move the limb without assistance. The nurse or attendant may occasionally place it in a more comfortable position.

The application of ointments or liniments is of no value, but an ice bag over the tender vein often gives great relief from pain. Frequent removal of the ice bag is necessary to avoid freezing. In other cases an occasional hot fomentation is preferred. After six or eight weeks the clot will probably be firm enough to allow the patient to move about a little. No massage should be allowed for at least three months.

For a week the patient should sit up in a chair for fifteen to thirty minutes daily. During the following week she should do no more than take a few steps about the room. The leg and foot usually become swollen after the patient gets up, and a warning concerning this is advisable to prevent disappointment or alarm. Some degree of swelling at the ankle is likely to persist for many months.

The use of an elastic stocking or a flannel bandage keeps the limb from undue swelling and is a great comfort.

ARTERIOSCLEROSIS

The subject of arteriosclerosis, or thickening and narrowing of the arteries, is a very complex one, and it can rarely be dissociated from primary diseases elsewhere. A relationship, the exact nature of which is still unsettled, exists between arteriosclerosis and high blood pressure. The public interest in the degree of blood pressure has become so great that it is a common experience to hear it discussed on commuters' trains, at lunch counters, across bridge tables, etc. It is true that this furnishes a proof that a "little learning is a dangerous thing," for many people talk of their blood pressure without any knowledge of the fundamental interpretation of it; nevertheless, the very fact of popular

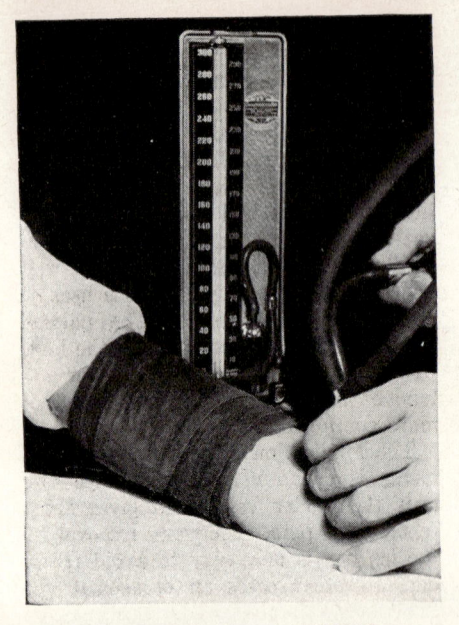

TO MEASURE BLOOD PRESSURE

The sphygmomanometer in use. Most people have seen this instrument but few understand it. An elastic bag is wrapped snugly around the patient's arm, and by pumping this full of air it is caused to press against blood vessels. When the pressure is high enough it halts the circulation by compressing the blood vessel, and this pressure is measured by the rise of a column of mercury in a graduated glass tube. The significance of blood pressure is more fully explained in the text.
© *Ewing Galloway*

interest and concern tends to show that arteriosclerosis is a disease giving an index to the general health, and forming a reflex of the victim's mode of life.

"A man," says an old proverb, "is as old as his arteries." Not long ago this was accepted by every physician as an exact statement of the truth. When "hardened arteries," or arteriosclerosis, presented themselves in the consulting room, a very gloomy view of the patient was always taken. But in recent years a great deal of new light has been cast on this rather mysterious disease, with the result that the gloom has somewhat lightened.

Sir James Mackenzie, for example, pointed out that "hardening" of the arteries is quite common in young and fit men and women. If their pulses are felt the blood vessel can be rolled under the finger against the bone of the wrist. Yet if these young people take a hot bath the hardening goes away at once and the artery becomes quite soft again, so that it can scarcely be felt at all. Clearly this is not a true hardening and should not be described as arteriosclerosis. It is due to a cramp or spasm of the tiny muscles in the wall of the blood vessel. The hot water causes these muscles to relax and so relieve it.

Causes. Not one but a hundred causes have been thought of to explain these vascular changes. If we consider for a moment that from the very day of our birth we are increasingly suffering from age, we can see how it is that many circumstances may contribute to the increased tension, to the overthickening of the walls of the arteries, to the subsequent degenerations and permanent hypertrophy of the muscular coats. The disease varies, too, according to its locality. All these points must now be enlarged upon.

High Blood Pressure. First, in the condition known as hypertension, the amount of blood pressure is generally above 160 millimeters of mercury. Clifford Allbutt called this form of high blood pressure hyperpiesia, and showed that it may occur in people who are active, highly strung, hard workers, living a life of stress and strain and generally doing the work of creation or of advanced and difficult performance under extreme difficulties, *e.g.* those of our modern civilization. In many of these cases the blood pressure may be permanently raised to as much as 180 millimeters, and the effect of advanced age need not be taken into consideration because often people in the twenties and thirties suffer in this way.

On examination there is little or no evidence of disease of the arteries; the heart is apparently normal. But it must

DISORDERS OF THE BLOOD VESSELS

always be remembered that hyperpiesia may lead to pathological arteriosclerosis with definite anatomical changes in the vessel wall. Thus, the victims of it may be expected to have hardened arteries of more or less senile type in early middle age. The one thing that may change the situation is change of habits, character, and method of living, but how many can hope to do this?

Excessive adrenal action (see Chapter 96) has a great effect on the sustaining of high blood pressure, and in view of the elucidation of the effect of adrenalin on the sympathetic system and on the opening of the capillary gates, it is probable that hyperpiesia is a reaction to the activities of the great capillary network that supplies the cells with blood.

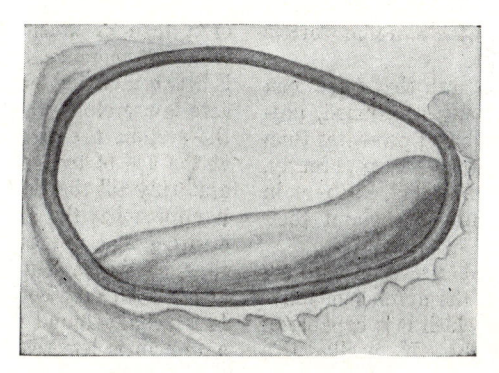

Here we may conveniently refer to the phenomenon of blood pressure.

Blood pressure may be defined as the expansive force exerted upon the walls of the blood vessels by their contents. It is usual in speaking of the blood pressure to ignore the pressure in the veins and to consider only that in the arteries. Pressure in the circulatory system is the resultant of the driving force of the heart's contraction prolonged in its action by the elastic recoil of the larger vessels and the obstructive effect of the smaller arteries and capillaries. Were it not for this steadying influence of elastic walls and peripheral resistance the blood stream would consist of a series of powerful spurts instead of the almost even flow which is the rule in health. The blood pressure also varies with the amount of blood in the vessels.

ATHEROMA OF A LARGE ARTERY
Cross section of an artery showing how calcium salts are deposited in the wall of a blood vessel in the same way that "fur" tends to collect inside a kettle.

When a man is excited his heart beats more strongly and at once his blood pressure rises. If he receives a large amount of fluid intravenously his blood volume increases and his pressure rises. If he goes out on a cold day the small vessels in his skin shut up, and again his blood pressure rises. Consequently blood pressure is never the same in anybody for two minutes on end. It fluctuates with every activity that is undertaken.

That fact is nearly always lost sight of by the public. The truth is that every man, during effort, has an enormously high blood pressure. It falls low enough when the effort comes to an end. An erroneous opinion of the state of the blood pressure when this is measured in a doctor's consulting room may be formed if the effect of excitement is not discounted. In these circumstances the pressure is always high in nervous people. A most dramatic fall of pressure will often follow the simple statement that there is nothing wrong with the patient's blood pressure. Anxiety is relieved, the heart quiets down and the pressure falls. Variations of blood pressure due to an increase or diminution of the circulating blood must also be remembered.

But it is obvious that if blood is to be moved about the body *en masse* it must, at times, flow in greater bulk along the vessels. There must be moments when all the blood channels of the body are full. These will be natural and normal moments of high blood pressure. At such moments, too, the heart will naturally be more active than usual, since there is more work for it to do in "moving" the blood mass. That, again, will tend to raise the pressure. Moreover, the least excitement or anxiety raises pressure. Thus, if a man begins to worry about his blood pressure, his blood pressure will tend to be high, and the more he worries the higher it will be.

The fact is also known that some men and women, as already mentioned, possess higher or lower blood pressures than others. These pressures are, apparently, necessary to their well-being, and remain more or less constant throughout their lives.

Records of blood pressure are expressed in terms of the number of millimeters of mercury which it is capable of supporting vertically. Naturally this figure varies according to the phase of the heart's activity at which the pressure is measured.

The figure taken at the instant of the heart's contraction, or "systole," is called the systolic pressure and is the maximum for the individual under investigation; the pressure reading taken during the resting period of the heart—"diastole"—is known as the diastolic pressure, and represents the normal distensile force exerted upon the vessel walls by the volume of blood within them while it is flowing in a steady stream. The difference between the systolic and diastolic pressures represents the driving force of the heart beats alone, and is known as the pulse pressure; its measurement gives an indication of the vigor of the heart muscle.

The factors upon which the height of the blood pressure depends, namely, the heart, the tone of the vessel walls, and the caliber of the small arteries, are all subject to control by the nervous system, and are liable to influences exerted by the secretions of certain glands or by chemical substances absorbed by the body or elaborated by its organs. Degenerative changes of obscure causation also play a part in bringing about alterations in the walls of the blood vessels by which their pliability is reduced and their power of expanding as each pulse wave passes along them is diminished.

In health the normal systolic pressure of a man of twenty-one is 120 millimeters of mercury, his diastolic pressure is between 65 and 80, and his pulse pressure is therefore about 50. In the child the systolic pressure is lower, about 70 at the age of twelve months, and rising gradually till the time of puberty, when it approaches the adult level. With increasing age the pressure very slowly rises, so that a figure of 150 to 160 in an old man may be regarded as normal. It is usually found that the pressure in a woman is less than that in a man of the same age, but there are physiological reasons why the woman shows wider variations at certain times. During exercise most people have a blood pressure of 180 to 200.

Two forms of instrument are in common use for measuring blood pressure—the mercury and the aneroid sphygmomanometer. They consist of an appliance by which a hollow airtight rubber bag is held in contact with

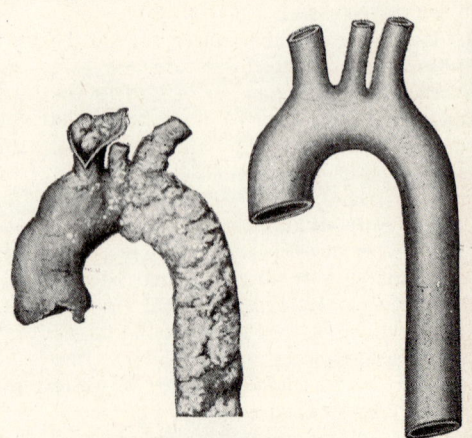

CALCIFICATION OF ARTERIES

In old age, arteries which are unhealthy may undergo calcification; that is, a deposit of calcium salts may accumulate in their walls. The walls of the aorta calcified (left), and a normal arch (right).

the arm by an armlet wound around the limb. To this bag is attached a rubber tube which has a small air pump at one end; by means of a T-shaped junction the armlet is connected with the manometer by which the pressure applied is recorded; the more accurate and constant form consists of a U-tube containing mercury, but for ease of transportation a small aneroid is very often used instead; its readings are of sufficient accuracy for ordinary purposes, but it is necessary to test the spring from time to time against a mercury manometer.

The doctor puts his finger on the patient's pulse and then slowly inflates the rubber bag by means of the airpump. Naturally, as the bag fills with air, it squeezes the arm, and so at last stops the blood from flowing down it. When that point is reached the pulse will no longer be felt at the wrist, because the "pulse" is that of one of the arteries of the arm. As soon as he feels the pulse disappear the doctor notes the figure to which the "hand" points or to which the mercury has risen. Then he gradually releases the air from the bag and, to check his first reading, notes the spot at which the pulse comes back again. That spot is called the systolic blood pressure, to distinguish it from the pressure in the vessel when the heart is resting between its beats, known as the diastolic blood pressure. Blood pressure can only be taken by an expert: an expert, too, is needed to interpret a special case.

Naturally it follows that excessive blood pressure is also a feature of cases which have progressed to the stage of arterial disease, associated as it may be with cardiac, renal, or other systematic disease causing permanent destructive changes in the arterial wall.

Old Age. What was said at the beginning of the chapter about old age may be referred to once more. After the age of fifty, the human being goes down the hill. His arteries bear evidence of the various uses to which they have been put. Some people inherit poor-quality elastic in the vessels; others play fast and loose with original good material; both end with premature old age.

Other Factors. There is reason to believe that infectious diseases may act as predisposing factors. Arteriosclerosis is apt to come on in patients with chronic foci of infection (tonsillitis, sinusitis, prostatitis) and after illnesses such as typhoid, malaria, and influenza. The frequency of arteriosclerosis in diabetics suggests a metabolic disturbance.

Syphilis. The effect of this blood disease is referred to below. Syphilis produces a particular variety of degeneration in the arterial wall.

Nature of the Condition. Depending upon the stage of the disease, we find different evidences on post-mortem examination. For instance, in the aorta there may be found small plateaus in the neighborhood of the branching arteries. So far as can be ascertained this is a local rising up of the tunica intima (the lining of the vessel). The patches are a dirty yellow in color. They become hardened by calcium salts later on and give rise to the condition known as atheroma, in which necrosis and ulceration may occur.

In the smaller vessels there may be widespread thickening of the intimal coat, elastic tissue is increased, and to a certain extent there is overgrowth of the middle coat. As time goes on the fibrous deposits increase, and in old age we are presented with the example of fully established arteriosclerosis, with tortuous vessels, walls degenerated and thinned, and deposits of chalky material all over, so that in the classical phraseology the radial artery at the wrist twists like a snake and is as hard as a pipe stem. The whole bore of the vessel may be filled up —a condition called endarteritis obliterans. On the inner surface of the aorta may be seen patches of chalky degeneration, as if an attempt had been made to mend a hole with rough cement.

So far as syphilis is concerned, the chief damage is generally in the middle and outer coats, a more generalized

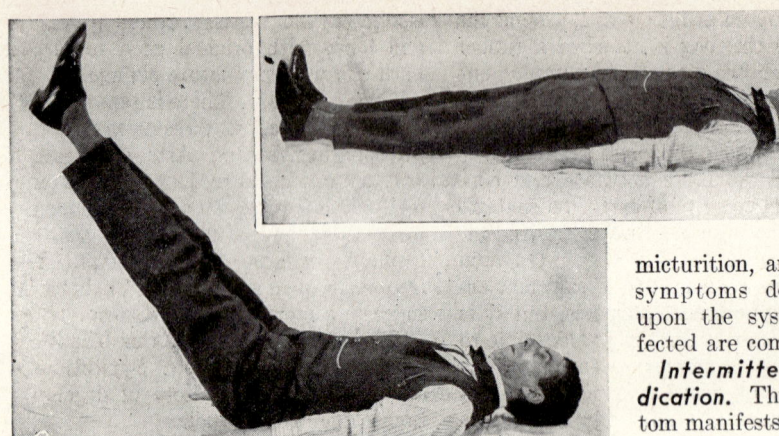

EXERCISE IN THREATENED ARTERIOSCLEROSIS
(1) The patient should lie flat on his back, arms at the sides, palms downwards, and with the muscles of the body well braced. (2) Keeping the body flat on the ground, the patient raises both legs to the height shown in the photograph, and holds them there for a moment before resuming the first position.

arteritis occurring in the first part of the aorta. This condition is entirely distinct from arteriosclerotic changes.

Symptoms. The dangers of high blood pressure are apoplexy (cerebral hemorrhage), nose bleeding (epistaxis) and heart failure, with severe anginal pain. Attacks of dizziness, coldness of the extremities, mental dullness, irritability of the mind, bad temper, frequency of micturition, and other symptoms depending upon the systems affected are common.

Intermittent Claudication. This symptom manifests itself by transient attacks of weakness with muscular cramps. It commonly affects one or both legs, though similar symptoms may occur in the arm. Moderate exercise may bring on an attack.

After walking normally for a short distance, the patient is surprised by a sudden pain and loss of power in his legs. He develops a limp and the limbs give way. In some cases the pain is very severe and it may radiate from the thigh to the ankle. Within a very short time both pain and weakness disappear as if by magic. The man, crippled a minute before, rises and resumes his walk in a perfectly normal manner.

With rare exceptions intermittent claudication attacks the male sex only, and it seldom occurs before the age of fifty years. The brief seizures result from a lack of sufficient blood supply in the affected limb. The hardened, constricted vessels cannot dilate and supply the increased need for blood that accompanies exercise.

This remarkable disorder is a sign, therefore, of unhealthy arteries. As the disease progresses the pain may become con-

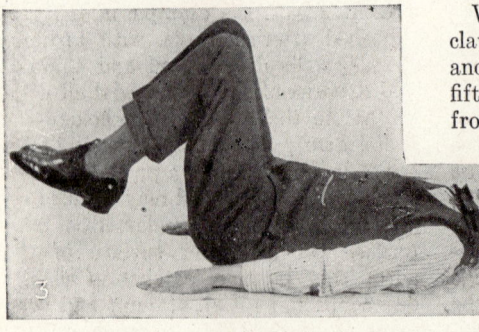

EXERCISE IN THREATENED ARTERIOSCLEROSIS
(3) A variant of the preceding exercise is to bend the knees sharply after reaching the second position, straightening them again before lowering them to the floor.

stant and remain even when the patient is at rest. Intermittent claudication should be regarded as a warning, and the patient should seek treatment without delay before worse things befall.

Treatment. The first attention of a sufferer from arteriosclerosis should be given to personal hygiene. He must see to it that the bowels are emptied well and completely each morning, and if possible again before retiring. This object can, no doubt, be achieved by taking laxatives; but this is an unsatisfactory way of attaining it. The constant use of cathartics is to be avoided as weakening and destructive of the bowel's own powers and the physiological rhythm of its activities. The right way is to educate the bowel to perform its own work in the proper manner.

This means a little care and patience in the first instance. The human bowel is supported in the body by the muscles of the front of the abdomen. These muscles, if toned up, help to keep the bowel active and in good position, but if flabby they allow the bowel to sag down and so hinder its action. Thus the first step in the avoidance of constipation is the production of a strong and supporting abdominal wall. There is a simple exercise which all may practise; it consists in drawing in the belly a few times, three or four times a day. This may seem a small matter, but such indrawing greatly strengthens the muscles and also gives the bowel a valuable stimulation. A second type of exercise is that of lying flat on the floor and raising the legs and trunk in the ways shown in the photographs on this and the facing page. This is a very valuable means of strengthening muscles, but in cases of arteriosclerosis should not be undertaken without medical advice.

Outdoor exercise and games suitable to the age and condition should be practised regularly. It is a great mistake to send unfit people to play strenuous games of golf. They may, with advantage, become golfers, but the process certainly ought to be slow and gradual.

It should, indeed, like all forms of exercise, keep pace with the patient's reserve. There are men who say, with reason, that golf has saved them from arteriosclerosis; there are others who believe that it has cured them of this disease. But there must be many who have done themselves harm by excessive exercise before they were fit to stand it.

Diet. The diet, generally speaking, should be frugal. Overeating is to be condemned. So also should be the use of

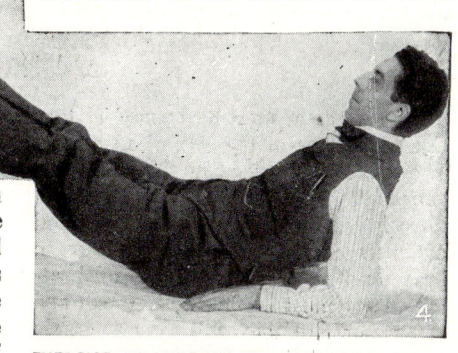

EXERCISE IN THREATENED ARTERIOSCLEROSIS
(4) A more difficult exercise than those on the opposite page. Rise on the elbows from the first position and, with the back at the angle shown, raise the legs. After some practice it will be possible to raise legs and shoulders simultaneously.

alcohol, which certainly aggravates these cases greatly. Water should be drunk freely between meals. Meat foods, including fish and chicken, should be taken sparingly—not oftener than once each day.

The patient must not overload his system, nor poison it, but rather try to return to simplicity so that his resistance may be strengthened, his muscles also strengthened, and his ability to take and enjoy exercise improved. He should wear light clothing, so as to obtain the stimulation of a cool skin, and he should, of course, sleep with open windows. Such measures as these greatly reduce the danger of complications and may even bring the arteriosclerosis under control entirely so that no shortening of life is caused by its presence. Obviously, the sooner the cautionary procedures are begun, the better.

Arteriosclerosis is very apt to be found in connection with Bright's disease. When the kidneys share in the damage the situation is, of course, more serious, since these organs then fail to get rid of the poisons circulating. It is obvious that hardening of the arteries must exercise an influence on every organ of the body, since every organ is entirely dependent for its supply of blood on these vessels. A hard artery is less efficient than a soft one; it is also more liable to break. An examination frequently reveals hardened and twisted vessels in the eye when arteriosclerosis exists, and sometimes loss of sight follows the breakage of such arteries. Again, hardening of the arteries of the brain may lead to apoplexy, which is due to a bursting of a brain artery. It may also lead to serious heart disease (angina pectoris), owing to gradual closing up of the small blood vessels which supply the heart. These, however, are consequences, not causes of the trouble. If the trouble is mastered early there should be good hope that the consequences will not supervene.

ANEURYSM

An aneurysm may be termed a dilation or bulging of the wall of an artery. The pressure of blood in the arteries is very high. These vessels carry the blood directly from the heart to the organs and members of the body, and so have to bear the full force of its powerful beating. They must be uniformly tough and elastic, or else they will tend to strain and then to bulge. If one part, however small, has any weakness, there will be a tendency to bulging at that part—in other words an aneurysm will begin to form.

Anything which weakens the wall of an artery anywhere may cause an aneurysm. The two commonest causes are injury and disease. The First World War furnished a very large number of injury aneurysms of various kinds. If a bullet or piece of shell grazed the wall of a blood vessel, the wall was weakened. After a time there was apt to be a bulging at this place. Thus, aneurysms were found by military surgeons in the arms and legs, the neck, the chest, the body—wherever, in fact, an artery runs and a bullet or shell fragment might strike.

Speaking generally, such aneurysms are not likely to prove fatal unless they occur in some very inaccessible place; for nature has gifted us richly in the matter of blood vessels. If one vessel goes out of action other smaller vessels

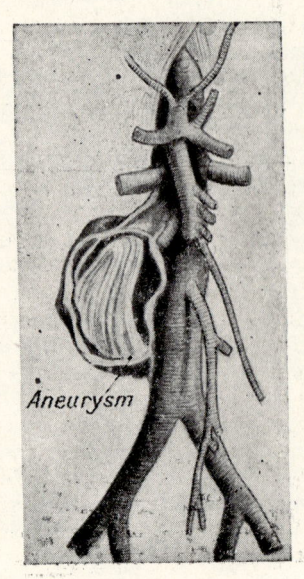

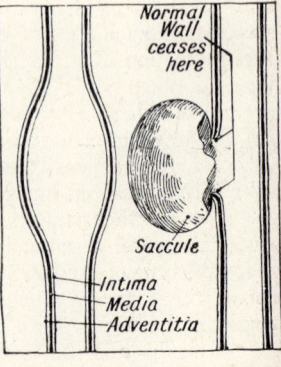

HOW AN ANEURYSM OCCURS

Above: aneurysmal dilatation shared by all the coats of an artery, and right: localized dilatation at a weak spot. Left: aneurysm in the abdominal aorta—layers of clot in suscessive deposits.

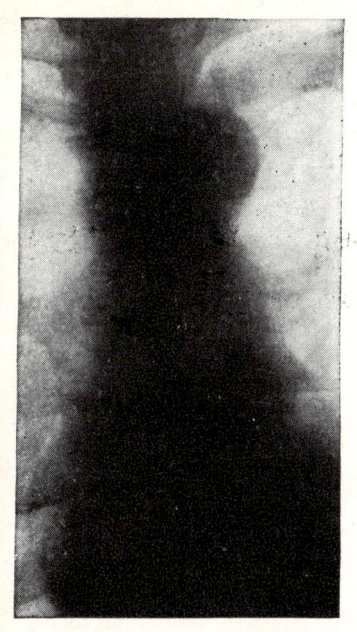

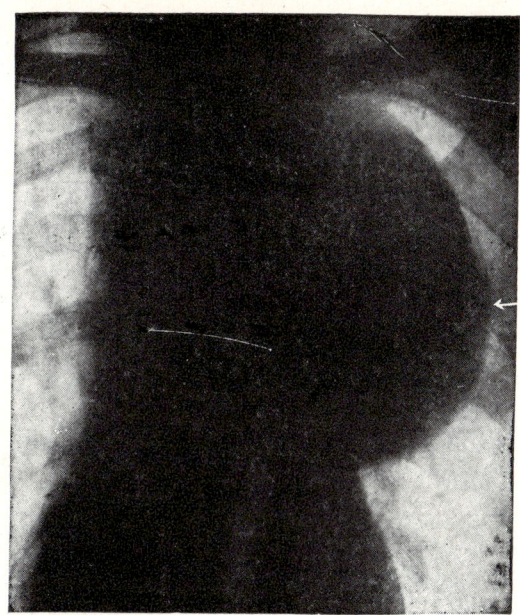

ANEURYSM OF THE AORTA REVEALED BY X-RAYS

Left: photograph of normal aorta, showing the arch and origin of the vessel from the heart. Right: aortic aneurysm, the large black shadow of which exceeds ordinary limits. With a fluorescent screen the vessels and the aneurysm can be seen pulsating.

open up and grow wider, and so carry on the circulation; this process is known as anastomosis.

The treatment of aneurysms of the limbs is, as a rule, to shut the blood vessels on which they are situated—a simple surgical operation. But this treatment cannot be employed when the aneurysm is situated in the greatest of all blood vessels, the aorta, which is the main trunk leading right out of the heart. There is no other way around in the case of this large and important vessel, which is so wide that it can accommodate two or even three fingers.

So far as ordinary civilian life is concerned, aneurysms of the aorta amount to about 90 per cent of all aneurysms. They are much more frequent in men than in women. The great majority of cases are due to disease of the blood-vessel wall, such as syphilis.

Sir William Macewen invented an operation for aneurysms of the aorta. He pushed long, thin needles right into the bulge in the blood vessel, and left them there for a few minutes. The needles were moved about by the current of blood and were thus kept pricking the lining of the blood vessels. If a blood vessel is injured on the inside, a clot of blood usually forms at the injured place, and Sir William Macewen's idea was to make clots form and so fill up the bulge. Electricity has also been used to bring about clotting with the same object.

Apart from this treatment, the usual way to deal with aneurysms of the aorta is to make sure that the patient leads a quiet life as free as possible from stress of all sorts. Complete rest in bed for some months on a very restricted diet is sometimes successful in delaying the progress of the trouble. In all cases the diet should be very light and moderate, and alcohol is to be forbidden. All muscular strain must be avoided.

Pain, which is often very severe, is due to the pressure of the bulging blood vessel on the nerves in its neighborhood. Other common symptoms of aneurysms of the aorta, also due to pressure on nerves, are a metallic tone of the voice and a cough resembling the sound made by a gander. When the case is very advanced the swollen vessel may be felt beating against the wall of the chest.

There is no doubt that the majority of aortic aneurysms are due to syphilis, affecting the small blood vessels which supply the wall of the aorta, leading to its degeneration. Treatment of the syphilitic infection will sometimes cause marked improvement in the aneurysm.

Aneurysms elsewhere than in the aorta are usually dealt with by ligature; that is to say, a strong thread is tied tightly around the artery, sometimes below the aneurysm, but much more frequently above it. The effect of this is to shut off or at least diminish the force of the blood stream so that the dilatation becomes filled up with clot and is obliterated; later the clot is replaced by fibrous or scar tissue. In the case of an aneurysm affecting a limb artery, the vessel can be tied above and below the dilatation, which is then removed like an ordinary tumor. The parts supplied by the artery which has been ligatured then depend for their blood supply on the collateral circulation provided by anastomosis.

DISEASES OF THE VEINS

Phlebitis. Derived from the Greek *phleps*, a vein, phlebitis means inflammation of a vein, and can be divided into two distinct varieties. There is a septic type associated with suppuration and a simple type which is not so associated. The former is much the more serious, and it may occur as a result of germs circulating in the blood and settling in a vein, or it may be due to the spread of a septic process from around a vein to the vein itself.

The simple type may be either acute or chronic. Causes of acute simple phlebitis are injury to a vein, gout (in which disease it may occur either during an attack of inflammation of the joints or independently of such attacks), the formation of a clot within the vein, *i.e.*, thrombosis, or in long confinement to bed with an acute illness such as typhoid fever. It may also occur as a result of anemia or may follow operations, especially those on the lower part of the abdomen. A special variety called phlegmasia alba dolens, or white leg, sometimes follows childbirth. The chronic variety is due to chronic inflammation around the vein.

Phlebitis may attack any vein in the body, but by far the commonest site is one of the veins of the lower limbs. In septicemia several veins may be attacked almost simultaneously.

Symptoms. Usually the first symptom noticed is pain along the course of the affected vein. If the vein is near the surface it can be felt as a hard cord and the skin over it may be reddened and swollen. There is usually a feeling of general discomfort and a rise of temperature seldom exceeding 102° F. in the nonsuppurative type.

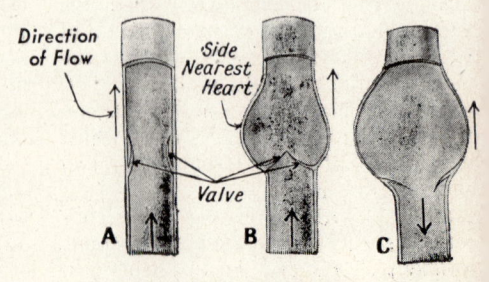

USELESS VALVES IN VARICOSE VEINS
The column of blood in a vein is supported by the valves, two flaps which open in the direction of the flow (A), and close against it, (B). Dilatation of the vein as it becomes varicose (C) makes the valves inefficient because the flaps can no longer meet.

DISORDERS OF THE BLOOD VESSELS

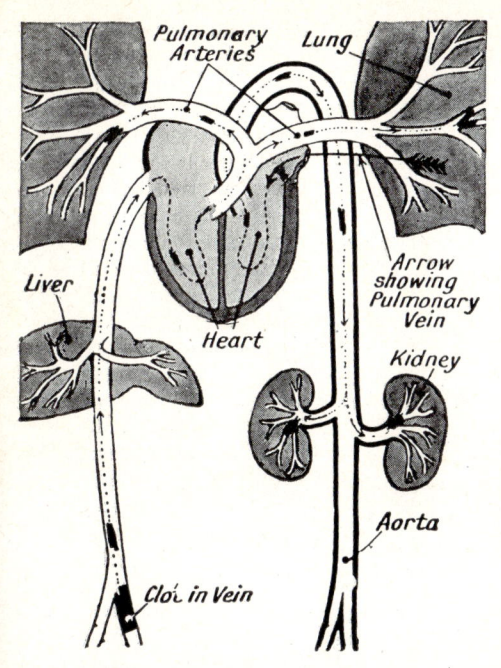

PHLEBITIS: INFLAMMATION OF VEINS
A possible result of phlebitis. Detached clot passes to the heart and thence to the lungs. Further clot forming in the lungs as a result of this can be carried to any organ.

The course of phlebitis depends almost entirely upon whether thrombosis occurs. In the septic variety this invariably happens, while in the simple variety it is frequent, but does not always follow. In the absence of thrombosis, the fever subsides in a few days and by the end of two weeks the signs have usually disappeared entirely.

In the chronic variety the signs are similar to those of acute phlebitis, but less severe and more prolonged, and there may be a series of relapses and improvements. The outlook here also depends upon whether thrombosis takes place. All cases must be regarded seriously, and careful treatment must be carried out.

Treatment. As soon as the condition is recognized the patient must be strictly confined to bed. If the phlebitis occurs in a limb, the affected limb should be raised so as to assist the return of blood along the vein. It should be wrapped up in a thick layer of absorbent cotton and the bedclothes should be supported to prevent pressure. All sudden movements, unnecessary handling, and rubbing must be avoided. Death has been known to follow such treatment.

Glycerine and belladonna gently painted on the affected part help to relieve the pain. The bowels must be kept acting freely. The diet will depend to a certain extent upon the cause of the phlebitis. Such conditions as gout and anemia must receive their appropriate diet.

This treatment must be persisted in until all signs have disappeared and the danger of thrombosis is over. Usually this will be about two weeks, after which time gentle passive movements of the limb may be started, followed in a few days by light massage and then by active movements. At the end of about four weeks the patient may be allowed up.

In septic phlebitis, clotting is always present and the treatment is that already advised for thrombosis in the earlier part of this chapter.

Varicose Veins. A vein is said to be varicose (Latin *varus*, twisted) when it has become dilated, tortuous, and lengthened. Many veins can be thus affected, but by far the most common lesions are found in the legs, and this is particularly true of the internal and external saphenous veins. These veins have to return a very large volume of blood to the heart against gravity. They will be dealt with first.

There is frequently a congenital weakness of the walls or an irregularity in the valves. Such valves are unable to withstand any extra call upon the circulation, and so become affected after very slight strains or even without any obvious cause at all. Naturally, any condition which leads to frequent or permanent distension of these structures will in all probability result in the ultimate appearance of the condition of varicosity.

Obvious examples are found in those callings which involve long standing, but tight garters are also culpable, while the pressure exerted by a pregnant uterus is one of the most common starting points of this condition among women. Other causes are found in the obstruction to and occlusion of deeper veins as a result of thrombosis, injury, or growths. But, in any case, once this venous distension has occurred it renders the valves of the veins incompetent, so that the weight of the superincumbent blood is not supported but excites still further pressure.

Signs and Symptoms. On examination these dilated vessels can be seen ramifying under the skin with a very twisted course. In marked cases there are large clusters which shine through the thin epidermis as bluish masses. Sometimes only the very tiny venules are obviously affected, and these are, of course, more serious in that little can be done to correct their state. Symptoms may be absent, but a common complaint is that of a feeling of heaviness and weariness. Swelling of the ankle with edema may be present. The congestion and stasis may lead to impairment of the nutrition of the skin, so that the slight rubbing of any area of irritation tends to render it eczematized. Even the smallest injury may cause a varicose ulcer to form. The treatment of these is discussed in Chapter 161.

Danger of Clotting. A more serious sequel is thrombosis or clotting, which is very liable to appear even after a light blow as well as during any more serious infective illness. If all goes well the clot may remain stationary and become converted into fibrous tissue so that the lumen is occluded and the condition thus automatically cured. It may even become calcareous and so form hard phleboliths or vein stones. Unfortunately the thrombosis may spread and fragments of clot may become detached, being carried around the blood stream as small solid particles or emboli which ultimately block a vessel in the lungs, kidneys or brain. Yet another possible complication is found in the fact that a dilated pouch may burst and give rise to an alarming flow of blood after it has received a blow or become involved in the ulceration.

Palliative Treatment. The exigencies of life demand that palliative rather than radical treatment should often be preferred by the patients. For this it is absolutely essential to remove tight and constricting clothing, and to avoid standing as much as possible. The legs should be elevated on a pillow at night or the foot of the bed raised. Gentle massage should consist of stroking movements only, these being performed only from the foot upwards and in such a direction as to aid the flow of blood. The bowels must be kept well open, the abdominal muscles kept firm and taut by special exercises, and the general health attended to.

Many victims find it helpful to wear supports in the form of crêpe bandages or elastic stockings. These must be applied first thing in the morning while the leg is not swollen, and so should be put on even while the patient is lying in bed. They should not be so tight as to cause local anemia and they should be sufficiently long to control all the veins involved. The elastic bandage is always applied by winding it spirally upwards.

Varicose veins can be obliterated by the injection of preparations of salicylic acid, sodium morrhuate, etc., into their

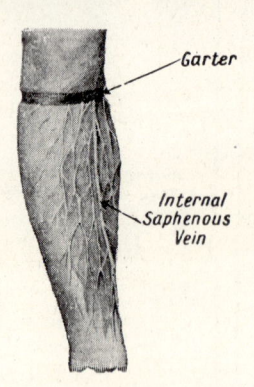

PRESSURE ON VEINS
The result of a garter or other constricting band; the veins swell and their valves fail.

DISORDERS OF THE BLOOD VESSELS

lumen. As a result of the injection the lumen of the vein is closed by the mild inflammation set up in its wall. Other and more healthy veins take over its function. This treatment does not involve a stay in bed and is painless, and in suitable cases very effective.

Radical Treatment. Radical treatment consists in the excision of the distended vessels. In one operation the upper end of the internal saphenous vein and its local tributaries only are removed. In others, and particularly when the veins are lower in the leg, small portions can be removed. Under modern technique, however, it is more general to dissect out and excise all those vessels which are obviously affected.

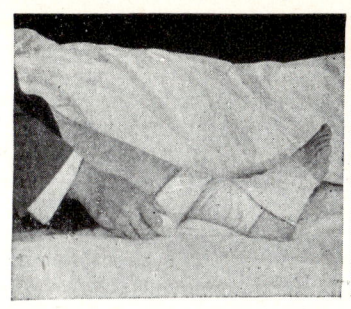

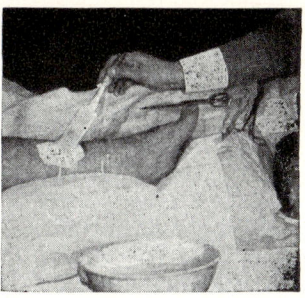

A woven elastic bandage should be put on before getting out of bed in the morning. Eczema or ulceration can be treated by applying appropriate medicated paste, if prescribed by the doctor, over the unhealthy portions of skin.

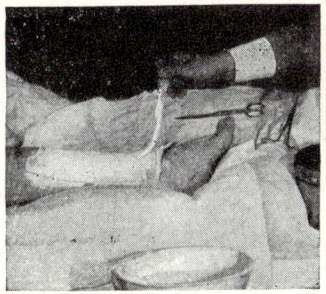

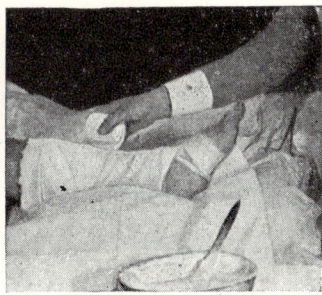

TREATMENT OF VARICOSE VEINS

A layer of gauze and paste may be used if deemed necessary. The final layer of paste is covered with gauze and with lint or absorbent cotton and the limb is then bandaged from below upwards.

Varicocele and Hemorrhoids. There are yet two other groups of vessels which are not uncommonly affected by varix. The spermatic veins are often found in such a condition and particularly those on the left side. This constitutes the state known as varicocele in which there can be felt a bunch of hard and distended veins in the scrotum. While many patients prefer to wear a suspensory bandage in order to lessen the aching pain, the only real treatment lies in operation, removal of the veins being effected through a short incision in the region of the junction of the scrotum and groin. Hemorrhoids, or piles (considered in Chapter 118) consist of a varicose condition of the veins surrounding the anus and the lower parts of the rectum; according to the location they are referred to as external and internal piles respectively.

RAYNAUD'S DISEASE

This disease is characterized by repeated attacks of interference with the circulation in various parts of the body, most commonly in the fingers and toes, and is probably due to spasm of the small arteries to the affected part. It may occur at any age, but usually begins in early adult life and affects females much more frequently than males. Heredity has a definite influence on its causation, and it is somewhat more liable to occur in persons of neurotic tendency.

The actual attacks are brought on by exposure to cold, which may be only of a mild degree, or occasionally by emotional disturbances. They naturally occur most frequently in the winter, and the disease is hardly ever met with in warm climates.

The parts most often affected are the fingers, with perhaps involvement of the whole hand, but the affected region rarely extends above the wrist. Next in order of frequency are the toes and feet, but the affected region seldom goes above the ankles; then the ears and the tip of the nose, but very rarely the chin. Both sides of the body are simultaneously affected.

There are usually three stages in an attack. At first the fingers, if these are the affected parts, become cold and white and have a waxen appearance, so-called dead fingers. There is a feeling of numbness and stiffness and perhaps tingling. This stage may last only a few minutes or up to an hour or more. In the second stage the affected parts become blue, sometimes almost black. They are extremely cold, tender to the touch, and slightly swollen. Pain of varying severity is present. After some time, which may

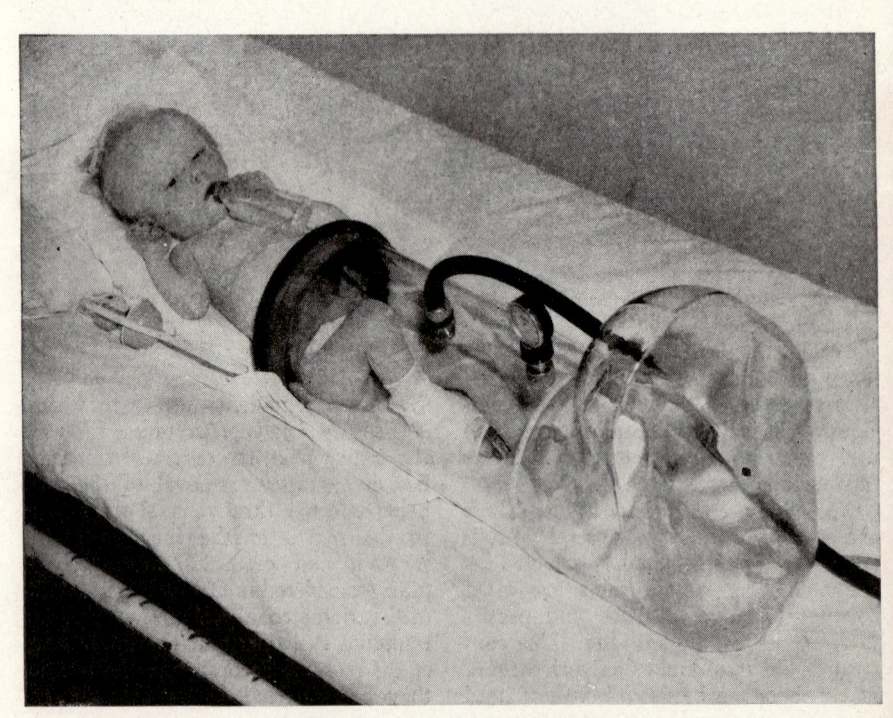

TO STIMULATE ARRESTED CIRCULATION

In severe cases of Raynaud's disease resort may be had to a pressure-suction boot in order to renew the flow of blood in the affected parts. Alternating high and low pressure is intended to dilate and compress the blood vessels, admitting and expelling blood until natural function is restored. The condition of the skin can be observed through the glass of the boot, and an alternate flushing and paling indicates the coming and going of blood. The boot shown is intended to accommodate one leg of an adult; the child is a patient at the Garfield Hospital, Washington, D.C.

© *Harris & Ewing*

DISORDERS OF THE BLOOD VESSELS

be several hours or even days, the arteries relax and blood flows into the parts again, making them hot, red, and swollen, with a throbbing pain. This gradually passes off and the part returns to normal.

Cases vary very much in severity, and in mild ones only the first stage may occur. Chilblains are really a mild form of Raynaud's disease. In severe cases, if the second stage is sufficiently severe and prolonged, gangrene may result. The part becomes quite black, very cold, and remains very painful. Small blisters filled with bloodstained fluid appear on it. Later a line of separation appears between the gangrenous and the healthy part, and the former is gradually shed.

Certain other symptoms are occasionally associated with Raynaud's disease, probably due to similar spasm of the arteries in other parts of the body. For example, some patients have periodical attacks of passing blood in the urine, due to affection of the vessels of the kidneys, as a result of exposure to cold, a condition known as paroxysmal hemoglobinuria. As a rule, Raynaud's disease involves no danger to life, but the attacks tend to recur every winter over a period of many years.

Prevention and Treatment. Treatment should in the first place be directed toward preventing the occurrence of attacks. The patient should always be warmly clad in the winter, with woolen garments next to the skin. Loose-fitting shoes and warm gloves should be worn out of doors. Wintering in a warm climate is an almost certain preventive of attacks. The diet should be arranged so as to prevent gastric disturbances, and the bowels must be carefully regulated. A considerable quantity of fat in the diet is helpful, or cod-liver oil may be taken throughout the winter. If the general health is below par, or if there is anemia, tonics containing iron and arsenic should be given. The hands should never be washed in cold water. Electrical treatment, such as galvanism, applied to the affected parts, has a beneficial effect.

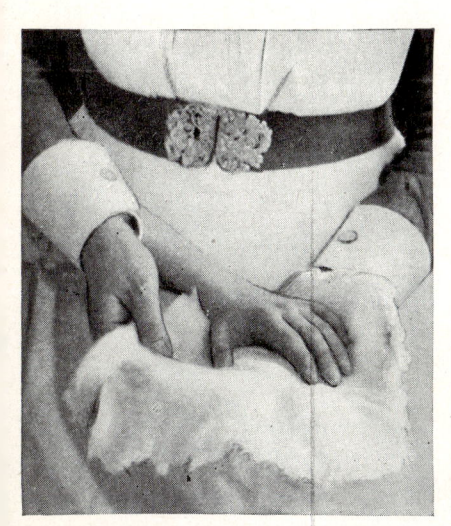

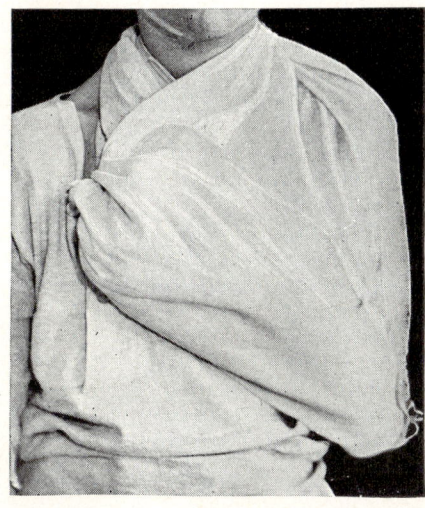

TREATMENT OF DEAD FINGERS AND ELEVATION OF THE AFFECTED PART
Left: when a tendency to dead fingers displays itself the hand or other part affected may be wrapped up warmly in a thick layer of absorbent cotton in conjunction with other kinds of treatment. Right: when it is actually the fingers that are affected, after being covered with cotton the hand is supported in a high position by a sling; for the toes, the foot is put on a cushion.

Drugs have little or no effect in most cases, except for the relief of pain, but occasionally calcium lactate or nitroglycerin seems to have diminished the frequency of attacks.

The treatment of an attack depends upon its severity. In mild cases, or in the first stage, gentle rubbing is all that is necessary. In more severe cases it is best to wrap the part in absorbent cotton. Sometimes an attack occurring in the hands or feet may be cut short by the application of an elastic tourniquet to the limb. It is put on tightly enough to cut off the arterial circulation, left in position for a few minutes, and then removed, allowing the blood to rush suddenly into the part. This may abolish the spasm, though it may be necessary for the application of the tourniquet to be repeated several times.

Cures have occurred following section of the sympathetic fibers to the affected limb. This operation produces vascular dilatation and prevents the occurrence of spasm.

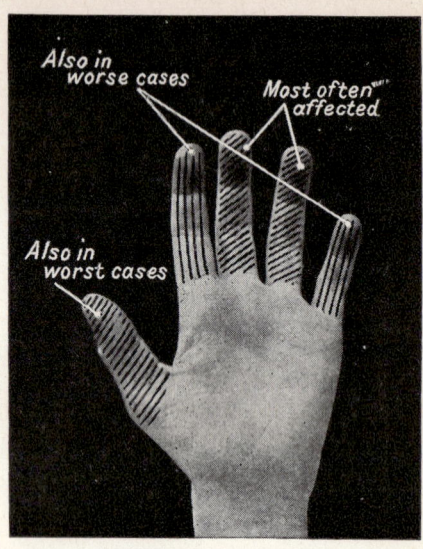

RAYNAUD'S DISEASE

Markings on the fingers in the illustration indicate the varying degrees of liability to the circulatory changes described as dead fingers; first, the ring and middle fingers, then the other two, and lastly the thumb.

Section XV Diseases of the Respiratory System

CHAPTER 106

DISORDERS OF THE NOSE AND NASOPHARYNX

Acute Nasal Catarrh — Chronic Nasal Catarrh — Rhinitis — Ozena — Hay Fever — Sinus Disease — Nasal Polypus.

THE nose, besides being part of the respiratory tract, is also the seat of the sense of smell, and a few words on the alterations of this function as the result of injury or disease may be useful. The olfactory nerve, or nerve of smell, is derived from the front part of the brain, and passes through a number of small holes in the bone of the skull into the nose, where it is spread over the mucous membrane of the upper and back part of the nasal cavities, its small terminal filaments being supplied with a special apparatus to which it owes its peculiar powers. In ordinary quiet breathing through the nose, the air hardly enters into the parts of the cavity gifted with the power of smell, but passes along the lower passages. If, however, the air is drawn in by the action of sniffing, in which the nostrils are compressed, it is driven up into the sensitive region of the nose. The air can also reach this region through the throat from the mouth, and all substances which have volatile or gaseous flavors or scents are recognized in this way by the sense of smell, as much as, if not more than by that of taste; this is especially true of wine tasting, etc.

If for any reason the air cannot reach the sensitive parts of the nose, the sense of smell is impaired. In some forms of paralysis or deformity of the nose the power of sniffing is lost; in cases of polypus the passages are blocked; in a bad cold in the head the mucous membrane is so swollen that the nose is obstructed. All of these are examples of loss of smell from mechanical reasons. Sometimes the mucous membrane becomes dry and insensitive, or its power of perception may be blunted by overstimulation, as with the formerly prevalent habit of snuff taking. A blow on the nose has been known to be followed by loss of smell, probably because the injury has cracked the bone forming the roof of the nose, through which the nerve fibers pass, and has torn these fibers. The same condition may result from disease, especially disease of nervous origin, as

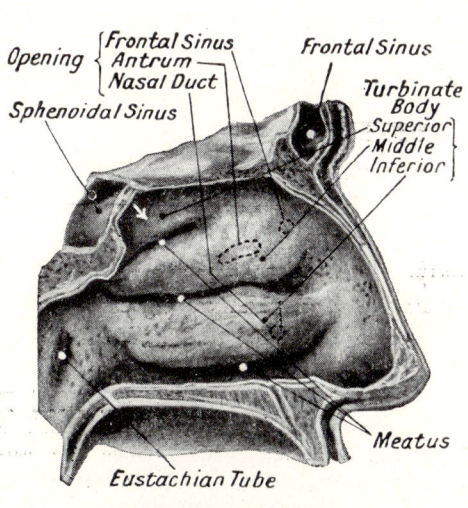

NOSE SEEN IN SECTION

Prominent here are the turbinated processes, covered with erectile tissue. These divide the cavity into four meatuses, or passages—uppermost, superior, middle, and inferior.

(1481)

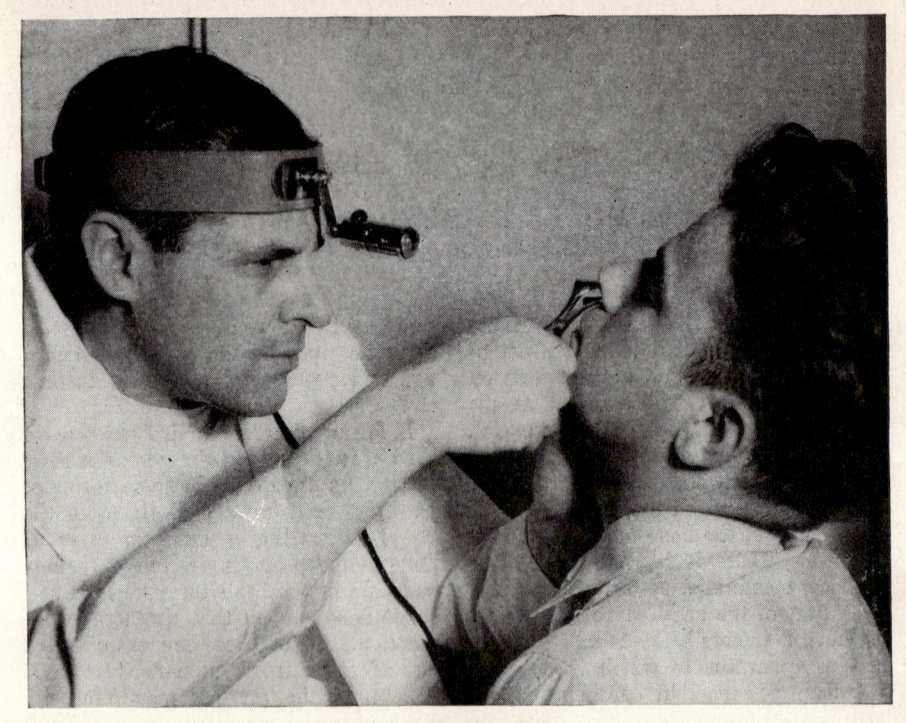

NASAL EXAMINATION

The instruments which the doctor uses to observe the nasal passages are simple—a light and a dilator. For examining the deeper passages reflectors arranged on the principle of the periscope, or even small cameras, may be used.

© *Ewing Galloway*

hysteria or brain affection. But perhaps the most common form of loss of smell is that which follows an attack of influenza. This may be complete for a time, but the sense of smell gradually returns as the general health is restored.

Acute Nasal Catarrh. The symptoms of coryza or "a cold in the head" are only too familiar, but although excessively unpleasant, the affection, if uncomplicated, is seldom at all serious. It consists of an inflammation of the mucous membrane lining the cavities of the nose, and as this is directly continuous with the mucous membrane lining other parts, the symptoms may vary according to the direction in which it spreads.

A feeling of chilliness, shivering, or even a chill ushers in many an attack of catarrh, and if the clinical thermometer is used a slight rise of temperature is discovered. Sneezing sets in, the nose feels stopped up and uncomfortable. The mucous membrane is swollen, full of blood, and very sensitive. It now begins to secrete a watery fluid, which requires constant blowing of the nose, so that the organ becomes red and sore, a condition which is aggravated by the irritating nature of the watery discharge. The catarrh may spread into the pharynx and produce sore throat with difficulty of swallowing; or it may pass along the Eustachian tubes and cause deafness and earache; or upwards into the cavities in the frontal bone, and give rise to heaviness and headache (sinusitis); or along the ducts to the eyes, and make them red, bloodshot, and watery; or into the larynx, with consequent hoarseness and cough; or into the mouth, making the tongue sore and the gums tender, setting up toothache and neuralgia; or finally downwards along the bronchial tubes to the lung, and end in a bad attack of bronchitis, or even pneumonia.

Preventing a Cold. Much can be done to prevent colds by raising the resistance to infection. This includes all the essentials of health—correct diet, bowel cleanliness, freedom from focal infections in the mouth, sufficient open-air life, adequate sleep, and avoidance of ill-ventilated, overheated rooms, and of chill and fatigue.

It has been shown that moderate exposure to cold air stimulates the secretion of the thyroid and adrenal glands, whereby the tone of the sympathetic nervous system controlling the internal organs and the elasticity of the blood vessels is maintained. It is a common experience that exercise in cold, bright weather stimulates the circulation and produces a general feeling of fitness, and there is no room for doubt that, to quote Leonard Hill and Mark Clement, the cause of the common cold "is not to be sought in meteorological conditions but rather in crowding in overheated and stuffy rooms, in ill-feeding and in 'coddling'." Probably the last-named cause is, in the majority of cases, the most important.

Animal fats and raw green vegetable leaves provide anti-infective vitamin. Sunlight, natural or artificial, is another aid to increased resistance. So is training the skin to react quickly to changes of temperature.

Tuberculosis treatment, sun bathing, and other measures by which regular exposure of the body to sun and air in all temperatures is carried out, have shown that not only are remarkable improvements obtained in conditions of disease, but that the increase of metabolism and production of body heat is a direct preventive of "colds." The expression "catching cold," is clearly an ancient and persistent popular misuse of the word cold.

Sitting with feet chilled by floor drafts and the head stuffy with the air of an ill-ventilated room, standing about in wet clothes or a cold wind until the body is chilled and shivering, are obvious causes of lowered vitality and reduced resistance to infection. Nor is it wise, when the body is heated by artificial means, to allow a cold draft to play on one part of it. These, however, are insufficient reasons for the still too prevalent fear of cold and open air. Clothing and personal habits should be adapted to changing climatic conditions and the open-air life should be practised as much as possible. Exposing the membranes of the air passages to infection by the viruses of catarrhal diseases is the great cause of these diseases, not drafts, and certainly not exposure of the healthy body to cold.

Certain local conditions predispose to the catching of a cold; deformed or unhealthy conditions of the structure of the nose and throat, such as

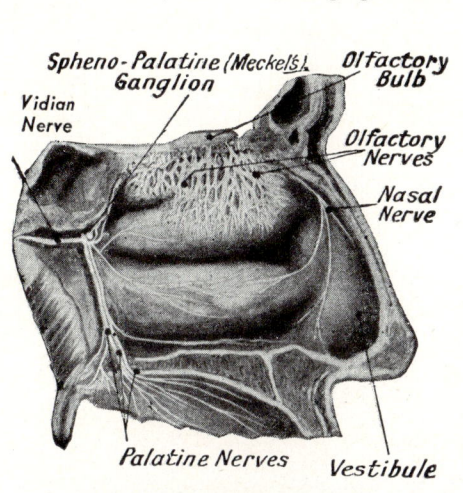

OLFACTORY NERVE IN NOSE

The branches of the olfactory nerve, which subserves the sense of smell, are distributed to the mucous lining of the upper third of the nasal cavities, being found both on the lateral and the central walls of these.

nasal obstruction, adenoids, and enlarged tonsils, are predisposing causes. Recurring colds, especially in children, should always arouse suspicion that there is chronic infection in the tonsils or back of the nose, and it is necessary to remember that a tonsil which is harboring virulent organisms is not always enlarged. If local disease of this nature is found it calls for prompt treatment. Highly susceptible persons can often be rendered less susceptible by a series of injections of a suitable vaccine given in the autumn and repeated during the winter. A so-called "stock" vaccine is usually employed. This preventive treatment will be more dependable when the nature of the infective agent is more definitely determined, as there is every hope it soon will be. Dochez and his coworkers have succeeded in isolating a virus which satisfies all the tests to which it may be put, and therefore it may be assumed that once definite conclusions are arrived at, the preparation of a specific anticoryza vaccine or serum will quickly follow. Thus it will be possible to provide both prophylactic and palliative injections for the "common cold."

Treatment. There are no measures which can be relied upon to stop a cold in its initial stages but bed rest for one to three days will in practically all cases shorten the duration of the illness and lessen the danger of complications. Some people always resort to camphor to check a cold; ten drops of the spirits of camphor in water or on a lump of sugar every half hour for three doses may be tried. A teaspoonful of the ammoniated tincture of quinine in water is also useful, although it is a remarkably unpleasant dose. Inhalations of eucalyptus oil are very soothing; it is well to use these when going to bed. A few drops of the oil are placed in a vessel of hot water, and the steam breathed in and out of the nose for a few minutes. Bathing the nose and forehead with very hot water is soothing, and relieves the feeling of congestion and lessens the discharge.

The instillation of a few drops of a 10 to 25 per cent solution of argyrol into each nostril is a widely used procedure but there is some doubt as to its bactericidal effect. When it is combined with adrenalin, some relief from the congestion occurs. In the later stages when the discharge is thick and mucopurulent, a 1 to 2 per cent silver nitrate solution is very beneficial.

If no success is met with in checking the cold in its first stage, when there is only a dry, sensitive, uncomfortable feeling in the nose, it is necessary to proceed to more active measures. Nothing now will relieve the symptoms so thoroughly as a good sweat, especially if the patient is at all feverish. He should go to bed and have something hot to drink—a cupful of hot gruel, a glassful of hot lemonade, or hot whisky-and-water with plenty of sugar. A hot bath, or putting the feet into hot water and mustard, has the same effect: it encourages perspiration and tends to draw away the blood from the head to other parts. Ten grains of aspirin or seven to ten grains of Dover's powder taken at bedtime cause

ORGANISM ASSOCIATED WITH NASAL CATARRH

One of the microbes most commonly present in conditions of respiratory catarrh is the Micrococcus catarrhalis, here seen in pure culture. It is magnified about 850 times.

a free sweat in the night, and the patient may get up in the morning without his catarrh. It is as well not to be in a hurry, however, to get up and about; better some extra hours in bed nursing a cold than the possibility of weeks with pneumonia acquired through going out again too soon.

The diet during the early and acute stages of a cold should be somewhat limited, and should consist of light solid and milk foods. This is particularly necessary if there is fever. In the later stages, however, the patient feels low and weakened, and it is then necessary to improve his condition and increase his strength by good feeding and perhaps a glass of wine. Warm simple drinks are usually very grateful to those suffering from a catarrh, and they find comfort in gruel, black-currant tea, and barley-water.

Chronic Nasal Catarrh. This sometimes follows repeated attacks of the acute form, but is much more often caused by the presence of an infection of one or more of the nasal sinuses. The lining membrane becomes thickened or even ulcerated, and from this comes the dirty, offensive discharge. It continues for a long time, and if not properly treated may spread deeply into all the nasal sinuses. A similar condition may be produced, though less commonly, by the presence of a foreign body in the nose, an accident most likely to be met with in children who amuse themselves by pushing buttons, peas, and such things up the nostrils. If these pass out of reach the child may forget their existence, and they are only discovered as a result of the investigation which is necessitated by reason of an offensive discharge being set up.

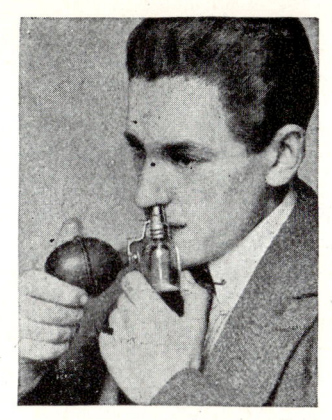

ATOMIZER
Inhalation through the nose while squeezing the rubber bulb will give great relief in the stuffy stages of a cold. See also page 1143.

To cure chronic nasal catarrh, healing applications must be applied to the cavities of the nose, and suitable treatment given to remedy the cause. For the latter, iron, cod-liver oil, and a high vitamin diet are useful. Locally, vapors may be used by inhalation, such as compound tincture of benzoin or menthol, or else sprays or nasal drops; or nasal solutions with the aid of a nasal douche. The last is certainly one of the most popular means of carrying out local treatment, and the nasal douche is easy to use. It is best not to use antiseptics, even mild ones, but rather to use alkaline solutions, such as bicarbonate of soda or even common salt, which dissolves the mucus. Since much injury and deformity may result from neglected cases, a doctor's advice should be obtained when possible.

Nasal Douching Apparatus. There are various forms of the nasal douche, and the simplest are the best. One of these is a peculiarly shaped little bottle, with a nozzle at one end and an opening at the other, through which the douche solution can be introduced; the nozzle is placed in one nostril and the solution poured into the nose, while the finger placed over the opening can control the flow. This douche is illustrated on page 1144.

Another form consists of a tube in the middle of which is a small ball. If the nozzle is placed in the nostril the flow of the solution can be started by squeezing the ball, and will continue to run by gravity. A simple pear-shaped nasal douche is very inexpensive and suitable.

Whichever form of nasal douche is preferred, care must be taken to use it

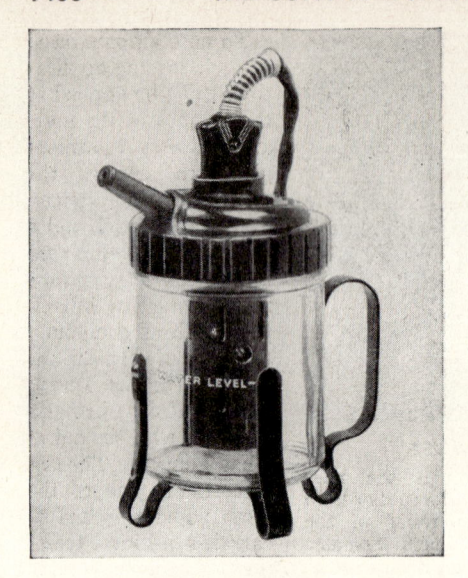

STEAM VAPORIZER

An electric heater and vapor nozzle are assembled into a unit in the jar cover. Medicine to be vaporized is poured into the jar, with water or other liquid according to the doctor's instructions, and heated until steam is produced. Substances which do not vaporize readily at ordinary temperatures can thus be inhaled to give relief from nasal inflammation or congestion. *Courtesy of DeVilbiss Co.*

very gently and the fluid must *not* be sniffed violently up. To use the douche the patient should bend the head slightly forward and open his mouth, breathing entirely through it. The nozzle of the douche is then introduced into the nostril and the fluid allowed to run freely. By breathing through the mouth the back of the nostrils is closed by the curtain of the soft palate, which is raised up into the opening, and the lotion will all run out of the other nostril, and none pass downwards into the throat. In this way the whole of the nasal cavities can be washed out thoroughly.

Rhinitis. This term is applied to all conditions of inflammation within the nose, a form of disease to which that organ is particularly liable. Probably the commonest form of rhinitis is an acute catarrh, more familiarly known as a cold in the head or nasal catarrh, already dealt with.

Chronic rhinitis occurs in many forms and leads to permanent changes in the mucous membrane of the nose. There are two main varieties, the atrophic and the hypertrophic. The former, as the name implies, results in wasting of the lining membrane; instead of being rich in blood vessels and somewhat velvety in appearance, it is pale, bloodless, and smooth. (See also Ozena, page 1487.)

Hypertrophic rhinitis is a disease in which the mucous membrane becomes thickened as the result of chronic inflammation. This gives rise to nasal obstruction, which is somewhat variable in its incidence. This is often relieved by a copious watery discharge, but the condition is chronic and obstruction is the main symptom.

The thickening is mainly confined to the inferior turbinal bone, but the adjacent part of the septum is often involved. The breathing space of the nasal chambers, at the best very narrow, requires but little swelling to close it; hence a small amount of temporary congestion, added to the hypertrophic condition already present, is sufficient to obstruct the nose completely.

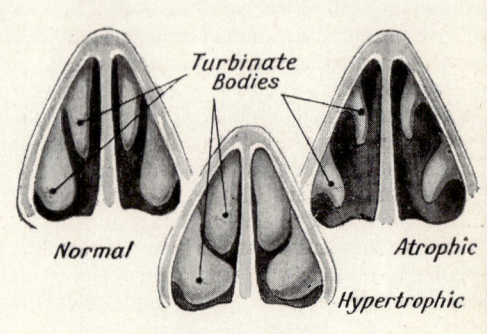

HOW RHINITIS AFFECTS THE AIRWAY

In hypertrophic rhinitis, from enlargement of the turbinate bodies, the airway is obstructed; while in atrophic rhinitis the airway is too large, so that inhaled air is not warmed and filtered.

Hypertrophic rhinitis is by no means an entirely local disease, the general health of the patient being at fault and resistance to infective catarrh lowered. There may be a neurasthenic element which renders the individual unduly susceptible even to minor degrees of the inconvenience.

Some patients are better in a dry, others in a moist, atmosphere.

Cleansing nasal douches are often of value, especially in the early stages. A solution for this purpose may be composed of a teaspoonful each of borax, bicarbonate of soda, and common salt dissolved in a half cupful of water; one part of this added to three parts of hot water will make a warm solution for douching.

In more stubborn cases it may be necessary to cauterize the mucous membrane, whereby the tissue is made to shrink. This simple procedure in experienced hands is often curative when combined with improved general hygiene.

The term rhinitis is also applied to suppuration within the nose. This may result from the presence of a foreign body in the organ, from disease of the bones, or from disease of the sinuses. In the latter circumstances polypi may be formed.

Ozena. The name of this disease is derived from the Greek *oze,* meaning a stench. There is thus immediately described one of its most obvious symptoms. Atrophic rhinitis, sclerotic rhinitis, and atrophic catarrh are synonyms indicating the same condition.

The majority of cases first begin before the age of twelve, and but few commence later than twenty-five. Women are affected five times more frequently than are men, and several members of the same family may suffer in the same way. The patient may complain of the smell from the nose, but it more commonly happens that she is completely unaware of the smell and complains only of the thick discharge from the nose or in some cases of a dry throat and cough.

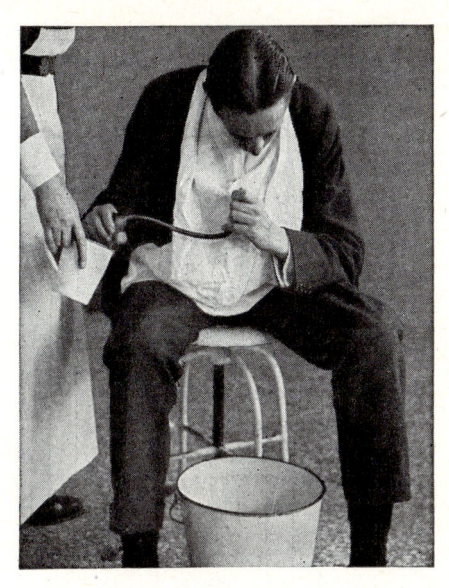

TREATMENT OF FETOR

In dry rhinitis, when decomposing crusts cause a highly offensive odor, it may be necessary to cleanse the nasal cavities with a syringe and a suitable solution.

Crusts separate from the mucous membrane and cause slight bleeding from the nose, which is always obstructed by the exudates to a greater or less extent. The mucous membrane and the glands degenerate and there is a diffuse scarring. The bones may also be attacked. The disease may spread to the throat or larynx and excite symptoms consequent on the atrophy in these regions. Some of the discharge is swallowed and its putrescence then gives rise to gastritis. The patient is inevitably shunned by society, for the stench is sickening. The absorption of the toxic material causes a general deterioration in health.

Congenital syphilis often produces changes in the noses of children which can only be distinguished from this condition with difficulty. Suppuration may occur round a foreign body, from adenoids, and from infection of the air sacs in the bones. Lupus, too, gives rise to somewhat similar exudates. Most of these conditions, however, are usually limited to one side of the nose, a limitation rare in ozena.

Although congenital deformities of the nasal passages and previous diseases may contribute to the onset of ozena,

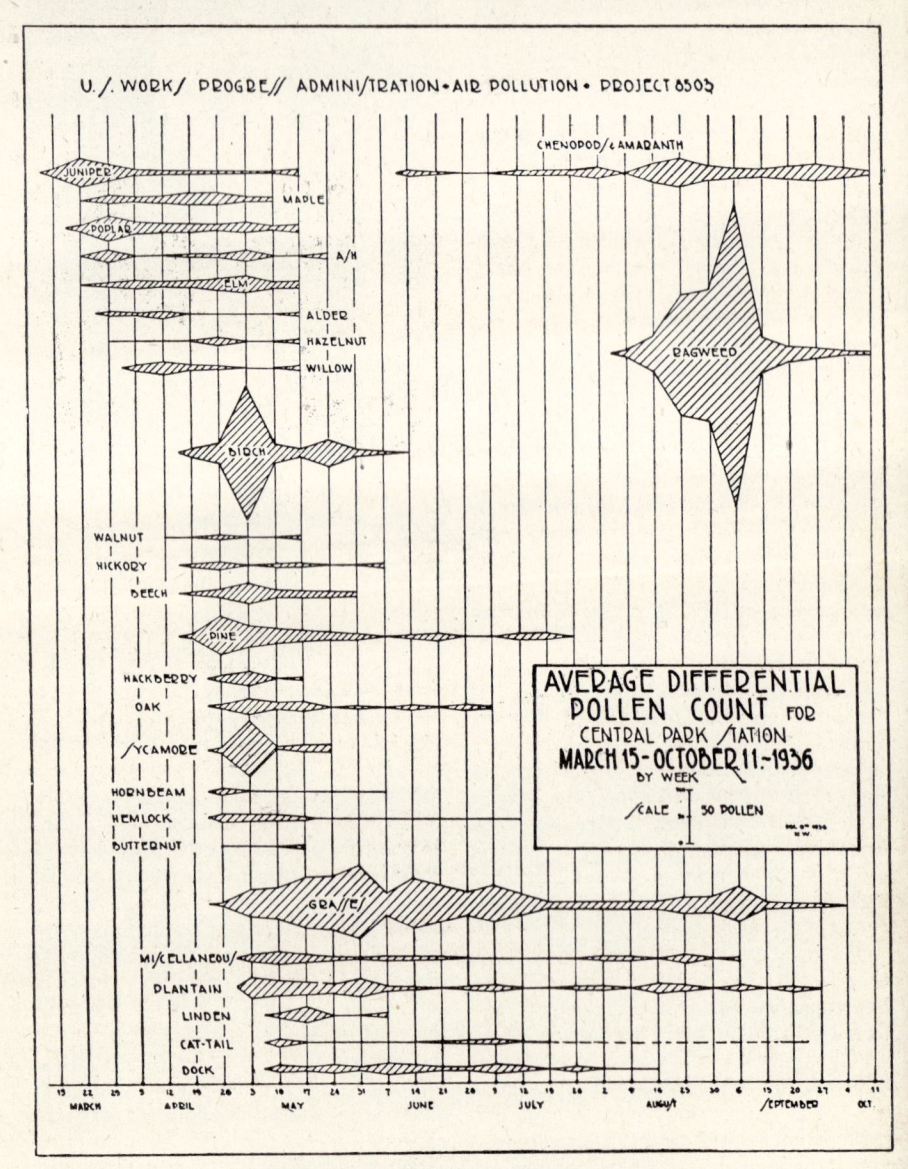

"HAY FEVER" RISK FROM SPRING TO FALL

A graph of the amounts of pollens counted in a city park. The month-to-month variation in specific pollens is probably similar to that for most cities. Pollen-sensitive persons will readily see why spring and fall are likely to provide them with the most uncomfortable weeks.

Courtesy of the American Journal of Public Health

they are not definite causes, nor has a specific organism been discovered.

Local cleansing with antiseptic solutions must be carried out with great patience and care. Sprays, inhalants, or douching by means of a glass syringe are the best methods of applying the solution. The general health, too, must be maintained, preferably by a visit to a seaside resort, which has a well-founded reputation in this disease.

Hay Fever. Hay fever or hay asthma is a peculiar form of catarrh to which certain persons are strongly predisposed. It is now know to be a form of allergy and is allied to true asthma. It runs in families, like the other allergic diseases, and although the cause of the predisposition is not yet definitely known, an extremely sensitive condition of the nervous system always accompanies it. The first attack often comes on in childhood, and rarely late in life, and girls are much more frequently affected than boys. The malady tends to become less troublesome after middle age. It is met with in most European countries, but reaches its highest incidence in the United States and England.

Hay fever is produced as the result of irritation of the mucous membrane by the grains of pollen from many grasses and from some plants and trees. This explains why the disease is only met with at certain times of the year. The pollination of trees in the early spring results in attacks of hay fever in those who are sensitive to one or more of the tree pollens. Those who are sensitive to the pollen of grasses suffer most in the late spring and early summer. About 75 per cent of hay-fever patients are sensitive to the pollen of one or more weeds, particularly the high and low ragweed. In these cases the attacks occur in the late summer and early fall. The little pollen sacs are extremely light, and are carried away by currents of air to great distances. Being inhaled, they settle on the mucous membrane of the respiratory passages, and, absorbing moisture from it, burst, and scatter minute granules over its surface. In some way the pollen proteins to which the individual is sensitive are absorbed into the system. Atmospheric conditions may affect the severity of the illness.

It is a bad time for hay-fever victims when the weather is hot and dry, and a heavy fall of rain is a cause of rejoicing, for it checks the complaint immediately.

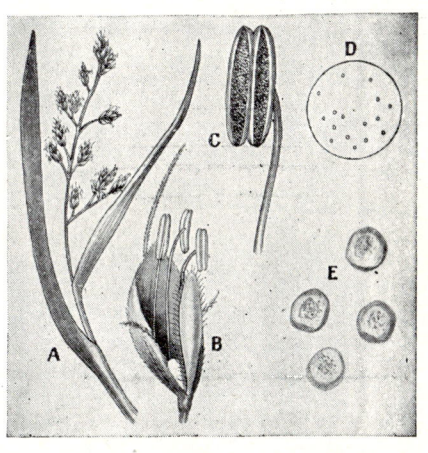

HAY FEVER: ONE OF THE CAUSES

Pollen of various plants is provocative of hay fever in susceptible persons. (A) Common grass in flower. (B) Flower enlarged. (C) Pollen grains being liberated by splitting of sacs. (D) Grains enlarged thirteen times and (E) further enlarged.

Symptoms. Directly the cause is applied the symptoms begin, and may affect, at different times or all together, the lining membrane of the nose, eyes, mouth, throat, larynx, windpipe, and bronchial tubes. The parts begin to itch and smart, catarrh is set up, violent fits of sneezing occur, the eyes water, the nose runs with a watery, irritating fluid, the head aches from a spread of inflammation of the cavities in the frontal bone, the nose becomes stuffed up, and the poor patient feels absolutely miserable. The eyes are bloodshot and swollen, the tears trickle down the cheeks from blocking of the ducts which lead to the nose, and the eyes are so irritable that it is almost impossible for the patient to avoid rubbing them and thus increasing the trouble. The catarrh spreads backwards from the nose and mouth to the throat, and up the tubes to the ears, causing a certain amount of deafness. If it spreads farther through the larynx and windpipe to the bronchial tubes it sets up an asthmatic condition, with difficulty of breathing, wheezing, and dry hacking cough, a certain amount of phlegm being brought up later on. The first attacks are usually limited to the eyes and nose, but the later ones involve the deeper parts, and are often accompanied by asthma (see Chapter 109).

If hay fever is left to take its own course it may last for four or five weeks and return whenever the patient is exposed to its exciting cause. A certain number of cases seems to be produced by bright sunlight or ordinary dust, or by certain vegetable and animal odors, but it is hard to prove the absence of pollen grains even then, as these small bodies can be carried to such great distances. Exercise is often found to increase the severity of an attack by increasing the frequency of respiration, and therefore the amount of pollen inhaled by the victim.

Treatment. The first step to be taken in the treatment of hay fever is to get away at once from the cause of irritation and escape the pollen grains; but this is not at all easy, for so many people are tied to work, pleasure, or duty that they must remain where they are and bear their trouble. If it is possible to go for a change, a sea voyage is of all measures the most satisfactory, for at a certain distance from land the air is quite free from irritating particles. The next best place is on the sea coast, and a place should be chosen where the prevailing winds blow from the sea; if land winds blow, the pollen is soon at its work again. If the place is protected by high cliffs there is more hope of freedom for the sufferer. High mountain resorts are sometimes beneficial to hay-fever patients, or large towns where grass and vegetation are conspicuous by their absence.

It is always a wise plan for hay-fever patients to keep indoors as much as possible during the hot parts of the day and go out in the evening when it is getting cool; it is well for them to remember also that it is not only the pollen of grasses but also that of certain flowers that causes the disease, and therefore they should have no flowers or plants in the house. But as these measures are often beyond the patient's power, or have proved ineffectual, we must next consider what can be done to give relief by other agents.

In the treatment of hay fever the attempt is made to build up a resistance or immunity in the patient against the specific pollen to which he is sensitive. The patient's sensitivity is first determined by eye and skin tests; that is, the doctor finds which pollens annoy the patient by subjecting the skin or the conjunctiva of the eye (or both) to various suspected pollens in extremely minute doses. Pollen extract is then injected subcutaneously at definite intervals of time. Treatment may assume one of three forms. Preseasonal treatment aims at producing an immunity in the patient before the season starts. Coseasonal treatment may be instituted if the patient first goes to the doctor for treatment during the season. Perennial treatment is treatment continued throughout the year. The first-named is the most efficacious and one of the methods employed may be outlined here. A start is made by injecting under the skin a dose of the extract equal to one-third of the smallest dose that has been found to excite a reaction in the conjunctiva. A course of injections is then given at weekly intervals and the strength of each is increased by 50 per cent over that of the preceding dose. Should a general reaction occur after any dose the subsequent dose must be substantially reduced. Treatment should be instituted about four months before the pollination is expected. The course may

DISORDERS OF THE NOSE AND NASOPHARYNX

have to be repeated for several years before there is enough immunity to enable the patient to react negatively to the pollen-extract test, at which time treatment may be discontinued.

Local treatment may be resorted to for symptomatic relief although this is usually not necessary if there has been adequate preseasonal treatment. One reliable preparation which is used for this complaint is adrenalin, the extract of the adrenal glands. A 1-in-1000 solution of adrenalin should be sprayed in the mouth, nostrils, and eyes, when it often acts like a charm, relieving the intense irritation in a few minutes. Five to ten minims injected hypodermically, or ten to twenty drops in water, by the mouth, are often likewise helpful. Ephedrine, which is prepared from the Chinese plant mahuang, acts similarly to adrenalin and many preparations of it are now on the market which are useful in hay fever. A ½ per cent cocaine solution applied to the eye relieves the congestion. Comfort and protection for the eyes may be had with dark glasses.

Asthma is a very frequent complication of hay fever. The only preventive measure is the prompt institution of adequate treatment. Sinus involvement may also occur as a complication.

SINUS DISEASE

Enclosed by the bones of the face are several cavities, containing air, which are known as sinuses. These are: the maxillary sinus or antrum, under the cheeks at each side of the nose; the frontal sinuses at the top of the nose over each eye; the ethmoidal and sphenoidal sinuses, tucked away deeper in the skull behind the nose. All these sinuses are situated in bones adjacent to the nose and communicating with it; they are liable to become full of infected matter, especially if the nose has been in an unhealthy state, through some such cause as a cold.

Occasionally bad teeth allow infection from an abscess to spread to the antrum and infect it. Sinus infection causes severe pain and is often an undetected cause of the health being persistently below par. If anything causes the condition to flare up into an acute one, a very painful and serious illness may result. Neglected sinus trouble may even lead to infection of the meninges or covering of the brain, the condition which is known as meningitis and is of serious import. The treatment of sinusitis is surgical if the attack does not clear up after treatment as for an ordinary cold. A specialist in diseases of the ear, nose, and throat should be consulted if it is suspected that there is chronic inflammation in any one of the nasal sinuses. Pain in the head or face will be the prominent symptom, and often there is a persistent discharge—especially a one-sided discharge—from the nose, or it may slip down the back of the nose by way of the throat into the stomach.

SINUSES OR CAVITIES IN SKULL BONES

In the frontal, maxillary and sphenoid bones there are spaces, known as sinuses, and all of these open into the interior of the nose, from which they may become infected. When this occurs the condition is referred to as sinusitis.

A bad smell or bad breath may sometimes be an indication of disease in one of the sinuses.

Nasal Polypus. In many cases there is a long history of chronic nasal catarrh with obstructive signs, and these are not elucidated until the specialist is asked to make an examination.

Frequently what is found is an overgrowth of the soft tissues lining the nose, so that multiple small grapelike bodies of pulpy consistency are formed, which hang down into the nostril, producing the signs referred to above. The actual cause of this condition is usually suppuration of the sinuses, mentioned on page 1491, or disease of the bone lying below the affected membrane, and there is almost always an associated chronic rhinitis of the hypertrophic type.

When traced to their short stalks and so to their origin, polypi are seen to spring from the ethmoid cells or other sinuses, but most commonly from the middle turbinate bone. The partition between the nostrils, which is termed the septum, invariably escapes.

Signs. Constant watery discharge, difficulty in carrying out nasal breathing, affection of the speech and voice, chronic headache, worst in wet weather; this is the picture of nasal polypus, a fairly common disease of the present day.

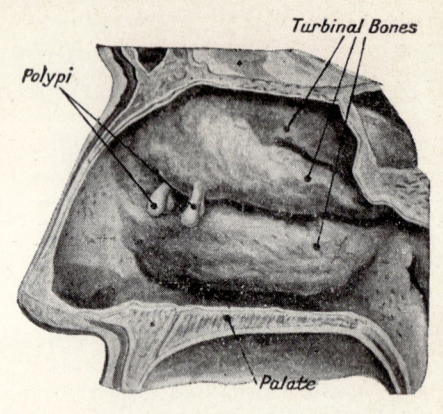

WHERE NASAL POLYPI ARE FOUND

The right side of the nose from within. The three turbinal bones are clearly seen; four small polypi are shown in relation to the middle one. The space between the middle and lowest bones, known as the middle meatus, is a frequent site of polypi.

Treatment. The usual method of removal is by applying a mixture of adrenalin and cocaine to the affected part; then a specially prepared wire snare is passed over the polypus and drawn tightly round the stalk. The latter may then be twisted until it gives way. Unfortunately, polypi growing in connection with sinus disease have a tendency to recur again and again.

CHAPTER 107

DISORDERS OF THE THROAT

Simple Sore Throat — Clergyman's Sore Throat — Relaxed Throat — Follicular Tonsillitis — Chronic Tonsillitis — Acute Tonsillitis — Quinsy — Septic Throat — Ulcerated Sore Throat — Infectious Sore Throat — Vincent's Angina.

THE "throat" is a somewhat indefinite term when used in this connection, and must be considered to include the pharynx and some or all of the surrounding parts, such as the palate, tonsils, uvula, larynx, and upper part of the trachea. It is liable to many different affections, and may be injured by substances swallowed, such as bits of bone and hard portions of food, or by drinking very hot fluids or corrosive poisons. The latter accidents produce acute inflammation, and may be followed by very serious symptoms, such as suffocation and difficulty in swallowing, due to the extreme swelling of the mucous membrane. Affections of the throat vary in importance from a slight catarrh to such severe conditions as are caused by scarlet fever and diphtheria.

The expression "sore throat" comprises in a general way all the inflamed and painful conditions which affect the part, but the symptoms of sore throat are present in many different complaints, the causes and course and treatment of which are quite distinct.

It must never be forgotten that practically all the infectious diseases begin with a sore throat, and when a sore throat is accompanied by a raised temperature the possibility of these being the early stages of an infectious disease must always be kept in mind.

The chief varieties of sore throat comprise: (1) simple sore throat; (2) clergyman's sore throat (pharyngitis); (3) relaxed throat; (4) follicular tonsillitis; (5) acute tonsillitis, abscess of tonsil, quinsy; (6) septic throat; (7) infectious sore throat.

Simple Sore Throat. In this complaint there is a condition of the mucous membrane of the throat very similar to that already described in nasal catarrh, and its most frequent cause is the same, namely, exposure to damp and cold; indeed, it is very often simply an extension of inflammation from the mucous membrane of the nose. It is predisposed to by any condition which causes general debility and ill-health, such as overwork or living in unhealthy, ill-ventilated rooms, and it most commonly affects young people. One attack strongly causes susceptibility to others, and many persons will always develop the complaint upon slight exposure to cold and damp or rapid changes of temperature. Rheumatic subjects are very prone to this form of sore throat.

Symptoms. The symptoms come on gradually, with slight fever, chilliness, headache, aching pains, and a general feeling of illness, soon followed by a sore, dry, uncomfortable sensation in the throat, with pain on swallowing, slight hoarseness, and tendency to cough. The inflammation is apt to spread to the surrounding parts, upwards into the nose, and downwards into the larynx and windpipe. If the throat be examined, it is found to be red and swollen; the mucous membrane, which at first is dry and irritable, soon produces a more or less abundant secretion, which is sticky and tenacious, and causes constant "hawking" and attempts to expectorate. Such attacks are not at all dangerous, and usually two or three days of care and confinement to the house are enough to effect a cure.

Treatment. The treatment is simple, and consists in the application externally of a linseed poultice, hot fomentation, or wet compress, and internally of soothing remedies. One of the best of these is glycerine and boracic acid which should be painted with a brush over the inflamed parts several times a day, and may be combined with the use of lozenges, such as the tablets of (1) chlorate of potash, borax, and cocaine, or (2) of chloride of ammonium, or (3) of niter. To some the use of a gargle is preferable, and for such people either hydrogen peroxide or Dobell's solution can be recommended. An aspirin gargle may give relief.

In slight cases medicine will probably be unnecessary. When fever is present it is well to take a good aperient and to remain in bed for two or three days.

During convalescence the food, which during the attack should be very light and consist of fluids, must be plentiful, nutritious, and sustaining; a glass of burgundy may be taken once or twice a day with meals, and generally great care should be exercised until the throat has perfectly recovered from the irritated condition.

Clergyman's Sore Throat. This form of sore throat is a chronic pharyngitis or inflammation of the pharynx, and in most cases there is a chronic laryngitis as well. It is usually due to bad methods of voice production or to a blocked nose. The disease is met with in those persons who are overworked, especially when their work necessitates constant use of the voice. It occurs frequently in clergymen, from preaching or reading aloud in church; in actors, from much and loud talking on the stage; in lawyers, from long speeches in ill-ventilated courts; in singers, from straining the voice for large audiences; in schoolmasters and professional men, from long lectures. There is little doubt that dust and dirt and irritating gases or chemical fumes increase the danger of voice strain, and that particular danger arises from using the voice when the throat is relaxed or when it has only imperfectly recovered from catarrh.

Symptoms. The early symptoms seem quite unimportant. The patient feels an uneasy sensation at the back of the throat, as if there were something in it, and this gives a constant desire to clear the throat by hawking; he also has a frequent inclination to swallow, as if to remove the irritation, but in neither way does he obtain relief. A little cough sets in, which is dry, irritating, and ineffectual. All these symptoms subside at once with a few days' rest, and if the throat be examined nothing very definite can be seen. But rest is seldom taken for a sufficiently long time, and the symptoms gradually grow worse; the throat becomes tired, and aches after speaking for shorter and shorter periods; the voice grows husky and indistinct,

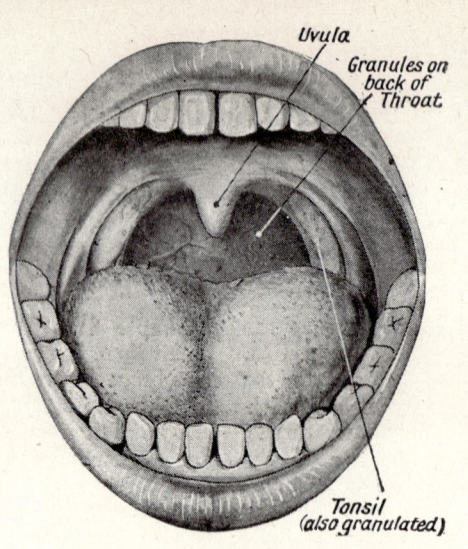

PHARYNGITIS OR CLERGYMAN'S THROAT
In the form of chronic pharyngitis, or inflammation of the lining membrane of the back of the throat, which occurs in public speakers, little red nodules are dotted over the throat, and the veins are dilated.

DISORDERS OF THE THROAT

and a chronic form of inflammation is set up in the mucous membrane.

The throat now shows distinct changes; the posterior wall of the pharynx—that is, the part that faces one when looking down the throat—is seen to be roughened and covered with small elevations, which are formed by the enlarged glands filled with secretion; the uvula is long, flabby, and relaxed; all the parts may be covered with thick mucus, which dries and crusts during the night and often makes the symptoms worse in the morning. In other cases the discharge is absent, and the throat looks dry and shiny, and may have raw patches or ulcerations on its surface. It now becomes impossible to use the voice, because doing so makes the symptoms severe; indeed, the voice may be entirely lost, and pain is complained of; the general health also suffers, and the patient grows debilitated and loses all interest in his work and ordinary pursuits.

Treatment. The treatment is rest; and rest will work a cure if it is taken for a sufficiently long period. But the disease is most tedious and difficult to cure; and it is, of course, a serious thing for a busy professional or business man to throw up his occupation altogether. But the longer the disease has been neglected the longer will the rest have to be to make sure of a cure. Rest in these cases, of course, refers to the throat and voice only, for rest of body is not at all necessary; indeed, the patient requires healthy exercise and amusement, and plenty of fresh air. Tonics, such as iron and quinine, with change of air and scene, sea bathing or a daily cold bath, and good feeding, brace up the general system and help the local measures. The use of tobacco is injurious, and should be entirely stopped. The indulgence in strong alcoholic drinks, except in great moderation, and the use of food too hot or too much spiced, should be avoided, and chronic constipation should be corrected with mild aperients. Of special drugs, probably the most useful is iodide of potash, in three-grain doses three times a day, but this has a lowering and depressing effect and should only be used under a physician's care.

Local treatment is of great importance, and may be employed in various forms.

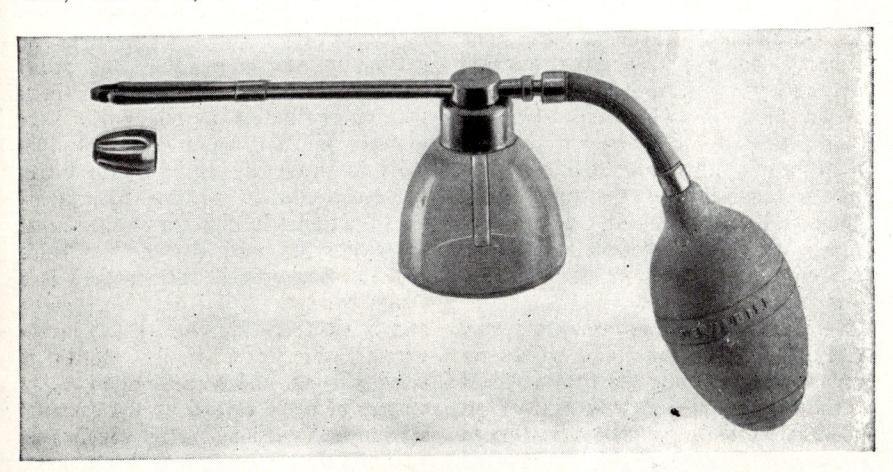

HOUSEHOLD ATOMIZER FOR NOSE AND THROAT

The low flat-bottomed jar of this atomizer makes it convenient to set upon a medicine-cabinet shelf and unlikely to be tipped over. The nozzle can be pivoted to discharge a spray either forward, upward, or downward, which makes it especially valuable for use in the back of the throat. The conical tip is fitted over the nozzle when it is desired to spray the nostrils.

Courtesy of DeVilbiss Co.

Drugs may be used mixed with glycerine, which renders the application thick and sticky; it should be painted freely on to the diseased surface with a large brush. A preparation of iodine in glycerine flavored with peppermint, may be strongly recommended; this should be painted on two or three times a day. Tincture of iodine is also useful; at first it should be diluted with an equal part of water, and, if it seems to suit, it may later be applied undiluted. Argyrol, in the strength of a drachm to an ounce of water, may also be used to paint the throat; it causes no pain or smarting. Gargles are of little value, as they probably do not reach the diseased part, and are very brief in their action. An oily mixture, such as chloretone inhalant, sprayed into the back of the nose by means of a spray or an atomizer, often relieves the pain for the time being. Compound benzoic acid, chlorate of potash, chlorate of potash and borax, and chloride of ammonium are all useful lozenges.

Externally a cold wet compress may be applied at bedtime, and on its removal in the morning the throat should be thoroughly sponged with cold water. In chronic cases it may be advisable to spend a winter and early spring in some mild and equable climate, or to take a thorough course of the waters at some spa.

As precautionary measures against relapse, work should be resumed gradually and with care, the health receiving strict attention.

Relaxed Throat. This is very frequently the condition left by an imperfectly cured attack of acute inflammation, but it may arise also quite independently. It is most common in people who are run down and out of health, or in those who live sedentary lives, and is not infrequently the result of smoking to excess, especially the smoking of cigarettes, according to some opinion.

Symptoms. The symptoms are a feeling of uneasiness at the back of the throat, a tendency to be constantly swallowing and to hawk up phlegm, which is always most troublesome on getting up in the morning, and grows less after breakfast. There is some little pain on swallowing, especially of a hard morsel. When there is persistent difficulty in swallowing, it is always better to have the throat examined thoroughly by a specialist in diseases of the throat to exclude the possibility of there being any ulcer or tumor. Often there is a cough which is of a hacking character, and is either fruitless or results in the expectoration of a small quantity of thick phlegm, and sometimes of a few streaks of blood caused by the constant straining. Occasionally the cough goes on until the patient retches or is actually sick. There are no symptoms of general constitutional disturbance, such as fever or quickened pulse, but the health is poor, the patient describing himself as feeling ill, without having

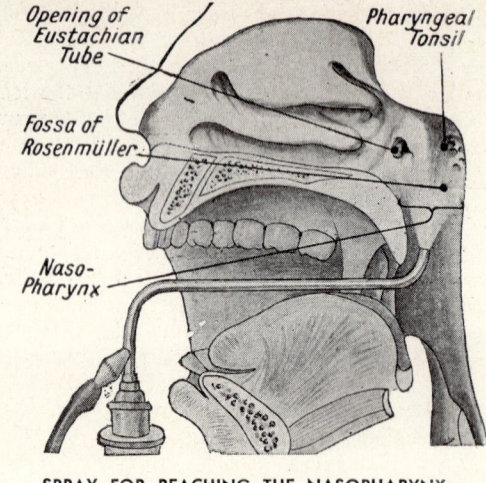

SPRAY FOR REACHING THE NASOPHARYNX
Sprays can be adapted to reach the more remote parts of the throat. Here an upward bend of the atomizer tube enables the spray to be distributed over the nasopharynx.

PROFESSIONAL-TYPE ATOMIZER AND BOTTLE

The cylindrical bottle of this device is intended to fit in a doctor's rack, where it rests on the ring of glass which is seen near the upper end of the bottle. The air may be supplied from a bulb or an air compressor. If it is necessary to warm the solution slightly, as is often desirable, the elongated bottle is easy to immerse in warm water without removing the sprayer head. The nozzle can be pointed upwards, downwards, or straight ahead.

Courtesy of DeVilbiss Co.

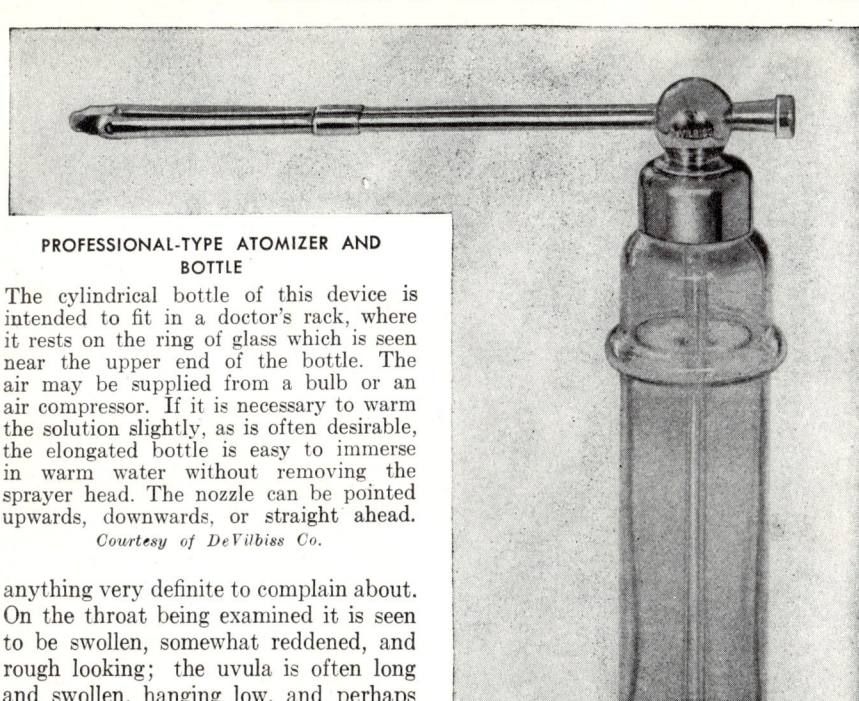

anything very definite to complain about. On the throat being examined it is seen to be swollen, somewhat reddened, and rough looking; the uvula is often long and swollen, hanging low, and perhaps touching the back of the tongue, and is the cause of much of the trouble. The back of the pharynx is sore and dry, and usually has much thick mucus sticking to it.

Treatment. There is often a good deal of difficulty in curing this affection, and the attention must be directed to improving the general health. Fresh air and exercise should be taken, and all coddling and sitting indoors given up at once. A healthy sharp walk is far better than sitting by the fire reading a book. As smoking is often a cause of this complaint, it should be given up altogether, or only indulged in with the greatest moderation; alcoholic drinks must be taken with circumspection. The bowels must be regulated, the digestion attended to, and any evident departures from health put right.

Local treatment must always be combined with the general. The best application is a preparation of iodine in glycerine (see under treatment of Clergyman's Sore Throat), which should be applied freely to all the affected parts with a large brush three or four times a day. Chlorate of potash lozenges and red gum lozenges are beneficial. Another useful astringent is tincture of perchloride of iron; a fluid drachm to an ounce of water makes a useful paint, but it is strong, and blackens the parts to which it is applied. However, it gives great relief at times. A spray is a very satisfactory way in which to apply the astringent. A solution consisting of an ounce of water with five to twenty grains of alum, or five to fifteen grains of tannin, or five to ten grains of sulphate of zinc, may be sprayed into the throat three times a day.

Follicular Tonsillitis. This name is given to a form of sore throat in which the crypts of the tonsils become filled with cheesy-white matter, and sometimes cause unnecessary anxiety because of their resemblance to the unskilled eye to diphtheria. The tonsils are enlarged, and on their surface are a number of smaller dirty yellow patches, round or oval in shape, but quite limited to the tonsils. These structures always secrete a small amount of thick fluid from their little glands or follicles, but when they are inflamed the discharge may be unable to escape freely, and then collects in the glands, which become swollen and visible to the naked eye. The discharge oozes out on to the surface of the tonsils, and produces the patches, but does not form anything like a true membrane as in diphtheria. The material, which has a yellow, creamy consistency, can be easily wiped off with a brush. It can also be squeezed out of the enlarged glands by pressure on the tonsil, and may in this way be distinguished from the membrane of diphtheria, which is only detached with some difficulty, and leaves a sore and perhaps bleeding surface behind it. These patches are also likely to be mistaken for ulcers, but there is no abrasion of surface as in the latter complaint. Treatment is the same as for relaxed throat, but the patient must remain in bed as long as there is any rise in temperature. The close association of follicular tonsillitis with rheumatic fever must never be forgotten.

After a severe attack of follicular tonsillitis, or if there are repeated attacks of sore throat and tonsillitis, the tonsils should be removed by dissection to prevent recurrence. This may be done either under local or general anesthesia.

Chronic Tonsillitis. A chonic inflammation of the tonsils produces the enlargement or hypertrophy of these organs so often met with in company with adenoids, and it is dealt with among the diseases of childhood (Volume VIII.)

Acute Tonsillitis. Inflammatory sore throat is a far more acute and serious illness than the forms of sore throat already described. It most commonly affects young people, but is not infrequently met with among the middle-aged. One attack produces a strong predisposition to others; some people who have this tendency strongly marked are liable to almost annual attacks, and develop in this way great delicacy of the throat. The spring and autumn are the seasons during which the affection is most prevalent, and this is probably due to the climatic conditions that then obtain. The usual exciting cause is exposure to damp, cold, and wet, and it is becoming increasingly evident that the germ responsible for such ailments is a streptococcus, allied to, if not identical with, the organism of acute and subacute rheumatic fever.

If the tonsils themselves are inflamed the affection is called tonsillitis; if there is an abscess in the tonsil it is called a tonsillar abscess; if, however, the surrounding tissues are involved the abscess is called a peritonsillar abscess or a quinsy.

Symptoms. The symptoms of acute tonsillitis vary in severity according to the case, but fever is always present to some extent, with its accompaniments of headache, chilliness, aching pains in the limbs, furred tongue, and loss of appetite. There may even be distinct shivering fits or chills, and the fever may run up quite high, perhaps to 104° F. The skin then is hot and dry, the face flushed, and the pulse very rapid, and there may be delirium at night. With these general symptoms the local trouble keeps pace. At first the throat is dry and sore and the mucous membrane red and swollen, and these symptoms rapidly increase until there is severe pain with great swelling, and swallowing becomes most difficult. The pain shoots up into the ears and along the jaws, so that it is painful to talk or move the tongue or open the mouth.

The tonsils are red and greatly swollen, and may almost meet in the middle line. The patient's speech is much altered, being thick and guttural. His throat feels as if it were blocked up and the effort of swallowing is so painful that it is with the greatest difficulty that he can be persuaded to attempt it. Fluids are really more difficult to swallow than soft solids, as the latter fill up the space between the tonsils more and require less movement of the parts. The swallowing is often so much impeded, and the movement of the palate so limited, that fluids are liable to pass upwards into the nose. If the neck is examined, enlarged glands may be felt running down on each side along the edge of the large muscle, and the whole neck is stiff and swollen, and painful when moved. The tonsils are not alone affected, for the uvula and soft palate and all the mucous membrane in their neighborhood are swollen and red, and the areas are covered with a thick mucous discharge.

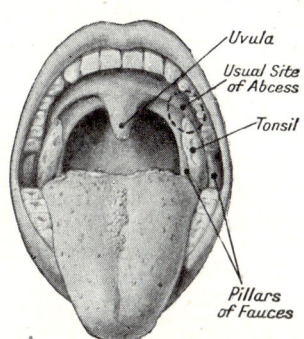

QUINSY: SITE OF ABCESS

The supratonsillar recess, indicated by dotted circle, is the most common site of suppuration in quinsy, but suppuration may burrow in various directions.

Treatment. Treatment of an acute attack consists in sending the patient to bed and administering one or two grains of calomel, followed by a saline cathartic some hours later. The application of hot fomentations or a linseed poultice to the outside of the throat or the application of an ice bag allays the pain, as does also the inhalation of steam from a jug of hot water. The throat should be sprayed with a warm normal saline solution or a weak solution of some antiseptic such as sodium hypochlorite. Sodium salicylate in doses of ten to fifteen grains four-hourly, or aspirin in ten-grain doses for an adult (half these doses for a child), helps to shorten the attack and give relief, and the latter drug, if sucked in tablet form, acts locally in relieving the pain of swallowing. Other treatment is that of fever in general. Food should be liquid or very soft. Milk is best avoided and use made of thickened broths, fruit juices, jellies, soft-boiled eggs, and well-sweetened drinks. Ice to suck is comforting. Semisolid food may follow as the inflammation subsides.

Possible complications of an acute attack are the spread of the infection to the peritonsillar area with formation of an abscess (quinsy) or to the tissues of the neck (cellulitis).

Quinsy. The symptoms of quinsy closely resemble those seen in acute tonsillitis, although the constitutional disturbance is even more severe. Soreness and dryness of the throat are usually, but not always, the first symptoms complained of. The pain on swallowing may be very severe, almost from the onset, the pain often shooting to the ears. The swelling of the palate and side of the throat may be so great that the mouth can only be opened with difficulty. When this is so, the patient may find the act of swallowing almost impossible, quite apart from the severe pain which is experienced whenever the attempt is made.

The onset is usually marked by shivering or chill, and pains in the back or limbs. The temperature rises to 104°, 105°, or even higher, and the pulse ranges from 110 to 130. Delirium at night is often associated with a high temperature. There is great weakness and prostration; the tongue is furred and constipation is usually present. The glands of the neck may become greatly enlarged, and this, too, may cause difficulty in opening the mouth.

On examination of the throat, one or both tonsils are found to be enlarged, dark red, and firm to the touch, while all the loose cellular tissue surrounding them is also inflamed (peritonsillitis) and boggy. Within a few days, usually from two to four, the enlarged tonsils become softer, and fluctuation can then often be obtained by placing one finger on the tonsil and the other at the angle of the jaw. The abscess swelling, which usually involves the soft palate, generally points towards the mouth, but exceptionally it may point towards the pharynx. It may burst spontaneously either through the tonsil or the soft palate, with instant relief of the pain.

The abscess, however, should not be left to burst of itself. A case of suffocation has been known to follow the rupture of a large abscess and the consequent escape of the pus into the larynx; while much suffering will be saved by operating as soon as fluctuation can be distinctly felt.

Treatment. Treatment then consists of two parts. In the first stage, before fluctuation has appeared, hot applications in the shape of poultices, fomentations, or a kaolin poultice should be applied to the neck and constantly renewed. Hot mouth washes, either of plain water or of a solution of hydrogen peroxide, should be given frequently and as hot as can be borne. The patient should remain in bed. Difficulty in swallowing nourishment may be lessened by first sucking a piece of ice. It is desirable to clear out the bowels with a dose of calomel, and it is usual to give either aspirin or sodium salicylate. Gargling with aspirin suspended in water before swallowing it relieves the pain considerably. As soon as fluctuation has appeared, or a feeling of softening external to the tonsil is perceived, an incision must be made over the abscess.

Only a local anesthetic is used; with a general anesthetic the pus may run down into the larynx after the abscess has been opened, and may set up pneumonia, abscess, or gangrene of the lung. A solution of cocaine may be sprayed into the throat. The patient should then sit facing a good light, and open his mouth as widely as possible. The tonsil itself is not incised.

After the operation the patient should gargle repeatedly with hot alkaline solutions, and use a mouth wash for some days. During the illness the diet must be liquid and as nourishing as possible. Convalescence may be slow, and such tonics as iron and quinine should be freely given. Repeated attacks of suppurative tonsillitis suggest the advisability of removing the tonsils, though this should never be done in the course of an attack except as an emergency measure.

Septic Throat. Septic sore throat is a communicable disease which frequently occurs in the form of epidemics among people using infected milk or milk products from the same supply. This disease also spreads by either direct or indirect contact with a person suffering from the disease. It is believed that the infective agent is a streptococcus capable of causing disease of a cow's udder.

The most prominent symptom exhibited, apart from the sore throat, is very high fever, which may run up to 103° or 104° F. Weakness and prostration are out of proportion to the local symptoms. The common complications are abscesses of the tonsils, infection of the middle ear, joint infection, erysipelas, pneumonia, and nephritis. Death may result from pneumonia or septicemia.

Rest in bed is most essential. The pain and soreness in the throat may be relieved by the application of cold packs and the administration of salicylates. Antiseptic gargles should be frequently used to disinfect the throat. Diet should be nutritive, of a fluid or semisolid nature and given in small feedings.

Great precaution is needed to prevent the spread of the disease to other members of the household. The discharges from the nose and throat should be destroyed at once by burning the paper napkins or pieces of cheesecloth used to receive the discharges. The dishes and utensils used by the patient should be kept separate and boiled for five minutes before being used by others. Persons in attendance should have nothing to do with the preparation of food for the well members of the family or the community.

Ulcerated Sore Throat. This is not a special disease in itself. An ulcer is a sore place, and is caused by the destruction of the surface of the mucous membrane, and this may occur in all forms of sore throat. It is especially common in the diseased throats such as occur in persons at work in hospitals. Ulceration is also common in many sore throats that form part of general diseases, such as scarlet fever, diphtheria, cancer, syphilis, and consumption. The white spots caused by accumulated secretion in chronic inflammation of the tonsils are very commonly mistaken for ulcers, but in this condition there is no raw surface, as can be seen if the secretion is removed by a gargle or a brush.

Infectious Sore Throat. Many forms of sore throat are due to the presence of germs, and by an examination of the discharge these can be discovered; and there are three forms of this affection which are undoubtedly infectious — namely, the influenza, scarlet-fever, and diphtheria forms.

The influenza throat has nothing particularly distinctive in its appearance, and must be recognized by the general symptoms and course of the attack. Scarlet-fever and diphtheria throats, on the other hand, have very definite characters by which to recognize them.

The scarlet-fever throat is similar in appearance to that of quinsy; the tonsils, palate, uvula, and pharynx are swollen and red, the tonsils are much enlarged and have patches of thick secretion dotted over their surface. Later, ulcers may appear or an abscess may form. What should be particularly noticed are the general symptoms, for in scarlet fever these are very severe; the pulse is quick, the temperature high, and the patient very ill. The appearance of the characteristic eruption settles the question. Scarlet fever is described in Chapter 98.

In diphtheria the same parts are affected and severe symptoms are present, but the temperature is not so high as in other forms of sore throat, although the patient feels ill. The characteristic point is the appearance on the throat, and especially on the tonsils, of distinct patches of membrane of a white, grayish or brownish color. The patches at first are small and separate, but they rapidly spread and join together. These patches of membrane can be removed only with difficulty, and if torn off leave a raw surface. The one means by which their nature can be cleared up and a definite conclusion obtained is by having some of the discharge removed by a doctor with a piece of absorbent cotton and having it examined by an expert. If the special bacillus of diphtheria is found, antitoxin must be administered without delay. The subject of diphtheria is considered in full in the section on children's diseases, Chapters 193-199.

Vincent's Angina. The term angina means choking, and is used for conditions in which a sense of choking or suffocation is a noticeable symptom. The condition known as Vincent's angina is one in which a thick membrane grows in the throat. It closely resembles diphtheria, but is noninfectious and not dangerous to life. As in diphtheria, there is an ulcerated throat and a foul-smelling membrane. The disease is due to a bacillus and is always secondary to infection in the teeth and gums. During the First World War it occurred in great numbers of cases and gained the name of "trench mouth." There is usually a slight degree of feverishness and some pain in the throat as well as swollen glands in the neck.

The condition is usually a short-lived one and clears up in a few days, but may be very troublesome on occasion. The mouth should be rinsed frequently with hydrogen peroxide and the gums swabbed with arsenic (Fowler's solution). The throat should be painted with iodine. The doctor may also use the arsenic preparation called neosalvarsan to swab the tonsils or inject intravenously. As soon as possible the teeth should be put in order. The general health may require toning up.

1502 THE CONCISE ENCYCLOPEDIA OF HEALTH

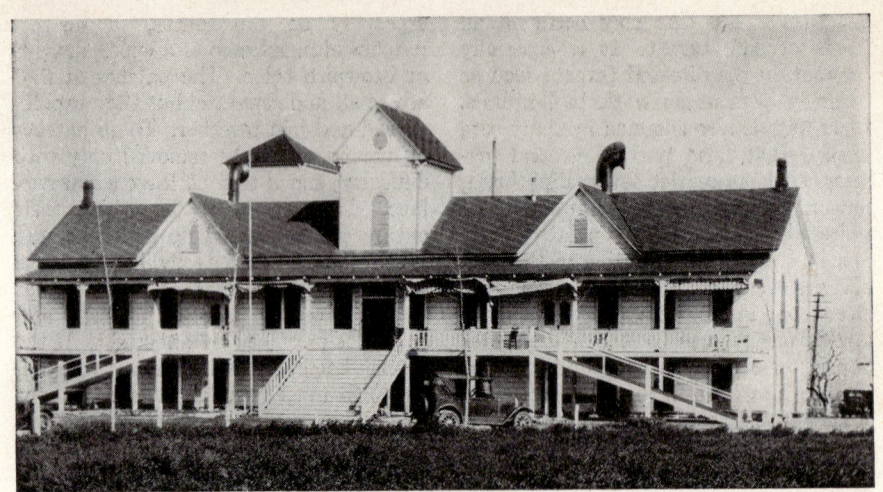

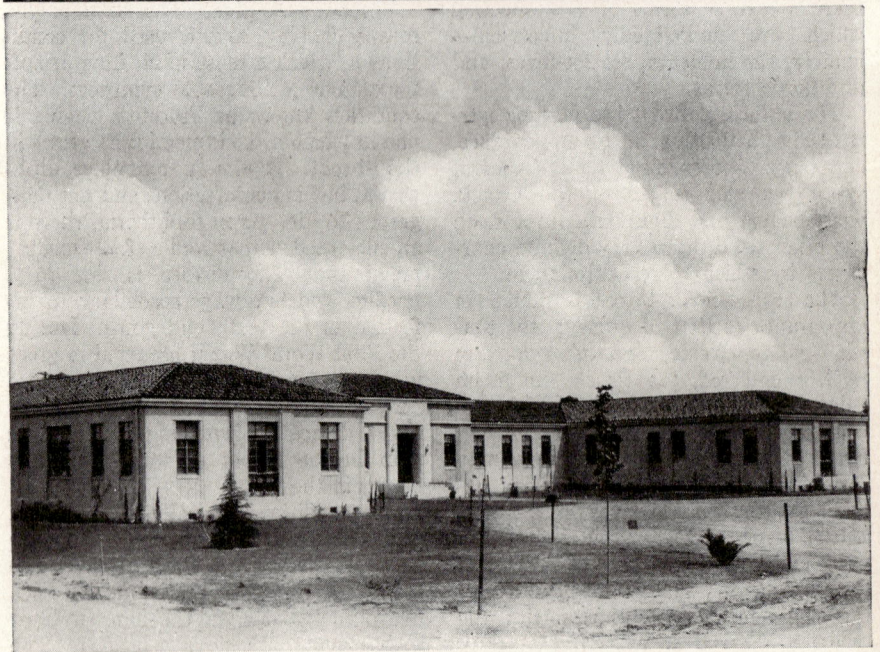

PROGRESS IN HOSPITAL DESIGN

During the nineteen-thirties Madera County, in central California, replaced its old hospital, which is shown here together with the modern building. Fire hazard was eliminated by the use of masonry instead of wood and by one-story instead of two-story design, which allows patients to be quickly and safely moved in and out of the building at or near ground level. Hence exterior ramps and porches, with their roofs, are unnecessary, and more sunlight is admitted to the interior. The ground plan, of units grouped around a court, also offers better exposure to sunlight, and moreover permits more effective separation of patients than was possible in a two-story block.

© *Harris & Ewing; Public Works Administration*

CHAPTER 108

DISEASES OF THE LARYNX

Laryngitis — Cough — Affections of the Voice — Aphonia.

DISEASES of the larynx are usually manifested by an alteration in the voice and by difficulty in breathing.

Malignant disease attacks the larynx most often in the form of cancer, which may either arise in that organ or spread to it from the adjoining part of the pharynx. Cancer in the former situation is known as intrinsic, and as a rule arises in relation to the vocal cords. It is not usually so malignant as when it originates outside the larynx, and is therefore more amenable to cure by operation.

Laryngitis. Inflammation of the larynx is most commonly caused by "catching cold," and is in many cases due to the spread of a catarrh of the mucous membrane of the throat. If during an ordinary cold the patient feels more ill and grows restless and anxious, it is probable that the larynx has become involved. The inflammation may also spread upwards along the windpipe from the lining of the bronchial tubes. Laryngitis occurs, too, as a complication of many general diseases, such as measles, scarlet fever, and influenza, and may in such circumstances be the chief source of danger. Accidents may produce it; the drinking of very hot water or the inhalation of noxious fumes being frequently followed by a very rapid and dangerous form of the complaint.

The mild form which accompanies an ordinary cold would popularly be called a "sore throat;" it is not at all a serious matter, and usually disappears in the course of three or four days under appropriate treatment; but it can be easily understood by those who have read a description of the anatomy of the larynx (see Chapter 49) that the inflammation and consequent swelling of the lining of this organ may produce very dire results. The body depends for its supply of oxygen upon the narrow chink of the glottis being kept open and free, and if this orifice be closed, tracheotomy (the surgical operation of making an opening into the trachea) will be necessary to prevent suffocation. In the old, the debilitated, the diseased, and in children, this affection must be looked upon as dangerous, and must receive careful attention. The most dangerous attacks are those that accompany the severe general diseases and those that are produced by swallowing boiling fluids, for in these a condition of inflammatory swelling often supervenes with great rapidity, and the patient's life is suddenly in jeopardy.

Symptoms. Fortunately the mild form resulting from cold is the most common,

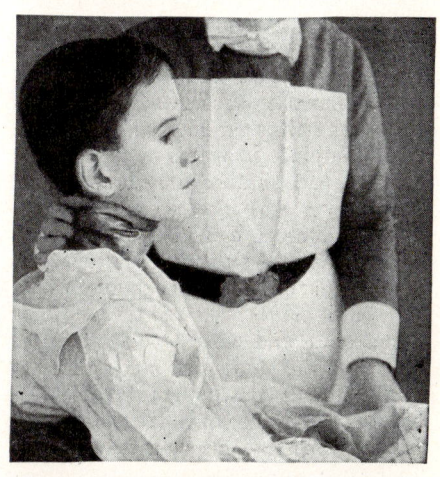

LARYNGITIS: APPLICATIONS TO NECK
Pain and hoarseness are usually benefited by hot or cold applications to the neck. A strip of lint is wrung out of water, applied, and covered with gutta-percha tissue and a bandage.

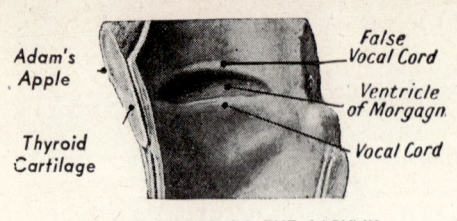

VOCAL CORDS IN THE LARYNX

Adam's Apple, Thyroid Cartilage, False Vocal Cord, Ventricle of Morgagn, Vocal Cord

The vocal cords are bands which are stretched between the arytenoid cartilages and the inner surface of the front part of the thyroid cartilage. Above the true cords are the false cords; both are seen here in side view.

and need excite no alarm. Changes in the voice are the most prominent symptoms. At first there is simply a slight thickness or huskiness, which is made worse by talking. This may increase up to loss of voice, the patient being able to express himself in an almost inaudible whisper only. There is a feeling of irritation in the throat, with a sensation of tightness or tickling in the region of the thyroid cartilage (Adam's apple), producing a constant desire to clear the throat and to swallow, both of which actions produce pain. The expectoration is small in quantity, and is at first only thin, watery fluid, like saliva, but it gradually becomes thicker and sticky as the inflammation subsides. There is usually some irritating, hacking cough, and the breathing increases somewhat in rapidity, and is rather difficult and noisy. Slight fever and increase of the pulse rate are present in most cases. Should the appropriate treatment be now carried out all the symptoms gradually subside, but if this is neglected the breathing grows more and more troublesome, the air enters the chest with much difficulty and straining, the patient becomes exhausted and blue and struggles to get fresh oxygen into his lungs; and probably, unless tracheotomy is performed, death from suffocation will then end the struggle. Laryngitis must therefore receive early and careful treatment.

Treatment. Place the patient in a warm room (at about 65° or 70° F.) and keep the air moist and at the same time fresh by careful ventilation. A bronchitis kettle (see page 1142) will both warm and moisten the air. Next apply a hot linseed poultice all over the front of the throat, and prepare a jug of boiling water with a few drops of eucalyptus oil in it, and let the patient inhale the steam. Clear the bowels with a cathartic and let the diet be light and simple—liquids and soft solids at first, such as milk, gruel, beef tea, bread and milk, and milk puddings. Give the patient warm milk, barley water, and black currant tea, and stop all talking. When he goes to bed let him have a hot bath, a hot drink, and a dose to make him sweat. This treatment will soon give relief, and probably by the next morning the symptoms will have begun to subside, but for a few days the patient must be careful to avoid catching cold.

Other inhalations may be found of value. In the early stages of laryngitis a teaspoonful of the compound tincture of benzoin may be placed in the bottom of a deep pitcher and one gallon of boiling water poured quickly upon it. The opening of the vessel is covered with an inverted cone and the mouth held opposite the smaller end. The steam should be inhaled for a period of five to ten minutes and the patient should remain in the house for thirty minutes to an hour after such treatment.

If the foregoing treatment is not rapidly followed by improvement it would always be wisest to get medical assistance, for we must remember that even in the most extreme cases the patient's life may be saved either by intubation or by the operation of opening the windpipe (tracheotomy), and also that some cases of laryngitis are due to hidden diphtheria, which is a most fatal form of this disease, and requires special treatment as early as possible to counteract the poison.

One attack of laryngitis greatly predisposes to others in the future; it may also end in a chronic inflammation very similar in its symptoms to those described as clergyman's sore throat. If the symptoms of hoarseness and irritation of the larynx continue for an unusual length of time it is wise to consult a medical practitioner, as they may be caused by conditions which domestic treatment cannot cure. Small tumors, either cancerous or innocent, occasionally grow on the cords, and can only be discovered and treated by a medical man who is accustomed to examining the larynx.

Cough. A cough may be defined as a violent expiratory effort. A deep breath is taken, the upper opening of the windpipe (glottis) is then closed, and is suddenly burst open by the forcible expulsion of air. With the sudden outward rush of air thus produced, any foreign body or collection of mucus is carried upwards into the throat and expectorated.

The most common cause of cough is the presence in the air passages of some irritant material. A cough is such a common affection, and is carried out in such an involuntary way, that we hardly realize how complicated is the mechanism which is necessary, and how serious it would be if any part of it were to break down and fail to act. It is necessary for the lining membrane of the air passages to be sensitive, and quickly to realize the presence of some peccant substance; the nerves which obtain this knowledge must convey it rapidly to the brain; that portion of the nervous system must be alert and ready to act; the nerves must convey back the intelligence to the muscles of the chest, abdomen, and larynx without delay, and all these many muscles must carry out an intricate combination of movements, or we should choke.

The causes of cough are as many as the forms of irritation of the air passages, but when we say we "have a cough" we usually mean we have a cold on the chest, or, in medical language, a slight bronchitis. This is the most frequent cause, but cough is a most distressing symptom in consumption and inflammation of the lungs. In throat affections it is usually very troublesome, enlarged tonsils or a swollen and flabby uvula producing the most irritating cough, which seems to give no relief, as it is impossible to expectorate these organs when they become the sources of such irritation.

Besides the various forms of irritation caused by affectations of the throat, windpipe, bronchial tubes, and lungs, there are others which to the uninitiated come as rather a surprise. For instance, the "stomach cough" in children is caused by some indigestible matter in the

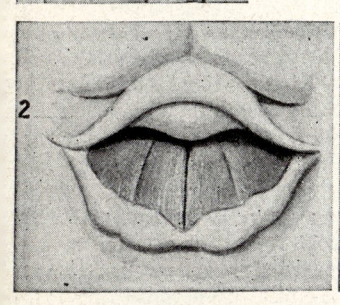

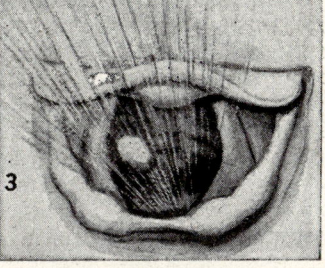

COUGH: THE PHYSICAL MECHANISM OF THE ACT
(1) In the first stage of a cough air is drawn into the chest; (2) then the vocal cords are firmly closed; (3) lastly, the breath is forcibly expelled from the chest, the vocal cords fly open and an irritating particle may be expelled.

Secretions blocking small Air Tubes

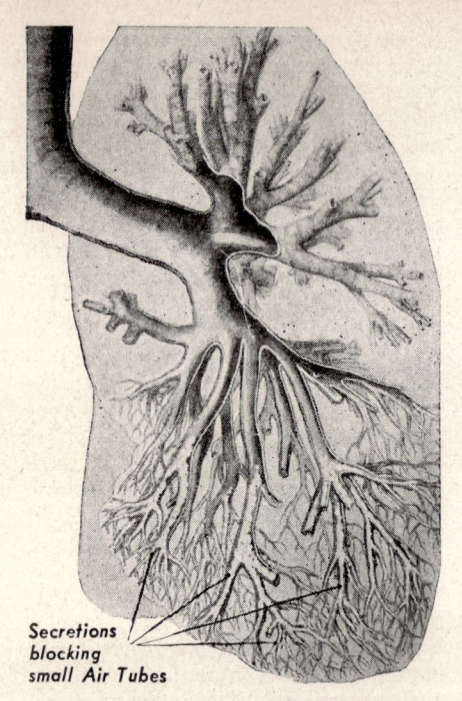

INSTANCE OF A USEFUL COUGH

The illustration shows how the smaller air tubes may be blocked by secretions so that their usefulness in breathing is destroyed. Here coughing should be encouraged in order to clear the tubes.

stomach, or by loaded bowels, acting on the nerves which control those organs. One of the great nerves—the vagus—gives off branches to both the stomach and the lungs, and it is through this close connection in nerve supply that the stomach cough is explained. For such a cough all sorts of cough remedies may be used without benefit, but a cathartic clears the bowels and remedies the irritation to which the "stomach" cough owed its origin.

In adults a somewhat similar condition is met with. A patient may have some slight irritation of his throat or windpipe which causes him little trouble, but some time after he has had a meal the trouble begins, and the cough continues incessantly, until he gets blue in the face and perhaps vomits up all the food he has taken. This condition requires no ordinary cough mixture, but will almost certainly be cured by the following treatment: Take half a teaspoonful to a teaspoonful of bicarbonate of soda and dissolve it in half a tumblerful of water, and sip it until it is finished or the cough is relieved. The treatment evidently acts either by relieving irritation of the stomach or by neutralizing excessive acidity.

Another branch of the vagus nerve is supplied to the ear, and may probably explain some interesting but rare cases of cough caused by ear trouble, in which a constant and irritating cough has been set up by a mass of hardened wax in one of the ears. When this is removed the cough is cured.

In hysterical and nervous people it is not at all uncommon to meet with cough which has a characteristic noisy "barking" sound, annoying indeed to the patient, but much more so to his friends. It is due to nothing but nervousness, and must be treated accordingly. In some stages of tuberculosis of the lungs the cough is dry, hacking, and ineffectual, but should be quite sufficient to arouse suspicion and lead to an examination of the chest, by which this disease may be diagnosed. In asthma, also, the cough has a peculiar character, which has been described as "suffocative." It comes on in violent spasms with the difficulty of breathing. In whooping cough the sound is sufficiently distinctive to enable us to recognize the disease. It consists of a series of short sharp coughs at the end of which the patient inhales deeply, making a crowing sound, or whoop.

Treatment. It is necessary to recognize which kind of cough is present in a particular case before it can be treated in a rational way. If the cause is in the throat, local treatment is of chief use. The inflamed tonsils and swollen mucous membrane must be soothed with sedative gargles or painted with thick liquids containing drugs. For cough associated with disease of the larynx and windpipe nothing is of such use as the inhalation of drugs with steam.

A few words on cough mixtures will be useful. It is no good to have a favorite prescription and use it for all cases of cough. It is necessary for the doctor to make a few simple observations first and decide what the medicine is to do, and then to prescribe accordingly. Let us suppose it is clear that the cough is not due to the conditions whose treatments have already been discussed. It is not due to throat or larynx, but is caused by a definite cold in the chest. Next we must consider whether the cough is dry (that is, without expectoration), painful, and accompanied with a soreness under the sternum, or whether it is loose, free, and with much expectoration. The former will require soothing, sedative medicine; the latter, stimulating drugs, which will hasten the clearing of the tubes. If sedative medicines were taken when there is much expectoration, the sensitiveness of the mucous membrane would be removed and the cough would be eased, but the phlegm would collect in large quantities in the tubes and obstruct the breathing. If the cough is dry and irritable, and the phlegm is brought up with difficulty and soreness is felt, sedative mixtures are suitable. They are most useful in the early stages of bronchitis. The acute inflammatory process is soothed by stimulating the secretion of protective mucus. In the later stages, as in subacute and chronic bronchitis, stimulating expectorants are needed to stimulate the mucous membrane to repair. The opiates (paregoric, morphine, and codeine) are anodyne expectorants and depress the cough reflex. They should never be employed when the mucus is excessive.

The cough mixture may be prepared in a thick and sticky form which is soothing to the throat. Such a preparation is called a linctus and relieves a cough due to an irritable throat.

If there is much expectoration, or the phlegm is thick and sticky, a stimulating medicine is required, and some of the best stimulating expectorants are squills, senega, and tolu combined with carbonate

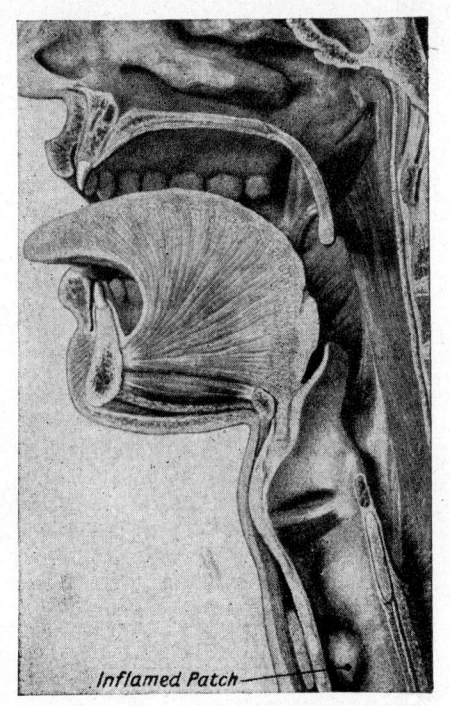

CAUSE OF A USELESS COUGH

A cough is sometimes due to irritation of the lining of the air passages, as shown above; in the absence of irritating material requiring to be expelled, such a cough should be checked.

of ammonia (the last being particularly useful).

When there is a large amount of watery expectoration, with constant cough and some difficulty of breathing, careful use may be made of ammonium chloride. If after a few doses the medicine has not given distinct relief, and decrease in the amount of expectoration, it had better be discontinued.

All cough mixtures must be administered with care, and discontinued as soon as possible, as they almost always contain drugs that are liable to upset the digestion, spoil the appetite, and even produce vomiting.

Many simple remedies are found useful for coughs, such as a piece of Spanish licorice, medicated glycerine jujubes, simple lozenges of chlorate of potash, tannin, or borax, combined with menthol or eucalyptus; black currant jelly, barley water, and linseed tea.

When the cough is sufficiently severe to require confinement to bed—and this is really always advisable if there is fever accompanying it—some local treatment should be employed. A hot linseed poultice to the throat and upper part of the chest will give great relief, and by the addition of a little mustard to it its effect may be increased. Rubbing the chest also may be tried, either with the compound camphor or the turpentine and acetic acid liniments.

AFFECTIONS OF THE VOICE

There are so many conditions which affect the voice that it is well we should know them and be in a position to distinguish those that are serious from those that are unimportant. The voice, as we have already shown, is produced by the vocal cords inside the larynx, but it is much affected in its timbre by the parts above, which act as resonating cavities and turn the voice sounds in different directions. These parts include the epiglottis, pharynx, nasal cavities, mouth, soft and hard palate, tongue, and lips. Affections of all these parts may therefore alter the quality and tone of the voice. The voice may be weak simply from want of force in the expiration, the air being driven outwards with insufficient power. This occurs in those cases in which the respiratory organs are affected. The voice may be tremulous, as in the feebleness of old age or in nervousness, in which the nervous system fails to control the muscles that must be used in vocalization.

In other cases the voice may be absent altogether, or only whispered sounds can be produced. This condition is caused by anything that prevents the vocal cords from being placed in apposition, such as loss of power over the small muscles of the larynx produced by disease or by some form of nervous affection.

One of the commonest alterations of the voice is that of hoarseness or a loss of the musical quality, caused by anything that interferes with regular and free vibration of the vocal cords, such as inflammatory or other swelling or thickening, growths, or paralysis. Since persistent hoarseness is often the first and only sign of a growth which may develop into a cancer, any person who keeps on being hoarse without any obvious reason should lose no time in paying a visit to a throat specialist or special hospital clinic.

We can divide the various causes of voice affections into two classes: (1) those that act indirectly upon the larynx through the nervous system; and (2) those which affect the larynx directly by disease of its various structures. These

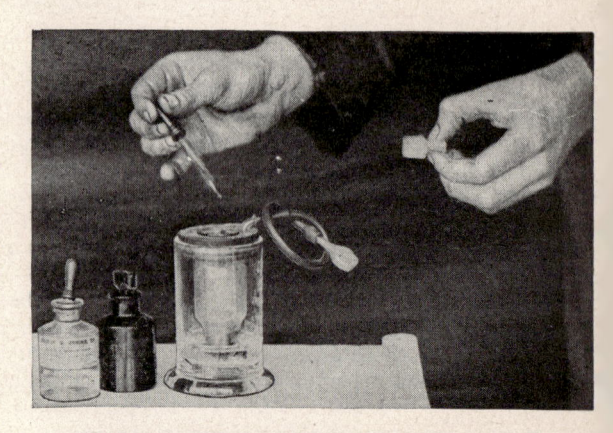

CHARGING THE AMMONIUM CHLORIDE INHALER
A small quantity of hydrochloric acid is put into the inner chamber shown in the diagram preceding. Sponge A is put on, and on this are dropped twenty drops of ammonia solution (see page **1510**).

classes correspond to what are called functional and organic causes.

Aphonia. The chief functional cause of voice affections is hysteria and its allied conditions, all of which are of nervous origin. Nervous loss of voice usually comes on quite suddenly, without any very definite reason. The patient is quite unable to utter a word, or he may be able to talk in a hardly audible whisper, and yet all the time he may be in perfect health, and quite free from pain or cough or any trouble which is symtomatic of an affection of the larynx.

This is called aphonia, or voicelessness, and is due simply to the psychological influences discussed fully in Section IX. A similar state is occasionally met with in men who have received a great nervous shock and whose nervous systems are broken down by work, worry, or dissipation.

Certain diseases of the nervous system also produce aphonia, such as tumors of the brain or injuries of the nerves which control the muscles of the larynx, but these can hardly be mistaken for the simpler forms we have been describing, as other prominent symptoms will be present.

The treatment of nervous loss of voice is usually very successful, many cases being cured on the spot by the application to the throat of some form of electrotherapeutic stimulation; but even if the first trial is unsuccessful the treatment should not be given up in despair, but continued daily for from five to ten minutes, gradually increasing the strength of the current. Often the voice returns for a time after this treatment and gradually goes again, but perseverance will usually be rewarded with success.

Another form of loss of voice is produced by overuse, especially if there is misuse also. It occurs in public singers, clergymen, and other public speakers, and its treatment consists of rest, all speaking and singing being absolutely given up, and only recommenced gradually and with great care after the passage of a reasonable length of time.

The voice is often much altered by conditions in other parts, the larynx itself being healthy. For example, a child who has adenoids or enlarged tonsils, or anyone with a sore or swollen throat, will talk with a thick, rough voice—"speaking through the nose," as it is called. The popular expression is an unfortunate one, for it is just those conditions which block the back of the nose and prevent the passage of the air

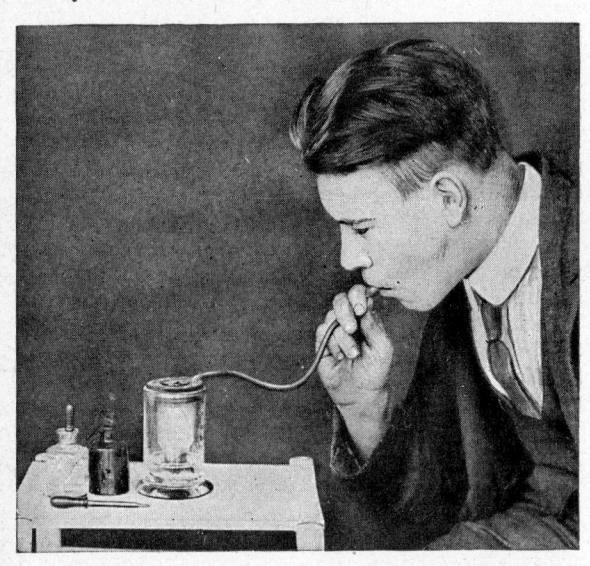

USING AMMONIUM INHALER FOR CATARRH
Immediately after ammonia has been dropped on sponge A (see diagram), the patient should suck air through the rubber tube. Freshly formed chloride vapor passes into the mouth and air passages. It should be inhaled deeply and then expelled through the mouth and nose, the "smoking" being kept up for ten minutes or longer.

through it that cause this change of voice. A highly arched or a cleft palate also gives a peculiar tone to the voice.

Each cause must receive its appropriate treatment, but we may here mention a few useful throat lozenges which have a good effect on the voice. Chlorate of potash tablets are excellent; they are much compressed and quite small, and may be kept comfortably under the tongue and allowed slowly to dissolve. Menthol and eucalyptus jujubes are sedative and softening to the swollen mucous membranes. Compound benzoic acid tablets encourage the secretion of mucus and moisten a dry throat, and are also soothing. A most useful class of remedies for hoarseness is formed by the various inhalations. Some of these have already been referred to; here it will be sufficient just to mention eucalyptus oil and compound tincture of benzoin (for inhalation with steam) and chloride of ammonium (in a special inhaler, shown in the accompanying photographs) as good sedatives for this purpose.

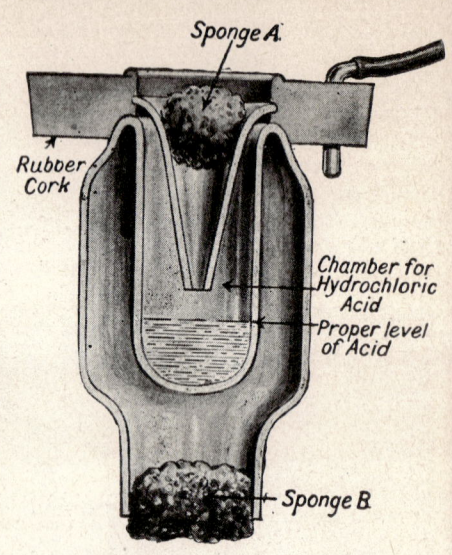

AMMONIUM CHLORIDE INHALER
Section of inner fitment of ammonium chloride inhaler, showing chamber for hydrochloric acid and sponge A, on to which ammonia is dropped. Sponge B alters the chloride vapor.

CHAPTER 109

DISEASES OF THE BRONCHIAL TUBES

Acute Bronchitis — Chronic Bronchitis — Bronchiectasis — Asthma.

BRONCHITIS, or as it is now more correctly termed, tracheobronchitis, since the trachea is affected in this condition, is an inflammation of the mucous membrane of the trachea and bronchial tubes, and in its mild forms is what we call a cold in the chest. Usually it is only the large bronchial tubes that are affected, and the disease is not then a dangerous one, but sometimes the small tubes are involved from the beginning of the illness, or the inflammation gradually spreads from the large tubes to the smaller ones, and the deeper it goes the more serious becomes the attack. The name of capillary bronchitis is given to the more serious condition, as the tubes then affected are so minute. This disease may gradually merge into bronchopneumonia from involvement of the lung tissue itself, which is in direct connection with the smallest tubes. We see, then, that cases of bronchitis vary in importance, according to the parts involved, from a slight cold to an inflammation of the lungs. Careful attention to a slight bronchitis may save a very serious illness.

Acute Bronchitis. The chief cause of bronchitis is exposure to cold and wet, and it is natural, therefore, that it should be a disease of the winter months, and of damp and variable climates. It is most commonly met with in those whose occupations involve much exposure. As the old and the very young are less able to bear exposure to cold, bronchitis affects them more often than the mature; it involves the delicate and debilitated more than the strong and healthy. Any chronic maladies, such as sinusitis, diabetes, or Bright's disease, predispose to it, and if a person has once been affected by it there is always a strong tendency to a recurrence, which can be avoided only by special care. Stout, fat persons are very prone to develop bronchitis in the winter. The mode of life in other ways also is a factor in the case, for those who live in overheated rooms, who work in ill-ventilated workshops, or who spend a good share of their time in any unhygienic surroundings generally run greater risks than those blessed with comfortable and healthy homes. Certain trades, too, are particularly dangerous from this point of view, for workers who are obliged to inhale much irritating matter, such as cotton, steel, or charcoal, develop a sen-

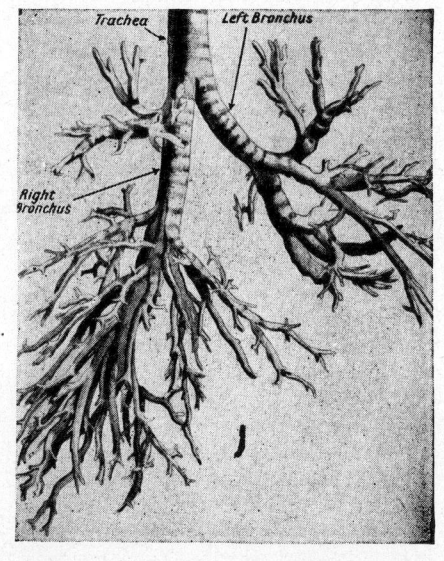

AIR TUBES TO THE LUNG
The system of air tubes resembles a tree with its branches turned upside down, the bronchi being the larger limbs and the bronchial tubes the branches. Inflammation of the tubes constitutes the condition known as bronchitis.

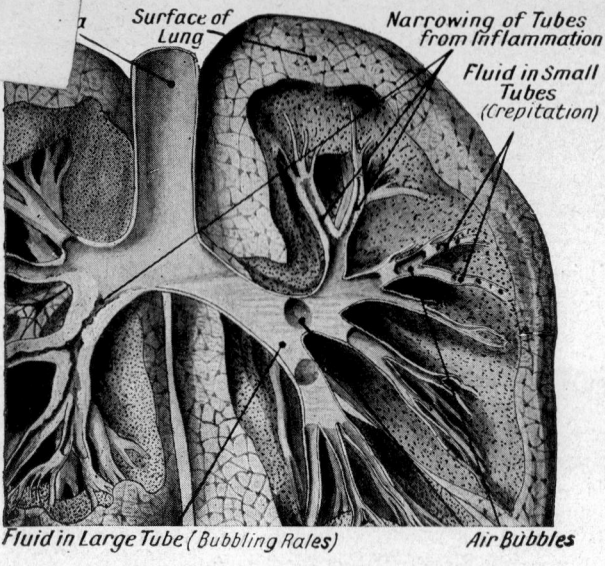

Surface of Lung
Narrowing of Tubes from Inflammation
Fluid in Small Tubes (Crepitation)
Fluid in Large Tube (Bubbling Rales)
Air Bubbles

RALES: SIGNS OF PULMONARY DISORDERS

In this diagram the conditions causing râles are shown, for clearness, in the larger tubes. Air passing through fluid in the smaller tubes causes crepitations; in the larger or in lung cavities, bubbling râles; passing through tubes that are constricted but dry, it causes whistling and snoring rhonchi.

sitive condition of the bronchial mucous membrane, which makes them a ready prey.

The effects of cold may act in many ways: the clothes may get soaked, and circumstances may prevent their being changed; the feet may get wet; the body may get chilled rapidly when hot, as after exercise; cold may be caught through insufficient clothes. This last condition is a particularly fruitful cause. A sudden change of weather from hot to cold, or from dry to damp, or change of wind from south to east, is followed by many cases of bronchitis; and although the complaint cannot be looked upon as "catching," yet climatic changes affecting many people at the same time may produce it in almost an epidemic form, and bronchitis is very often a complication of the ordinary epidemic infectious diseases, such as measles. In fact, the chief danger of measles is that the accompanying bronchitis will develop into broncho-pneumonia.

Symptoms. The symptoms, therefore, which usher in an attack of bronchitis are simply those of a cold. There are shivering and sneezing, chilliness and a feeling of illness, headache and a little fever, a slight cough and soreness of the chest. Generally there are nasal catarrh, sore throat, watery eyes, and slight hoarseness, the inflammatory trouble evidently affecting all the mucous membranes and gradually spreading lower along the air passages. If the temperature be taken on going to bed it is found to be slightly raised, perhaps 1°, to about 100° F.; the pulse is more rapid than normal, but only by about ten beats; the respiration is quickened to a rate of twenty-five a minute.

This is the time for the employment of prompt and efficient treatment, for if the cold be neglected the symptoms get worse; the cough grows more troublesome, and comes on in fits excited by slight causes, as a gust of cold air, movement or talking; soreness in the chest is more severe, is felt beneath the upper part of the sternum, and is much increased by coughing.

In the early stage there is no expectoration, the mucous membrane being dry, swollen, and sensitive, but phlegm soon begins to form. At first it is only slight and consists of a thin, watery fluid; after a time, however, it grows free, thick, and yellow. It may be so thick and sticky that the greatest difficulty is experienced in coughing it up, and the violent straining may cause little streaks of blood to

DISEASES OF THE BRONCHIAL TUBES

be mixed with it. This is alarming at first, but does not indicate any danger, being due to some minute blood vessels of the mucous membrane having given way.

If, now, the inflammation spreads into the smallest tubes, even more serious symptoms develop, and there is real cause for anxiety. This complication is more common in children than in adults. The breathing gets much more difficult and labored, the respirations are increased in rapidity, inspiration is carried out with great energy, many extra muscles being brought into use; it becomes almost impossible to breathe while lying down, and the patient has to sit propped up with pillows in bed, or even in a chair. The cough grows more violent and exhausting, the expectoration is most profuse, and is got rid of with the greatest difficulty. The temperature may rise and the pulse grow quick, and the patient become collapsed and exhausted. The mucus collects in the tubes, expectoration ceases, blueness of the face and extremities appears, and death may result from suffocation and prostration. Fortunately, a fatal outcome occurs in only a small number of cases, and ordinarily the symptoms never become so serious.

Treatment. An ordinary mild attack of bronchitis lasts from ten days to a fortnight, but in the severer cases it is a much longer illness. The knowledge that a neglected attack may become so serious should put us on our guard, and even the mildest cases should be carefully treated, and no risks run by going out of doors. It is far better to be overcareful than to treat the matter lightly and suffer accordingly. It is always the wisest course to stay indoors with an attack of bronchitis, however important one's engagements. A few days in a comfortably warm room will often cure the attack. The temperature of the room should be kept at about 65° F., and the bedroom should also be kept warm, as nothing is so bad as going from a warm room into a cold one, for in this way the cough is sure to be made more troublesome, and may cause a sleepless night. A good plan is to have a hot bath, or to put the feet in mustard and water, go to bed early, and have a hot bottle to warm the bed.

If the chest feels sore, put on a hot linseed poultice (see Chapter 86) or give it a good rubbing with camphorated oil until it is red. A hot drink—a glassful of hot spirit and water or a basin of gruel—will help to make one sweat and do one good. During the night care must be taken not to throw the clothes off, or all the good may be undone.

If these measures have not successfully checked the attack, the patient must remain in bed and continue the linseed poultices. A fresh poultice should be put on every four hours; each should be kept on for two hours, and a piece of absorbent cotton should be put over the chest during the intervals. The poultices may be applied either to the back or to the chest, the advantage of putting them on the back being that the weight of the poultice is less felt and the breathing is not so impeded. For a poultice to be of any good it must be thoroughly hot. Stimulating liniments act in the same way as poultices by bringing the blood to the skin and thus relieving the inflamed parts within; they should be rubbed on the chest, both back and front, until the skin is well reddened.

Inhalations give great relief. In the early stage, when there is little expectoration, plain steam is useful, or a tablespoonful of compound tincture of benzoin may be added to the pint of hot water. Later, to assist in the expectoration of the phlegm, it is better to use oil of pine or pure terebene, or iodine and creosote. A pitcher, teakettle, or jar is the most convenient form of domestic inhaler, and each inhalation should last for from five to ten minutes.

Another useful form of treatment is the bronchitis kettle (see page 1142), which both warms and moistens the air of the room, and almost acts like an inhalation. It must be so arranged that its spout conducts the steam well into

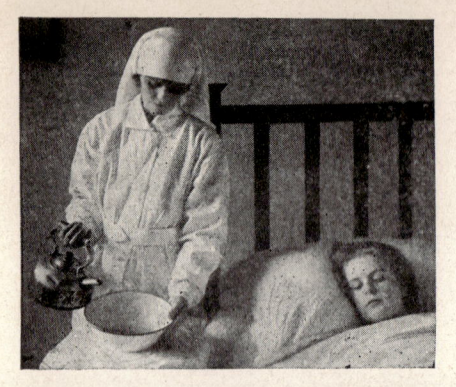

ARRANGING A BRONCHIAL INHALATION
One way of giving an inhalation is to pour some tincture of benzoin or other soothing remedy into a small basin and fill it up with boiling water. This should be set near the patient.

the room and as near the patient as is convenient. A little eucalyptus oil added occasionally to the water conduces to its usefulness. The effect of steam in bronchitis is to soften and loosen the phlegm and render it more easy to expectorate.

Diet. The food should be light and nutritious, and should consist chiefly of fluids. If there is much fever, or if the cough is troublesome, solid food is quite inadmissible. Plenty of beef tea and milk and milk foods must be taken, and from three to four pints of fluid nourishment will be required in the twenty-four hours. The complaint is an exhausting one, and as much food should be taken as the digestion will permit; in this way the weakness of convalescence may be lessened. As far as possible the food should be taken at regular intervals, a cupful every three or four hours. Stimulants are not usually necessary, but if the attack is a bad one, and the patient weak or exhausted, they are advisable, and about four to six tablespoonfuls of good brandy in the twenty-four hours would be a suitable quantity; it can be given mixed with the milk, or with some effervescing water. As convalescence begins the food must be increased in quantity and strengthened in quality, starting with a little boiled fish, some chicken or meat jelly, and going on to ordinary food gradually, lamb or mutton being the first meat to attempt.

Drugs. As the expectoration gets more plentiful and thicker a stimulating mixture should be given. The most commonly used drugs for this purpose are ammonium chloride, terebene and terpin hydrate. When the cough is very distressing an opiate is usually added to the mixture.

It is well not to begin a sedative cough mixture too early, as by relieving the sensibility of the mucous membrane and easing the cough it may allow the phlegm to collect in the tubes. It is particularly useful in the later stages of the attack, when the cough may be troublesome and the expectoration small in amount. During the illness care must be taken to keep the bowels acting regularly; a dose of salts or aperient water will be all that is required.

Complications. It must never be forgotten that there are many serious complications which may arise during a sharp attack of bronchitis, and that these are difficult to recognize and treat successfully. It is always wise, therefore, in all but the mildest cases to call in a doctor.

The special tendency of this complaint to return makes it of great importance to assure a very thorough recovery from the first attack, and to adopt very careful precautionary measures for the future by keeping the body in a good state of health. Warm clothing should be worn, and it is advisable that the undergarment be of some absorbent material, such as wool, both for winter and summer; in this way the body will be protected from chills. The utmost care is necessary to avoid all exposure to cold, dampness, or sudden changes of temperature, and to take great care when going out in wet windy weather, fogs, or night air. The mouth must be closed and only the nose used for respiration. The danger of breathing cold and damp air is not always understood, but it is important to know that this is as fruitful a cause of bronchitis as exposure of the chest and body. Where circumstances permit, much benefit will be obtained by spending the winter in a warm, equable climate. One winter passed without a cold in the chest may mean complete recovery from the catarrhal tendency.

If the tendency to winter catarrhs and bronchitis is pronounced in a young person, the nose and throat should be examined. Often the removal of septic tonsils, the straightening of the nasal septum, or drainage of an infected sinus will act as a charm in clearing up bronchitic chests.

Chronic Bronchitis. This is often the result of an acute attack which has been imperfectly cured, or it may be left after repeated attacks. It is the cause of the winter cough of elderly people, and is then a regular visitor every year. Some persons never fail to have a cough every winter, which troubles them more or less through the whole of the cold season, and leaves them only when the summer is well established. The disease commonly affects those whose occupations expose them to all weathers, and is one of the commonest reasons for the poor seeking admission to hospitals.

Symptoms. The previous history, then, is that the patient has had many attacks of bronchitis, and for years has had a cough in the winter, which begins about October and, unless he is very lucky, does not leave him until May. Directly the cold weather sets in he catches cold, and the cough begins. It is very violent, comes on in frequent paroxysms, and shakes him to the foundation. The attacks are brought on by the slightest exertion—by speaking, by breathing cold air, or even by moving from one room to another. The cough is often particularly troublesome when going to bed, probably because the bedroom is colder than the living room, and when getting up in the morning, because phlegm has collected in the bronchial tubes during the night and must be cleared out of them before the cough will cease.

The expectoration is usually very free, and varies in character considerably, sometimes being thick and yellow and very difficult to expel, or transparent and watery, and occasionally tinged with blood. Besides the cough there is usually some shortness of breath, which is brought on by slight exertion, such as going upstairs or even walking. It is bad at night, makes it almost impossible to go to sleep when lying flat, and is only relieved when the sufferer is propped up in bed with pillows or is sitting up in a chair. Both cough and breathlessness are much increased by fogs, cold wind, and dampness.

The general health is naturally much affected. The patient grows thin and weak, his heart fails, his circulation becomes sluggish, his legs swell, and his complexion is dusky. All his symptoms improve in the summer, but each winter he loses more ground, which finally cannot be recovered, and he becomes a chronic invalid. Various complications ensue; the chest becomes barrel-shaped and enlarged from emphysema (see later); the heart becomes weak and dilated, and occasionally a chronic inflammation of the lungs sets in, which may prove fatal.

Treatment. The treatment of chronic bronchitis must be directed to relief rather than cure. The disease, when it has reached at all an advanced stage, is really incurable, and it then becomes necessary to relieve as much as possible the various symptoms as they arise, and to preserve the general health by careful hygiene and suitable surroundings. The preventive measures advised for acute bronchitis are all of even greater importance in the chronic form, and every means must be taken to maintain the strength and avoid catching cold. After a time it becomes almost impossible for the chronic bronchitic to venture out at all in severe weather; he must shut himself up as soon as cold sets in, and remain a prisoner to the house until the warm weather returns. The only way to avoid this privation is to winter in a warm and equable climate. When the expectoration is profuse a dry climate is best, with a stimulating air; when it is scanty, then a moist, warm, soft, and relaxing air should be chosen. Pine woods in the neighborhood, sea air, and shelter from mountains are all useful auxiliaries. Everything should be done to assist the digestion and encourage the appetite. A certain amount of exercise out of doors, when the climate permits, or of massage when confinement to the house is a necessity, will help in this direction. The food must be good, nourishing, and taken in as large quantities as possible. Stimulants in moderation are usually required. Fatty foods are useful; among them cod-liver oil and halibut-liver oil must be included. Tonics are required, such as iron or quinine and the various malt preparations—malt and cod-liver oil are of special value.

For the various symptoms external and internal measures may be employed. Counterirritation by stimulating liniments often eases cough and reduces expectoration. Turpentine and acetic acid liniment, or turpentine liniment with a teaspoonful of weak tincture of iodine to each ounce, and compound camphor liniment are all useful; they should be rubbed in thoroughly, back and front, night and morning, and continued for a long time.

Drugs often prove of much value when employed by inhalation. In some cases, tincture of ipecacuanha is found very useful; it is mixed with twice as much water in a spray apparatus. The spray should be drawn well into the chest with a deep breath. At first this measure must be employed with care, only a few breaths being taken at each sitting, but as the patient grows accustomed to the drug it may be taken with greater freedom. Creosote, terebene, and compound tincture of benzoin may be used in hot water, the steam being inhaled; or they may be mixed with mineral oil and then inhaled in the form of a cloud. For this purpose a special apparatus is required, called an atomizer or nebulizer (see Chapter 87). Chloride of ammonium is also used in a special form of inhaler, and consists of white, unirritating fumes (see Chapter 108).

The special medicines which may be used for chronic bronchitis are the balsams and iodide of potash, especially the latter, of which three grains may be taken three times a day, in the form of tablets dissolved in water.

BRONCHIECTASIS

Bronchiectasis is a condition characterized by the formation of cavities of various sizes, resulting from dilatation of the air tubes or bronchi. These become filled with excessive secretion which stagnates and putrefies. From time to time the contents of the cavities are coughed up; the expectoration is extremely offensive in odor and taste, and the breath is very objectionable.

One cause of bronchiectasis is the inhalation of some small foreign body down the windpipe into the lung (see illustration). This passes along the bronchial tubes until it comes to rest in one of the smaller tubes, giving rise to inflammation and softening of its walls as the result of infection with the germs which are carried into the lung. The bronchial tube then gradually dilates, owing to the pressure of the air caused by the strain of coughing. The spread of the inflammation into the substance of the lung around the bronchial tube leads to the formation of scar tissue, which as it contracts down, still further tends to dilate the tube by pulling on its already softened walls.

Bronchiectasis in most cases arises as a complication or a sequel of a disease of the lungs. The method of causation is similar to that just described. The most important of these are bronchopneumonia, pneumonia, tuberculosis, bronchitis, and chronic pleurisy. In rare cases the disease is congenital.

DISEASES OF THE BRONCHIAL TUBES

If bronchopneumonia or pneumonia does not resolve completely, *i.e.*, if the products of the inflammation which made the lung solid during the acute stage of the illness are not completely absorbed, scar tissue forms in the lung. This tends to contract and so may give rise to dilatation of some of the bronchial tubes, and a condition of bronchiectasis, the dilatation being uniform or on one side only of the tubes, may ensue. In the same way, in the more chronic or fibroid form of pulmonary tuberculosis, bronchiectatic cavities may appear in the lungs.

The detection of bronchiectasis in its early stages is a matter of some difficulty, but it is of the utmost importance that knowledge on the subject should be widely disseminated, for in the early stages every hope may be held out that efficient treatment will effect a cure. Hence it is proper to give here a description of the early case of bronchiectasis.

Symptoms. The symptoms vary depending on how the condition originates and how rapidly it progresses. The early clinical course may be that of a protracted bronchopneumonia or may be a sequel to measles, whooping cough, or influenza. The slight toxemia may manifest itself by easy fatigue, lack of tone, and sometimes fever. The symptoms may subside and not reappear until another infection occurs, but even a mild cold may renew them.

A feeling of false security is thus engendered. After an interval of a few weeks or longer, however, a cough develops which is accompanied by a little expectoration. This expectoration is at the beginning small in amount, often not more than a teaspoonful, and occurs usually on getting out of bed in the morning, or with any change of posture, as in stooping or lying down. The matter coughed up has a peculiarly offensive smell. Directly this warning is noticed no time must be lost before treatment is begun, or it will be too late for this to be successful.

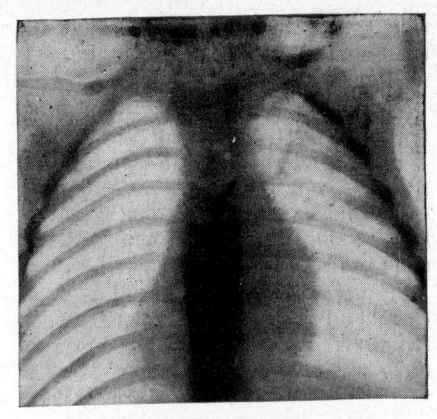

ONE CAUSE OF BRONCHIECTASIS
X-ray photograph revealing a screw caught at the junction of the bronchi. Inflammation ensues and leads to dilatation of the tubes, which may result in the formation of a cavity in the surrounding lung tissue.

The condition of a patient who has a fully developed and extensive bronchiectasis is most distressing. He is very short of breath, has a paroxysmal cough, and brings up large quantities of evil-smelling sputum. As much as a pint or more may be coughed up in twenty-four hours. Any change of position of the body, such as getting out of bed or lying down, will lead to expectoration and a partial emptying of the cavity in the lung.

Usually by this time several cavities are formed and both lungs are affected. The cavities are generally situated in the lower parts of the lungs, and not at the top, as occurs most frequently in tuberculosis. In the last stages of the disease great weakness and prostration result from the loss of appetite and from the poisons generated from the putrefying matter in the lungs. Periodical bouts of fever occur, corresponding at first with the retention of secretion in the cavities, but in the later stages the temperature is almost constantly raised. Secondary abscesses may arise in other parts of the body, a very favorite site being the brain, and cerebral abscess, when it occurs, is always a fatal complication. In other cases the infection may spread to the pleural sac, giving rise to an empyema (see the Surgery section for this condition).

The fingers in bronchiectasis undergo a peculiar change known as clubbing. The finger-tips become swollen, bulbous, and usually somewhat blue, with curving of the nails. In long-standing cases the toes are similarly affected, and the joints of the wrists and feet may swell.

Treatment. In cases resulting from an inhaled foreign body an examination should be made under the X-rays in order to locate the presence of the foreign body. By means of a surgical operation, in which an instrument known as a bronchoscope is used, the foreign body can frequently be removed. Its removal shortly after its inhalation will take away the cause of bronchiectasis in this group of cases, and the disease will thereby be prevented.

It is sometimes necessary for the establishment of the diagnosis to inject iodized oil into the bronchial system. In the X-ray film taken after this procedure the bronchiectatic cavities can be visualized.

If the lungs are examined carefully in a child who has had an attack of bronchopneumonia it is often found that the air entry to one lower lobe is weak, and some sticky bubbling noises (râles) can be heard as the patient breathes very deeply in and out. These signs indicate that there is an early formation of fibrous or scar tissue at the bottom of the lung. Such a case, if left untreated, may well develop bronchiectasis.

The only reasonable hope of prevention is the avoidance and careful management of acute respiratory infections. Inflammatory foci in the upper respiratory tract, especially the sinuses, must be eliminated.

A complete cure is only obtainable through the surgical extirpation of the diseased portion of the lung. This operation is an extensive one and can only be used in certain cases.

An important technique used to aid the escape of suppurative material from the bronchi is postural drainage. The patient hangs his head over the edge of the bed or may simply bend over the back of a chair with the head as low as possible. This should be made part of his daily toilet and should be done twice a day, fifteen to twenty minutes each time. In very severe cases removal of the secretions by means of the bronchoscope may have to be resorted to. Attempts have been made to disinfect the cavity in the lungs by means of inhalations of antiseptic substances, especially of creosote. This may be placed upon the pad of a mask, worn almost continuously throughout the day over the mouth, the pad being moistened from time to time with a few drops of solution. Antiseptic expectorant drugs such as creosote, terebene, benzoin, etc., are also of some help.

Another method of creosote administration is that which is known as the creosote bath. The patient is placed in an atmosphere containing a high percentage of the creosote vapor, which he inhales. A small room with a concrete floor and bare of furniture should be set aside for the purpose. A small quantity of commercial creosote is placed in a metal tray over a lamp or other heater which stands upon the floor. The lamp is lit, care being taken not to have a sufficiently big flame to ignite the creosote. The patient, wearing a gown or other garment which covers the whole body, and with his eyes protected by closely fitting goggles and his nose by plugs of absorbent cotton, is then shut in the room, and as the creosote volatilizes, the vapors are breathed deep down into the lungs. Coughing ensues as the result of the irritation, and large quantities of offensive sputum are brought up from the cavities in the lung.

The "bath" is usually given for about five to ten minutes, and two or three such treatments are administered during the week. Gradually the treatments may be prolonged until at the end of a few weeks the patient may be taking a daily bath lasting for half an hour. Care is required in the selection of cases for this form of treatment, as it is found to be too drastic for those of weakened constitutions.

The administration of autogenous vaccines, prepared from organisms in the sputum, affords a certain amount of relief in some cases, but the results are for the most part unsatisfactory and it is clear that such a form of treatment will not lead to an obliteration of the cavity.

ASTHMA

This disease is described here in company with other affections of the organs of respiration because its symptoms closely connect it with them; but it is now known to belong to the group of diseases known as the allergic diseases, in which an individual or a family becomes so sensitive to certain substances that these substances constitute a poison to them while being perfectly harmless to other persons. These people are said to be anaphylactic to, or allergic to, the given article or articles, and to have an idiosyncrasy to it. The chief allergic diseases recognized as such at present are asthma, hay fever, urticaria, eczema and angioneurotic edema. There is a definite tendency for them to be hereditary, though sometimes an idiosyncrasy comes on after a severe shock to the nervous system, such as an operation or the birth of a child, or a long period of nervous strain. In these allergic diseases the nervous system appears to be unduly irritable, and in the case of asthma this irritability shows itself by its action on the bronchial tubes.

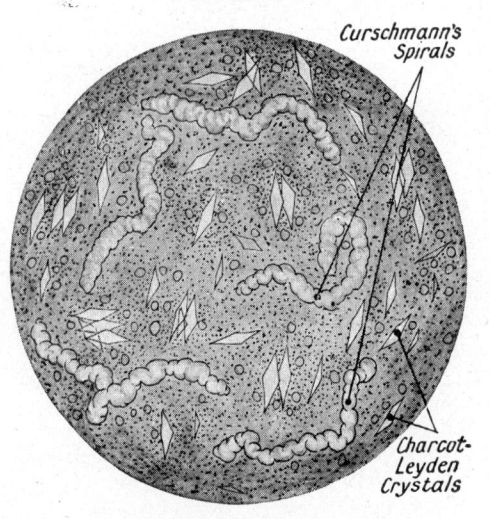

SPUTUM ABNORMALITIES IN ASTHMA
The rough pellets occurring in the sputum of asthma, when examined microscopically, are seen to contain Curschmann's spirals, supposed to be casts of small air tubes, and Charcot-Leyden crystals; the latter are found in leukemic blood, etc.

Causes. Asthma is liable to run in families; it is also distinctly hereditary, asthmatic parents begetting children with a predisposition to the complaint. But it occurs, too, in many people in whom there is no evidence whatever of inheritance, and the causes of this acquired form are legion, so we can only attempt to give a general outline of them. It affects both sexes, but is slightly more common in men than women. It occurs at all ages, but the first attack most commonly comes on in childhood, and not infrequently the complaint sticks to the individual for years, the attacks recurring in spite of treatment; but those cases that begin early in life are often outgrown when maturity is reached. It may be difficult to tell beforehand what will bring on an attack in any particular case, but a person who has suffered for some time can generally do so as regards himself from previous unpleasant experiences. There are two distinct divisions into which the causes can be grouped, the first being sensitivity to proteins introduced into the body from the outside and the second being sensitivity to those that arise within the body as bacterial products emanating from foci of infection. Combinations of the two may exist.

It is a curious thing that the very slightest change of locality may set up an attack, or may remove one when it exists. Some people can live on one side of a street and not on the other, at the back of a house and not at the front; some are free from the trouble in inland air, others at the seaside; some in elevated and others in low-lying localities; some in a smoky town, which they find suits them better than even pure mountain air.

Of the second class of cases, those sensitive to bacterial products, the focus of infection is usually in the sinuses or teeth, but may be anywhere in the body (lungs, kidney, Fallopian tubes, etc.).

Hay fever, eczema, and urticaria are all at times associated with asthma, they may occur in different members of the same family, or in the same member at different times. An attack of eczema or urticaria may subside only to give place to an attack of asthma, and may reappear as the asthma passes off. Some affection of the nose or larynx may be the origin of an attack—some sensitive part in the nasal passages which is irritated by the inhalation of solid particles or noxious emanations. These are perhaps sufficient examples of the strange vagaries of this complaint.

Symptoms. The symptoms of asthma come on in paroxysms at indefinite periods. The patient goes to bed feeling perfectly well, and sleeps comfortably for several hours; then, early in the morning, he wakes up with a feeling of oppression and discomfort; his breathing is difficult and noisy. He falls again into a troubled sleep, only to wake still more oppressed. He again dozes, but can sleep no longer, for all his energies are required to struggle with his breathing. He sits up in bed, or is forced to get up, and he places himself in the position he has discovered by previous experience to be most helpful, and brings into play all the muscles of his body that can in any way help his respiratory efforts.

His breathing is noisy and whistling, and is accompanied by a loud humming sound. The air is drawn into his chest with the greatest difficulty; he cannot speak or move; his face gets pale, anxious, and covered with sweat; he grows dusky or even blue in the face. The condition is one to excite alarm, but probably is worse to look upon than to endure. However extreme may be the difficulty of respiration, it never ends fatally during the attack, for after a longer or shorter period of struggle the symptoms gradually abate, and the sufferer recovers his usual health. The attack may vary in duration from half an hour to several days, and usually ends by the expectoration of a certain amount of mucus, which seems to give relief, and the patient can then eat, sleep, and go about as usual.

The expectoration in asthma is peculiar, for it consists of semitransparent masses, like little balls of jelly, during the first two or three days of the attack, and in the later stages of ordinary phlegm.

These attacks occur at irregular intervals, and after a time leave their mark upon the sufferer's frame. He grows wasted and anemic, develops a severe stoop and the barrel-shaped chest of emphysema (see the illustration on page 1562).

The immediate cause of all this trouble is usually a spasmodic contraction of the small muscular fibers of the bronchial tubes, by which the size of the air passage is diminished. Another variety of asthma is caused by a sudden swelling of the mucous membrane lining the tubes, very similar to the sudden swelling of the skin which occurs in urticaria. It is only when the swelling or spasm passes off that the patient is able to breathe again with freedom.

Treatment. The treatment of asthma is divided into two distinct parts: the treatment of the immediate attack and the measures to be taken to avoid future attacks.

With regard to the acute attack, it is well for asthmatics to find out between attacks which drug, among the many used, best agrees with them, and to keep a supply ready by the bedside or in some convenient place. If skilled attention is at hand or if the patient can use a hypodermic needle on himself, an injection of adrenalin or ephedrine under the skin immediately after the first symptoms are felt may stop the attack almost instantaneously. Ephedrine sulphate tablets are very helpful to some people; others like a strong cup of coffee or an amyl nitrite capsule, such as is carried for angina pectoris (see page 1459). Many people find that stramonium inhaled in the smoke from a stramonium cigarette or burned in a plate is very helpful in controlling an attack. An abundance of fresh air often relieves the shortness of breath.

When the acute attack is over, preventive treatment is of great importance. The patient will have found that sleeping in certain places or particular climates, or inhaling certain smells, or indulging in certain articles of diet, will bring on an attack, and he must avoid

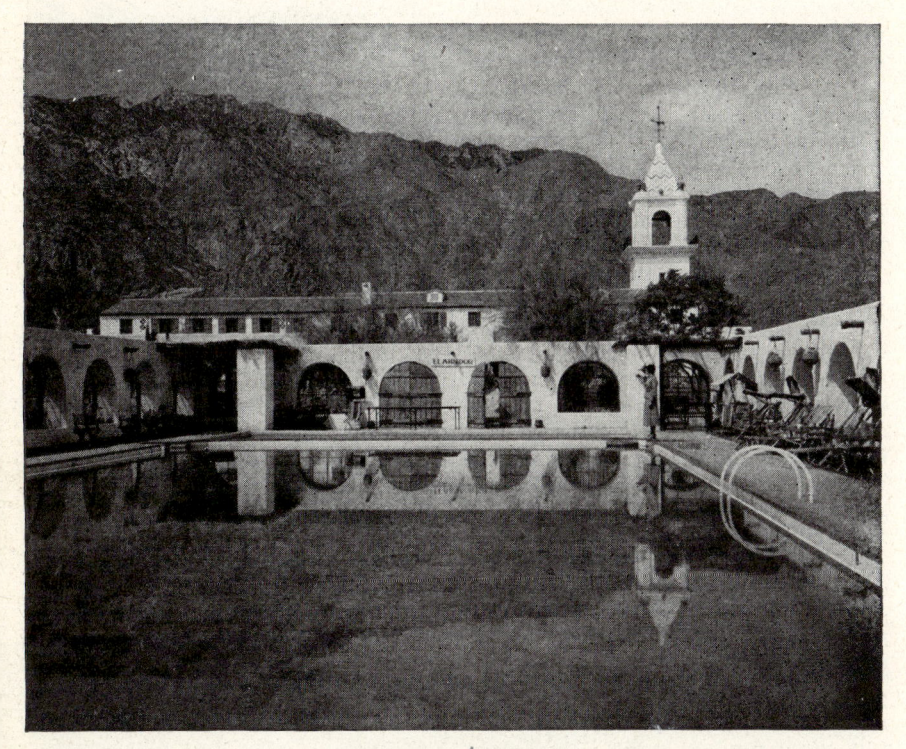

RELATIVELY POLLEN-FREE

Sufferers from asthma have for centuries found relief by going to various localities known to give relief. It was not until the causes of asthma were recognized that other treatment was possible. Today, although asthma yields to anti-allergic measures, many people continue to seek resorts for relief. These resorts have one feature in common—a low pollen count in the atmosphere, whether by reason of desert or high mountain location. Palm Springs, here shown, has such an atmosphere as a consequence of being located inland in California, beyond the richly vegetated coast region and shielded from it by intervening mountains.
© *Ewing Galloway*

the cause, whatever it be. As food idiosyncrasy is a common cause, the diet must be carefully managed. By careful consideration the individual may be able to work out exactly what articles of food are harmful to him, and these should be resolutely avoided. Tests can be made to discover if there is any susceptibility to the materials with which the bed is furnished, such as horsehair, feathers, down, all of which are causes of trouble to some people. The domestic animals may also be a stumbling block; cat asthma, in fact, is fairly common, and in part explains the instinctive dislike that many people have for cats.

In summer time there are many pollens about which while causing hay fever in one person may cause asthma in another. Extracts of many of these substances have been prepared and can be rubbed into a little scratch on the arm in order to see whether the patient is unduly sensitive to them, as shown by the fact that the scratch will become surrounded by a red ring if there is sensitivity. The patient may be found sensitive to substances which cannot be completely avoided, either because they are so widespread or because they are essential, and in these cases an attempt is made to desensitize the individual. A person sensitive to house dust will find it practically impossible to avoid contact with this offending agent. The house dust is prepared in a form suitable for injection and the patient is then given subcutaneous injections starting at first with very minute doses and gradually increasing to a relatively large dose.

The principal meal should be taken in the middle of the day, and only a light one in the evening. The general health must be maintained by good habits, by healthy exercise, fresh air, cold bathing, freedom from worry, and careful avoidance of all the risks likely to lead to an attack of bronchitis.

No particular climate can be recommended, but the patient must choose that which experience has shown suits him best. If one place disagrees with him he must try a change of air, always remembering that it is not necessarily the theoretically healthy climate that will give him relief. In some cases relief has been obtained by removal of the patient to a state like Arizona, New Mexico or Florida. There is, however, growing belief that climatic treatment is overrated.

All asthmatics should have the nose examined to see that there is as good an airway as possible. Adenoids or nasal polyps, if present, should be removed so

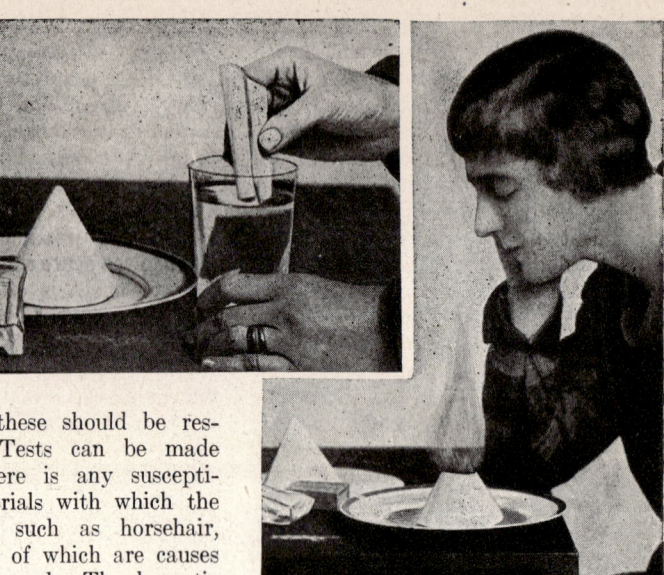

NITER PAPER FOR ASTHMA
Above: soak a circular piece of absorbent paper in two ounces of niter (saltpeter) in a tumbler of water. When dry, fold it in cone form; light at top and inhale fumes, as shown below.

as to avoid the risk that they may become foci of infection.

A wide variety of drugs have been used in the treatment of asthmatic attacks. No single one is ideal. Many, such as morphine, papaverin, and atropine are only to be used by a physician. Certain simple measures applied by the patient himself may give relief.

In many cases the application of drugs directly to the mucous membrane is found very useful, and this can be carried out by employing smokes, sprays, or clouds containing the drugs. A very useful smoke which is both cheap and easily made at home is that of niter paper. It is prepared by dipping a piece of fairly thick ordinary blotting paper in water in which niter (nitrate of potash) has been dissolved, and drying it. There is no difficulty in making the solution, as it requires as much niter as the water will dissolve. These papers are sometimes made stronger and more efficacious by adding some chlorate of potash to the solution. They are soaked in boiling water to which has been added equal parts of the niter and chlorate of potash in as large quantities as the water will dissolve, and using much thicker blotting-paper. The papers will keep for any length of time, and will not lose their virtue. The way to use them is to fold the paper across the middle and stand it up on a metal plate, or the cover of a tin box, and light it at its upper corners. The milder papers gradually smoulder; the stronger burn more quickly and give off, in doing so, thick fumes of smoke, which fill the air of the room and cause a feeling of drowsiness when inhaled. The best time to use them is when going to bed.

Many other smokes are produced by burning the dried and powdered leaves of plants, those most frequently used belonging to the order Atropaceae, such as belladonna, Datura stramonium or D. tatula, the two latter being generally included in asthma powders. The leaves are powdered up, mixed with a small quantity of niter to make them burn, and a teaspoonful is placed on a plate and set alight.

Tobacco often succeeds in warding off attacks, and can be used in a pipe, cigar, or cigarette, but for preference a pipe. Mild tobacco is quite efficacious, and is less likely to produce sickness, but in confirmed smokers the stronger tobaccos may be required. For women and children a few whiffs of a mild cigarette may be all that is necessary. Various asthma cigarettes can be recommended—for instance, notably cubeb cigarettes.

When using smokes for asthma it is well to inhale the smoke well into the lungs, and not simply to draw it into the mouth and puff it out again. If while the patient is using stramonium the throat gets very dry or the pupils dilated, it is an indication that the remedy should be discontinued.

We may complete our list of preparations which are employed as smokes by adding the following: Dissolve half an ounce of niter in half an ounce of boiling water; add half an ounce each of lobelia, stramonium leaves, and black tea, all well powdered. Mix well together, dry, and add one minim of oil of anise. Half a teaspoonful or more of this is to be burned on a plate, and the fumes inhaled six or eight times a day, the bedroom being fumigated with the same.

Most of the preparations that are inhaled as smoke act better if they are taken early in an attack or as a preventive, rather than when the asthma has become well established. This may partly be explained by the great difficulty the patient has, when the asthma is bad, in inhaling anything at all. The difficulty of breathing prevents the smoke from being drawn at all deeply into the chest and being brought in contact with the part where it can act with benefit.

Coffee is an excellent remedy, and should certainly be tried by every asthmatic. It should be taken hot, strong, black, and in small quantity. A small quantity of brandy, whisky, or gin with a little very hot water may check an attack. In those cases of asthma which are so severe that the patient finds it difficult either to swallow or inhale, it may be necessary to administer drugs by injections under the skin, and morphia or atropine may be used, but this form of treatment must only be carried out, as mentioned before, under a doctor's supervision. Sometimes relief is obtained by plunging the hands or feet into hot water, or by holding the breath as long as possible and then taking a gentle inspiration. A mustard leaf can be applied over the breast bone and left on for ten minutes.

In those attacks which are brought on by irritation of the mucous membrane of the nose, a spray of cocaine of the strength of 2 per cent may be employed.

To sum up: In order to check a threatened attack of asthma we must first try to discover the cause. It it can be determined and then can be completely eliminated no further trouble will result. If it can't be eliminated then the patient should undergo desensitization. In some cases a simple change in diet is all that is necessary.

Constipation should be combated by taking a good cathartic, or by clearing the bowel with a soap-and-water enema. If an immediate attack is threatened when the stomach is irritated or overloaded by the last meal, take an emetic: a tablespoonful of ipecacuanha wine, or some mustard and water, followed by a couple of tumblers of warm water. When an attack is inevitable, as comfortable a position as possible should be adopted—sitting up in an easy chair with a table to rest on is probably as good as any—with suitable remedies close at hand. If previous attacks have been experienced, try first the remedy, such as adrenalin, which is known to give the greatest amount of relief. A cup of hot black coffee and plenty of fresh air will make for more comfort.

CHAPTER 110

DISEASES OF THE LUNGS

Collapse — Dilatation — Consolidation — Congestion — Cancer of the Lung — Pulmonary Abscess — Pneumonia — Serum Treatment — Pneumonia as a Secondary Condition — Complications and Sequelae — Bronchopneumonia — Consumption — Home Treatment — Home Prevention of Infection — Sanatorium Treatment — Aftercare — Special Forms of Treatment — Public Prevention — Emphysema — Treatment.

BEFORE describing the symptoms and treatment of the principal disorders to which the lungs are subject, something may be said about certain general effects of disease in these organs.

Collapse. The lungs are normally spongy, resilient organs, filling up the chest cavity and in close apposition with its walls. In certain conditions, however, a state of collapse of the lungs occurs. This may affect the whole of one lung or only portions of one or both of these organs. When the whole of the lung collapses it lies as a small airless mass in close contact with the spinal column.

This collapse may be brought about actively or passively. Active collapse is so called because the lung becomes airless, as it were, of its own accord, without there being any obstruction to the entrance of air to the main bronchus, or any external pressure in the pleural cavity, as occurs in passive collapse of the lung. The contraction of the lung in active collapse is thought to be due to a nervous reflex, whereby the diaphragm, one of the most important muscles of breathing, is put out of action. Active collapse was first observed to occur in severe cases of diphtheria; later it was noticed after operations upon the upper part of the body, and during the war it was a frequent complication of chest wounds.

When the lung is thus suddenly put out of action by this process of deflation the patient usually experiences a sensation of shock. The temperature rises, the pulse rate and respirations are quickened, and there is some difficulty in breathing. Examination of the chest shows physical signs very similar to those found in cases of lobar pneumonia, but owing to the collapse of one lung the heart is displaced towards the affected side of the chest, which is not the case in pneumonia. The condition is not generally serious, and after one or two days the collapsed lung is found to re-expand.

In passive collapse of the lung the whole lung may contract and become airless, as the result of some foreign body, such as a nut, being breathed into the windpipe by accident, and passing down until it is arrested in the mouth of the main bronchus going to one of the lungs. In this way air is prevented from entering, and the air which is entrapped in the lung is gradually absorbed by the circulating blood until the lung is rendered solid and airless. Passive collapse of the lung may also be due to pressure in the pleural cavity, the space which lies between the lung and the chest wall. Thus a large pleural effusion, or the presence of air in the pleural cavity, will compress the lung and prevent the entrance of air. The lung then becomes collapsed (see illustration, page 1558).

Small areas of lung may be deflated when there is obstruction to the entrance of air to small groups of bronchioles. This is especially liable to occur in association with bronchitis, bronchopneumonia, consumption, whooping cough, and diphtheria. These small areas of

(1525)

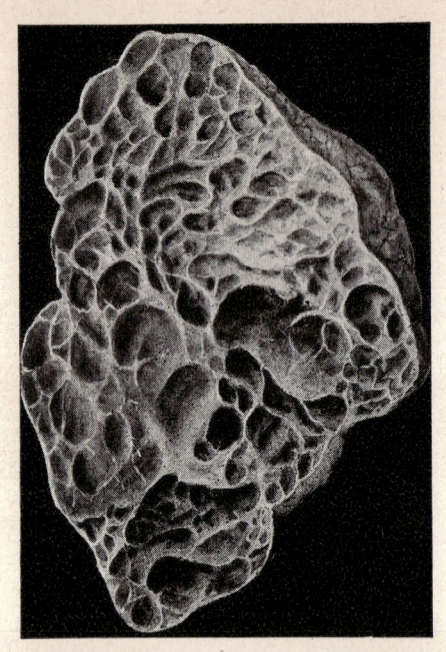

DILATATION OF LUNG IN EMPHYSEMA
In the portion of lung here shown the air spaces are very large, with the effect of diminishing the quantity of blood exposed to aeration as compared with normal lung, in which the spaces are minute.

collapse do not usually give rise to serious disturbance.

Dilatation. The first breath of a newborn child opens out the lungs, a process somewhat resembling that of blowing up a balloon, and the air enters all the innumerable air cells. Physiological dilatation of the lungs is thus produced, and persists normally throughout life. Overdilitation occurs only as an abnormal condition.

In certain diseases the air cells become markedly distended; the partitions separating one from another may give way so that several adjacent cells fuse and form a larger cavity. Such a condition produces a state of dilatation of the lungs which is referred to as emphysema (see page 1561). The dilatation may be general or may affect only localized portions of the lungs. In emphysema the chest assumes a barrel-shaped appearance.

As a result of the dilatation of the lungs the air exchange is greatly reduced and breathlessness follows. The ears, lips and cheeks have a bluish color and cyanosis (see page 1431) occurs.

The localized form of dilatation of the lung does not give rise to such noticeable alteration in the shape of the chest. The lung, or portion of lung, dilates as a result of collapse, contraction, consolidation (see below), or destruction of either a neighboring portion of the same lung or of a large part of the opposite lung. This variety of dilatation is therefore considered to be compensatory in nature, and examples of it are met with in consumption.

When one lung becomes shrunken and contracted as the result of the formation of scar tissue, the unaffected lung generally dilates. The heart and contents of the mediastinum, or space in the middle of the chest, are pulled over to the shrunken side, and the healthy lung is expanded to fill up the space left by the mediastinal displacement. This dilatation of the healthy lung increases the patient's difficulty in breathing.

Localized areas of dilated lung are also met with in association with chronic bronchitis or with bronchopneumonia.

Consolidation. As already stated, the lung in health is a spongy organ, composed of numerous spaces or vesicles containing air. In certain diseases these air spaces are obliterated, and a portion of the lung becomes solid. Such a condition is known as consolidation of the lung. It may occur in a variety of conditions, and may form part of an acute or of a chronic process.

The best example of an acute illness which is due to consolidation of the lung is lobar pneumonia. Here one or more of the main divisions of the lungs, known as lobes, is affected by an acute inflammation. The blood vessels become much dilated and pour forth fluid derived from the blood into the air spaces. This fluid clots, as blood does when shed, and thus the affected part of the lung becomes airless and solid. As the patient recovers the contents of the air spaces are absorbed.

A similar process takes place on a small scale in the condition known as bronchopneumonia or lobular pneumonia. Here small patches of the lungs become temporarily solidified, resolving again as the patient recovers. According to the amount of lung consolidated, so will the breathing be embarrassed.

Tuberculosis of the lungs gives rise to areas of consolidation in the lungs. The finding of the germs of consumption in the sputum demonstrates the real nature of such an illness. Another important form of consolidation of the lungs is met with as the result of a sudden complete obstruction of a main bronchus by a foreign body or by external pressure. This is known as massive collapse. Here one lung, or a large portion of it, contracts and becomes airless and solid.

The chief distinguishing feature between collapse of the lungs and a septic pneumonia which also may follow on bronchial obstruction is that in the former condition the heart is displaced towards the affected side of the chest, as the collapsed lung is smaller than normal, whereas in pneumonia the affected lung is slightly increased in size, and no change in position of the heart takes place.

Consolidation of the lung may follow the formation of what is known as a pulmonary infarct, usually due to the detachment of a clot of blood, called an embolus (see page 1461), which has been formed in a vein or in some other part of the body. This reaches the lungs, where it blocks the circulation through one of its branches. A wedge-shaped piece of lung supplied by this branch of the artery undergoes the changes known as infarction, and so becomes solid.

Fibrosis of the lung, due to chronic irritation, may lead to the formation of patches of scar tissue. These tend to contract and so to produce small areas of solid lung.

Congestion. Hypostatic lung congestion, known also as low pneumonia, occurs in any enfeebling condition, especially in old age, fevers, particularly typhoid fever, debilitating states of the brain, apoplexy, and coma. The patient becomes short of breath, blue, and cold. This condition is often a fatal termination of an illness. To prevent such a state arising in old persons suffering with apoplexy or a broken leg, and in patients who have contracted typhoid fever, the best treatment is to move the patient at intervals of two hours from one position to another and to stimulate the heart by appropriate medication.

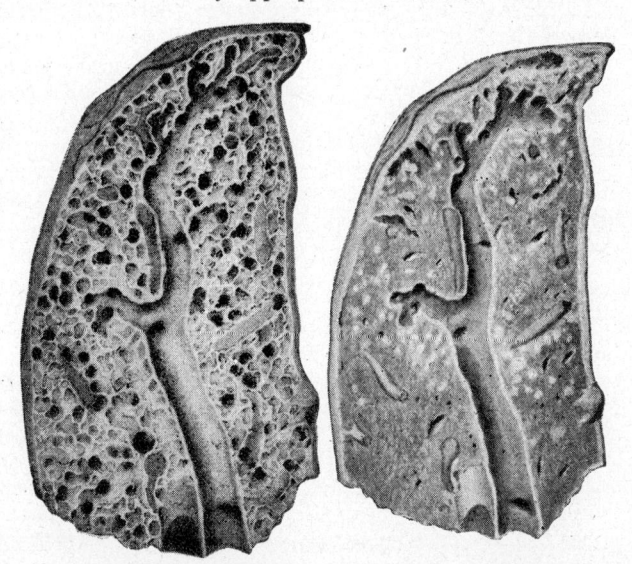

CONSOLIDATION OF LUNG: LOSS OF SPONGINESS
Above, left, is an illustration of the normal appearance of a piece of lung; an air tube is seen communicating with a large number of air cells with thin walls, the whole resembling a sponge. Right, a piece of consolidated lung, resembling a portion of liver.

By these measures the flow of blood through the fine capillaries of the lungs is aided by the action of gravity, and if the patient can be induced to take deep breathing exercises the lungs become well ventilated, the minute cells of the blood are able to take up a full supply of oxygen, and the nutrition of the tissues is maintained.

Cancer of the Lung. Cancer is a disease which may affect the lungs. When it begins primarily in the lung the onset is usually very insidious. The patient often complains of a troublesome, persistent and ineffective cough which is not relieved by a sedative cough medicine. In other cases pain referred to the side of the chest may be the first symptom noticed. The patient gradually loses weight and becomes weak and easily exhausted. As the growth spreads in the lung the cough increases, and is then accompanied by expectoration. The sputum frequently contains blood and is rather dark in color.

At this stage there are usually definite signs of disease in the lung. Examination with the X-rays reveals the areas of solid lung tissue which are the sites of the cancerous growth. The disease is now being treated surgically, but cases usually come to the attention of the doctor only after the cancer is so well established that there is little hope for a cure.

Pulmonary Abscess. Abscesses in the lung are most likely to occur in individuals who are debilitated, or whose resistance is lowered as the result of chronic overindulgence in alcohol, or by malnutrition or diabetes.

An abscess in the lung may follow an attack of pneumonia or may result from the inhalation of some foreign body, as described under the heading Bronchiectasis (page 1516). Those who are unconscious whether from a blow or from alcohol may inhale septic material from the mouth into the lungs. Pulmonary abscess may also result from injury to the chest wall and fractured rib, in infection of the blood such as pyemia, and also in amebic dysentery.

A pulmonary abscess is always a serious condition, giving rise to profound constitutional disturbance. The patient feels ill, his temperature rises, the breathing becomes rapid, and there is often marked sweating and pain in the chest. If the abscess makes its way into one of the larger air tubes, some of its contents are expectorated, and the breath and sputum are then noticed to be very offensive. It is important that the condition should be diagnosed as soon as possible, as early surgical treatment is often of great value. It is necessary, however, to distinguish it from bronchiectasis.

PNEUMONIA

Pneumonia, or inflammation of the lungs as it used to be called, is an affection of the true lung tissue, as distinct from those of the bronchial tubes and the pleura. As a rule one lung only is involved, and it is its lower part or base which is most commonly affected. Both lungs are, however, sometimes inflamed, either together or in succession, and the illness is then termed double pneumonia.

The disease may begin in various ways. It may come on suddenly without warning or previous ill-health, the lung alone being affected, and it then forms the typical variety of inflammation of the lungs, or acute lobar pneumonia. More commonly the pneumonia follows on an acute upper respiratory infection such as a cold. If the disease affects patches of lung tissue and causes inflammatory changes in the smaller bronchi (bronchioles) it is called bronchopneumonia, or lobular pneumonia. These cases are always accompanied by a bronchitis. The cells become blocked up with mucous secretion, until large portions of the lung are rendered airless and useless for respiration.

When the lungs are acutely inflamed a large quantity of thick fluid is poured into the air cells, which become filled up and airless, and the lung is then said to be consolidated. By various means a physician is able to recognize consolidation of the lung and thus diagnose the disease, but these means are not at the disposal of an unprofessional person. The symptoms are, however, sufficiently characteristic, in most cases, for all to be able to recognize this disease.

Causes. Pneumonia is a very distressing and dangerous infectious disease. It is caused by a germ, the pneumococcus. This germ is found normally in the noses and throats of most people and is one of the chief offenders in causing colds and so-called chills of all sorts. As a result of its prevalence we have acquired a high degree of immunity to it, and it is only when the germ is present in a particularly virulent form or in unusually large numbers, or when the individual is run down and debilitated for some reason, that it becomes powerful enough to attack the lungs and cause pneumonia. It is remarkable that a healthy, out-of-doors robust person will often put up a poorer fight against pneumonia than will the more feeble and delicate person. Since the disease is caused by a germ it is infectious, though not to the same extent as the childish infectious diseases such as measles. But at the same time it sometimes becomes almost epidemic in certain localities.

Pneumonia is most prevalent in the winter months between November and Easter, which is the time when people are liable to suffer from lowered vitality, owing to cold and lack of sunshine. It is more frequent in towns than in the country, probably because the conditions of overcrowding, bad ventilation, and herding together in buildings favor the spread of the germ. On the whole it is more a disease of youth and old age than of middle age. The greatest number of cases occur before the age of forty, then there is a lull, and then pneumonia carries off a large proportion of old people, especially those who are already far down the hill with diseases such as diabetes, cirrhosis of the liver, etc. It used to be thought that alcoholic excess was actually a cause of pneumonia, but this is not so.

Symptoms. For two or three days after catching cold the patient experi-

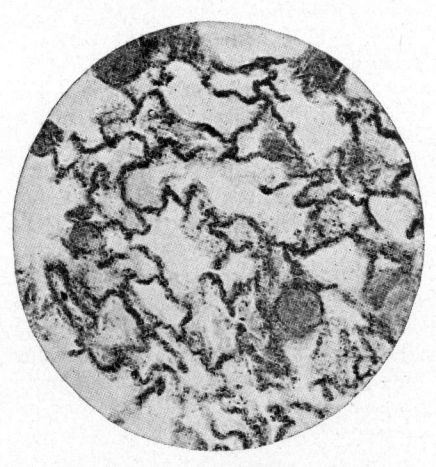

PNEUMONIA: CONGESTIVE STAGE

First of a series of microphotographs showing lung affected by early pneumonia; the black, undulating lines are the walls of the air sacs distended with bloods cells. Magnification in each of the stages about 55 diameters.

ences a feeling of general malaise, with some slight rise of temperature and restlessness. He feels out of sorts and miserable, loses his appetite, and has headache and pains about his body. These symptoms may be so slight as hardly to attract attention at the time, and are only remembered when the more serious ones make their appearance. The onset of pneumonia usually, therefore, seems sudden. The patient is attacked with a violent shivering fit; he trembles all over, his teeth chatter, and he feels exceedingly alarmed at the evidently serious state he is in. There is found to be a high degree of fever, the temperature being perhaps 104° of 105° F. The pulse is rapid—100 to 120 beats a minute; the respirations are frequent, perhaps two or three times as frequent as normal; the skin is hot and dry; the cheeks are flushed, the head aches, the tongue is dry, there is great thirst, the appetite fails, and vomiting often comes on.

But all these symptoms may occur in other highly feverish diseases, and it is necessary to find something distinctive about them to guide us as to what part of the body is involved. The one symptom which will help in this case is the relation of the beats of the heart to the movements of breathing. In health there are about four beats to every respiration, but when the respiratory organs are affected by disease this relation is much altered; the respirations are increased much more than the heart beats, and this is particularly marked in pneumonia. If, therefore, an acute illness comes on with a chill and high fever, and at the same time the respirations are increased more markedly than the pulse rate—for instance, respiration being from 50 to 60, and the pulse only from 100 to 110—we should immediately suspect some disease of the respiratory organs, and more particularly pneumonia.

The other symptoms confirm this suspicion. There is usually some pain in the side, more marked if pleurisy is present, and the pain is increased by coughing. The breathing is not only rapid, but is short, shallow, restrained, and carried on with much difficulty. There is a short hacking cough, which at the outset is dry, but in a little time is accompanied by expectoration. This expectoration is a very characteristic symptom; it is transparent and jellylike, and exceedingly sticky. At first it is clear, but very soon becomes colored with blood, getting tawny, then reddish or rust-colored. Occasionally it looks like plum juice from being mixed with dark-colored blood; at other times it is pale yellow or saffron-colored. But the rust color is commonest, and constitutes one of the most certain indications of the presence of penumonia.

The temperature in this disease runs a peculiar course. We have already seen that at the very beginning of the attack with the initial shivering fit it rises very high, and it remains at this height for from four to ten days, with slight intermissions in the morning, the evening temperature being always higher than the morning. Then one day a sudden

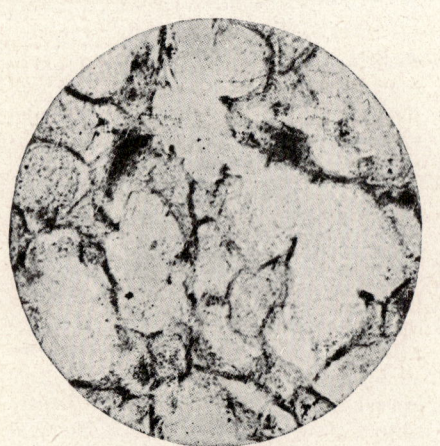

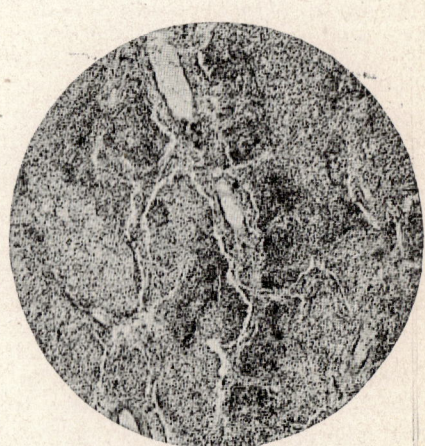

THE LUNG SOLIDIFYING AND CONSOLIDATION NEARLY COMPLETE

In this later stage (left) the air sacs are more or less filled with blood cells, the walls of the sacs being less congested than in the top figure. The microphotograph on the right portrays a stage still later. The lung tissue has become practically solid, due to filling of the air sacs with blood cells and fibrin. In the center of the picture an outline of the air sacs can be seen.

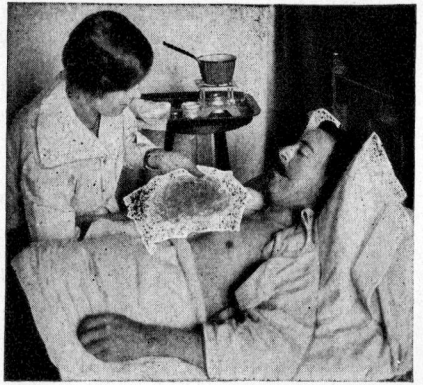

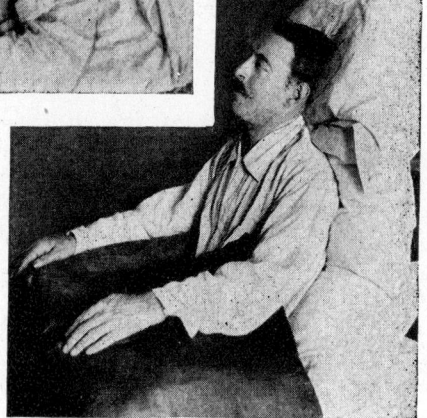

DISEASES OF THE LUNGS

the patient is likely to wander in his mind and be delirious, especially in the evening or during the night, but this is not a serious matter.

This account of the symptoms ought to be sufficient to enable one to recognize pneumonia, and to realize how serious a complaint it is, and how important is a doctor's assistance in its management. It is also one of the diseases in which good nursing is of paramount importance and plays a prominent part in the recovery of the patient.

Course of the Disease. When the crisis occurs all the symptoms abate. The fever may rise and fall, but never reascends to its original height; the cough gradually grows less, the pain disappears, the expectoration ceases, and the patient gradually passes on to a state of convalescence without complication. In many cases, however, the recovery is very slow. No definite crisis occurs; the temperature returns to the normal only after many days of rises and falls. Recovery may be satisfactory and complete. On the other hand, complications may occur. The other lung or another lobe may become inflamed, and all the symptoms be increased or return—a serious matter, but not by any means hopeless, for, even so, many patients make a good recovery. However, in

fall occurs, and the temperature runs down to normal, or even below it.

This rapid fall corresponds with what is called the crisis (see page 1252), and is a peculiar feature of pneumonia. The patient seems very ill and in a most critical condition, with high fever, rapid breathing, and quick pulse, when suddenly, without any warning or apparent cause, a wonderful change occurs: the temperature falls, the breathing improves, the pulse becomes less rapid, and the patient shows a general improvement.

This crisis is believed to result from the formation in the body of an antitoxin, and is a common termination of pneumonia. It may occur on any day of the illness or may never occur at all, but it usually takes place on the fifth, sixth, or seventh day from the first onset or chill, and in all probability in the late afternoon. At the height of the disease

IMPORTANCE OF CORRECT POSTURE

A pneumonia patient should not be allowed to lie flat on his back, or on one side, as circulation through the lungs is thereby impeded. He should be propped up, and the hands should rest on cushions in order to lessen the strain on the heart. The pain in the chest may be relieved by a kaolin poultice, as shown above. It is better not to use an oxygen-consuming heater, however, such as the one shown. After application a pneumonia jacket of gamgee tissue may be put on and the patient once more propped up.

the very young or the old and feeble, and sometimes in healthy adults, the strength is insufficient to meet so great an emergency; the heart grows weak, the pulse feeble, rapid, and irregular; the lung is so seriously damaged that insufficient oxygen is obtained; the patient becomes blue and exhausted, and a fatal issue ends the case. In some instances suppuration occurs in the lung, and produces an abscess, or gangrene sets in and destroys the lung, or the inflammation clears up imperfectly, and chronic disease of the lung is left, which may end in the development of consumption. As already noted, good nursing is of the utmost importance, and, whenever circumstances permit, the services of two graduate nurses should be obtained without delay, one for the day and the other for the night.

Treatment. The patient should at once be put to bed, clothed in some woolen garment and preferably between blankets. The room should be as large and airy as possible, and the temperature maintained at about 60° F.; it is not necessary to keep it quite so high as for a case of bronchitis. Fresh air is most important, and the room must be well ventilated. The window should be kept open, and draft avoided by arranging a screen so as to protect the patient. He must be kept absolutely quiet and still, and getting out of bed for any purpose must not be considered for a moment. He must not be allowed to lie flat on his back, or on one side, as circulation through the lungs is thereby impeded. The chest must be covered up with a jacket made of gamgee tissue. A hot linseed poultice gives relief to pain and cough, and should be applied at regular intervals of four hours; it should be kept on for two hours and then taken off, and the chest quickly dried and covered up with the gamgee until the next poultice is due. A kaolin poultice is also helpful and does not require renewing so frequently. In many cases treatment with the ice bag is adopted instead of poulticing. Upon the physician's judgment will rest the decision as to whether or not the case should be treated at home. If hospital care is advised the patient should be removed at once. In the event that the patient remains at home the following dietary and nursing suggestions may be followed.

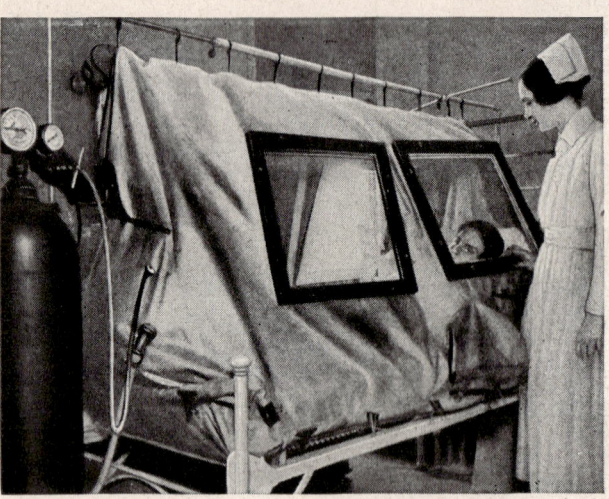

OXYGEN TENT FOR TREATMENT OF PNEUMONIA
The apparatus consists of a gas-tight tent made of rubber and balloon fabric provided with air-tight windows for observing the patient. Oxygen enters the tent under regulated pressure from the cylinder at the foot of the bed. The used air is extracted through the larger tube. Oxygen, though not itself curative, is valuable in providing a rich atmosphere during attacks of breathlessness. Devices of this sort are being constantly improved; light tents of transparent material have come into use.

Suitable Diet. Plenty of fluid should be given by the mouth in cases of pneumonia. In this way the kidneys are kept

DISEASES OF THE LUNGS 1533

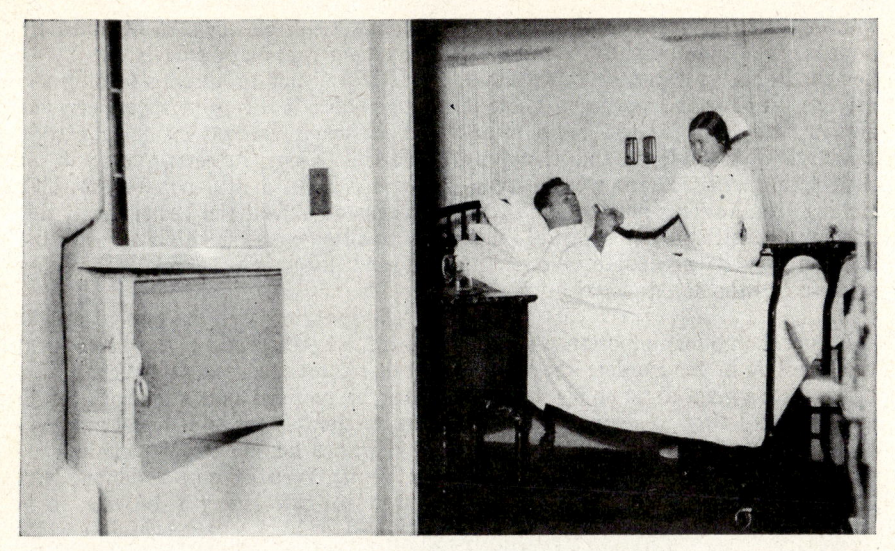

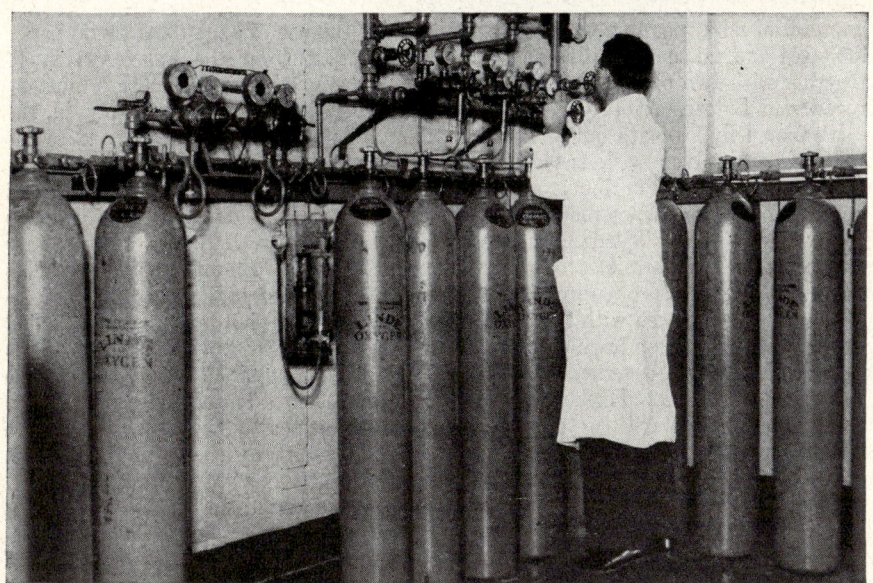

OXYGEN ROOM AND BATTERY OF OXYGEN TANKS

The inevitable inconvenience of the oxygen tent is not compatible with the need of a very sick patient for complete rest and peace of mind. Many hospitals have therefore arranged sealed rooms, supplied with additional oxygen, in which normal activity can be carried on with due regard for increased fire danger. When the door has been closed air can enter only through the ventilating system; part of the battery of oxygen tanks which feeds this system is shown below. Note the airlock in the wall of the oxygen room through which small objects, food, etc., can be passed in or out without opening the door; this helps to maintain a constant concentration of oxygen.

© Keystone View Co.

working freely, and the circulating poisons are more rapidly eliminated. Lemonade, barley water, and plain water may be used for this purpose. There is always a tendency for acid bodies to accumulate in the blood, and these, by their action on the nervous centers controlling respiration, increase the frequency of breathing. Infusions of saline solution may be needed to combat the acidosis and the accompanying dehydration.

It is of the utmost importance to keep the digestion in good order; the patient has to meet a great drain on his strength, and the only way to maintain it is to take plenty of simple, easily digested nourishment.

The most suitable dietary for a patient during the acute stage of lobar pneumonia is as follows: For breakfast, a cupful of milk, possibly colored with a little tea and taken from a feeding cup, together with two or three slices of thin bread and butter. At 11:00 a.m. some calf's-foot jelly, tomato juice, or meat juice may be given with two or three rusks or crackers. For lunch a cup of beef tea or meat extract may be taken, followed by a lightly boiled egg and some thin bread and butter. At 4:00 p.m. the patient should take a cupful of milk, which may be flavored with tea or cocoa as or if desired. Some invalid food may be given for supper, together with a rusk or bread and butter. During the night small quantities of milk or beef tea or jelly should be given every three hours if the patient is awake. Drinks of fresh fruit juices diluted in a little water are of considerable value. Not more than a pint or a pint and a half of milk a day is usually required, as excess tends to set up flatulence and indigestion. In extremely acute cases nothing but a fluid diet is possible.

The bowels must be kept regular with laxatives, or the digestion will suffer. Medicines are of quite secondary importance to good nursing, but various symptoms may require drug treatment as they arise. Some relief to the general feverish condition may be obtained by the administration of salicylates.

It is well not to attempt to stop the cough unless it is very persistent or painful, or keeps the patient from getting sufficient sleep. A certain amount of cough is necessary to remove the thick phlegm, and if it is checked suddenly this may collect in the small air tubes of the affected lung and in this way cause trouble.

The sputum which the patient coughs up contains the germs of the disease, and is therefore a source of danger. This must be received into a special sputum cup, preferably made of metal and covered with a lid. It should contain some antiseptic, such as phenol diluted with water to the strength of one in a hundred, or lysol, a teaspoonful in a pint of water. When the expectoration is very sticky the use of squares of tissue paper to wipe it from the lips saves much exertion for the patient. These must be immediately burned, preferably in the annex to the sickroom, or carried to the incinerator in a closed container.

Sleep should be secured by giving at night a sedative drug, such as bromide or paraldehyde. If the cough is very distressing or if there is great restlessness a small dose of codeine is often invaluable. If the patient is delirious he should be sponged with tepid water, and an ice cap may be applied to the head. As the cough becomes looser the expectoration may be helped by the use of drugs such as ammonium carbonate and potassium iodide given as a mixture.

Cardiac stimulants should be reserved until the heart or pulse shows signs of requiring them. The most beneficial, of course, when the indications arise, is digitalis.

Alcohol, best in the form of well-matured brandy, should not be given as a routine measure, but reserved for signs of heart failure or for profound toxemia with collapse, or when food is refused or there is great restlessness. Up to three or four ounces in twenty-four hours may be given in doses of half an ounce.

Sometimes the breathing becomes much impeded, and, in spite of the violent and rapid breaths the patient may take, the blood grows more and more impure from insufficient supply of oxygen, and the face becomes dusky and blue. This is a serious condition, and requires energetic treatment; a cylinder of oxygen should be obtained and the patient made to breathe the gas through applicators which fit into the nostrils. Oxygen therapy is usually instituted whenever cyanosis or delirium exists or whenever the patient is in a severe toxic state. A more certain way of administering oxygen is by means of an oxygen tent. These are in common use in hospitals and give great relief to pneumonia patients. Some hospitals even have special oxygen chambers.

To reduce fever, if it is very high, nothing is better than sponging the body over with tepid water. Great care must be taken to avoid chill, and one portion must be treated at a time. By this means also the symptom of sleeplessness may be relieved. If the pleuritic pain is severe, strapping the chest (see page 1566) will afford relief. Another useful measure is to immobilize the affected lung by allowing a shot bag to rest on the chest.

As the symptoms gradually subside the patient may be allowed to get out of bed, but he must do this with care, for he is sure to be very weak, and fainting attacks are likely to come on. The first occasion must be for but a few minutes while the bed is being made comfortable, the time being gradually increased as the strength returns. With convalescence he must return to an ordinary diet gradually.

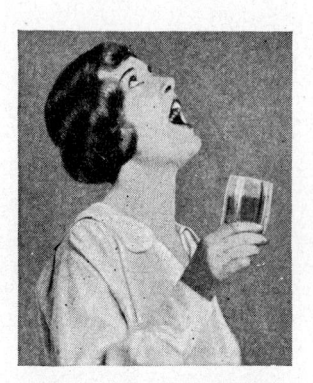

PNEUMONIA PRECAUTION
All persons who come in contact with a patient suffering from pneumonia should exercise a constant personal disinfection. The throat should be gargled with antiseptic solution and the nose washed out.

Diathermy has been successfully used in the treatment of lobar pneumonia, giving prompt relief both locally and generally. Two electrodes of equal size, about eight inches square, are applied one in front and one behind in such a way as to bring the diseased area between them. Treatment should be given for a period of twenty minutes and repeated every six hours, the effect being to relieve the difficulty in breathing, lessen the cough, and calm the nervous system.

Serum Treatment. There are thirty-two main types and several subtypes of the pneumococcus capable of producing disease in man. For many of these types specific antisera have been prepared from horse and rabbit blood. The type of the causative agent can usually be determined by bacteriological examination of the sputum. The specific serum is then administered intravenously if the patient reacts negatively to skin and eye sensitivity tests. The dose is repeated at varying intervals of time and the results are usually very dramatic. There is no doubt but that serum therapy has been the greatest advance made in the treatment of pneumonia.

Some patients will react to the administration of serum and develop what is known as serum sickness. This is characterized by malaise, fever, urticaria, and generalized aches and pains. Fortunately it is not a serious complication.

Pneumonia as a Secondary Condition. Lobar pneumonia may occur in the course of certain diseases. Thus in enteric fever a pneumonic consolidation of the lungs may occur early in the disease or later during the third or fourth week. In either case the changes in the

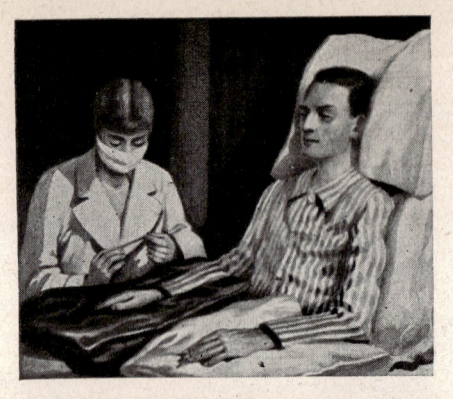

HOW TO PREVENT GERM TRANSMISSION
Those in attendance on the patient should wear a gauze bandage mask to prevent inhalation of the pneumococci. A long gown should be donned when entering the sickroom and not worn in any other part of the house.

lungs may be produced by infection with the typhoid bacillus, either alone or associated with the pneumococcus. Similarly, in typhus fever, in plague, and in influenza, signs of lobar pneumonia which are caused by organisms other than the pneumococcus may be found.

Hypostatic pneumonia, as already mentioned, is a condition in which congestion of the base of the lungs occurs in patients who have been kept lying in bed for a prolonged period, and in whom the circulation is poor. In addition to the congestion, the lung is infected with germs such as the pneumococcus or the streptococcus, and the base of the lung then becomes solid. Hypostatic pneumonia is therefore especially liable to occur in any prolonged immobilization in bed.

Complications and Sequelae. Instead of the consolidation of the lung proceeding to resolution as described earlier, a very serious complication may ensue. This is the formation of an abscess in the lung itself. The outlook in such cases is grave in the extreme. In other instances, and happily very rarely, the lung may become gangrenous, a complication which is almost invariably fatal.

The complications of pneumonia may affect the abdomen, causing inflammation of the peritoneal lining, or peritonitis; inflammation of the mucous membrane of the large intestine, or colitis; and inflammation of the kidneys or nephritis. These various complications are separately described in their appropriate sections. Jaundice may occur either as the result of an inflammation affecting the smaller bile ducts in the liver, or else be due to an excessive destruction of the red cells of the blood owing to the poisons formed by the germs of pneumonia. Meningitis is another very serious complication which is almost invariably fatal. Delirium may occur apart from meningitis, and is often noticed just after the crisis, especially in alcoholic patients.

One of the most frequent complications is the development of fluid in the pleural sac. This is usually of a thick nature, due to the formation of pus, and is then called an empyema (see the Surgery section). The empyema usually forms during the early stages of convalescence, and causes the temperature to rise again after it has fallen to normal, or prevents it from reaching the normal line. The fluid has to be removed before the temperature subsides.

The heart, or its covering membrane, the pericardium, may be affected in lobar pneumonia. Pericarditis is usually a serious complication which increases the distress of the patient and enfeebles the action of the heart. In the early stages, when the membrane is acutely inflamed, a sharp pain is experienced over the front of the chest. The pain usually disappears if fluid subsequently develops as a pericardial effusion. The heart muscle may also be poisoned by the toxins produced by the disease, and dilatation of the heart or heart failure may ensue. This is one of the causes of death in lobar pneumonia.

Pneumococcal inflammation of the joints, or arthritis, may prove a very painful and crippling complication. Inflammation of the ear is not infrequent in children, and is characterized by severe earache, which is later followed by the discharge of pus when the drum of the ear bursts. The parotid gland may swell up during an attack of pneumonia.

A clot of blood may form in one of the main veins of the leg; this is known as thrombosis, and often leaves a permanent swelling or weakness of the limb.

Fibrous or scar tissue may gradually but progressively form in that portion of the lung which was the seat of the lobar pneumonia. In course of time, as this contracts, it may be accompanied by a dilatation of some of the air tubes and bronchiectasis (see page 1516) ensues.

People who have had one attack of pneumonia are unfortunately very apt to contract it again.

BRONCHOPNEUMONIA

This form of pneumonia arises in adults during an attack of bronchitis by the spread of the inflammation along the mucous membrane. It is necessary to describe this condition separately from lobar pneumonia, because its onset is quite different, and its treatment varies in some important particulars.

Bronchopneumonia is produced by all those conditions described in Chapter 109 as causing bronchitis, especially those which bring on great exhaustion, such as measles, whooping-cough, influenza, and diphtheria. It is a complication of bronchitis very likely to occur when the general system is reduced and exhausted, and it is to this fact that its special dangers are to be traced. In lobar pneumonia there is a severe active inflammation, often occurring in one who has power of reaction and recuperation, but in bronchopneumonia there is a slowly progressive inflammation, spreading insidiously in a debilitated and exhausted organism.

Symptoms. The symptoms come on almost unobserved in the course of an ordinary attack of bronchitis, and the only definite evidence of its presence is that all the pre-existing symptoms become worse and the general state more serious. The well-marked chill of pneumonia is absent, and there is no sudden rise of temperature or increase in the rate of pulse and respiration. The pulse, already quickened by bronchitis, grows somewhat quicker and weaker, the respiration rather more rapid and more difficult, the expectoration thicker and streaked with blood, the cough more troublesome. The temperature rises gradually, never reaching the height of lobar pneumonia; the illness runs no definite course, and is terminated by nothing like a crisis. The digestive organs are disturbed; vomiting is common, and is often accompanied by diarrhea, either of which conditions may easily be brought on by indiscretions in diet or by irritating medicines. The case is very liable to run a downward course. The breathing becomes more rapid and shallower, the cough is less vigorous, and the phlegm collects in the small bronchial tubes and air cells. The difficulty of breathing becomes extreme; the face grows blue, and the hands and feet cold and swollen; the strength fails and the patient passes into a state of semiunconsciousness, and may die from sheer exhaustion and from suffocation due to the accumulated mucous discharge.

The disease is a dangerous one, and is particularly likely to end fatally in the old and the debilitated, who have insufficient strength to pass through so prolonged and exhausting an illness. Therefore every case of bronchitis in people over sixty must be looked upon as serious and treated with care. Convalescence is prolonged and tedious.

Treatment. The treatment must differ from that of pneumonia in being more active, stimulating, and sustaining. In the latter disease a great deal can be left to the recuperative power of the system, but in this the system is weak-

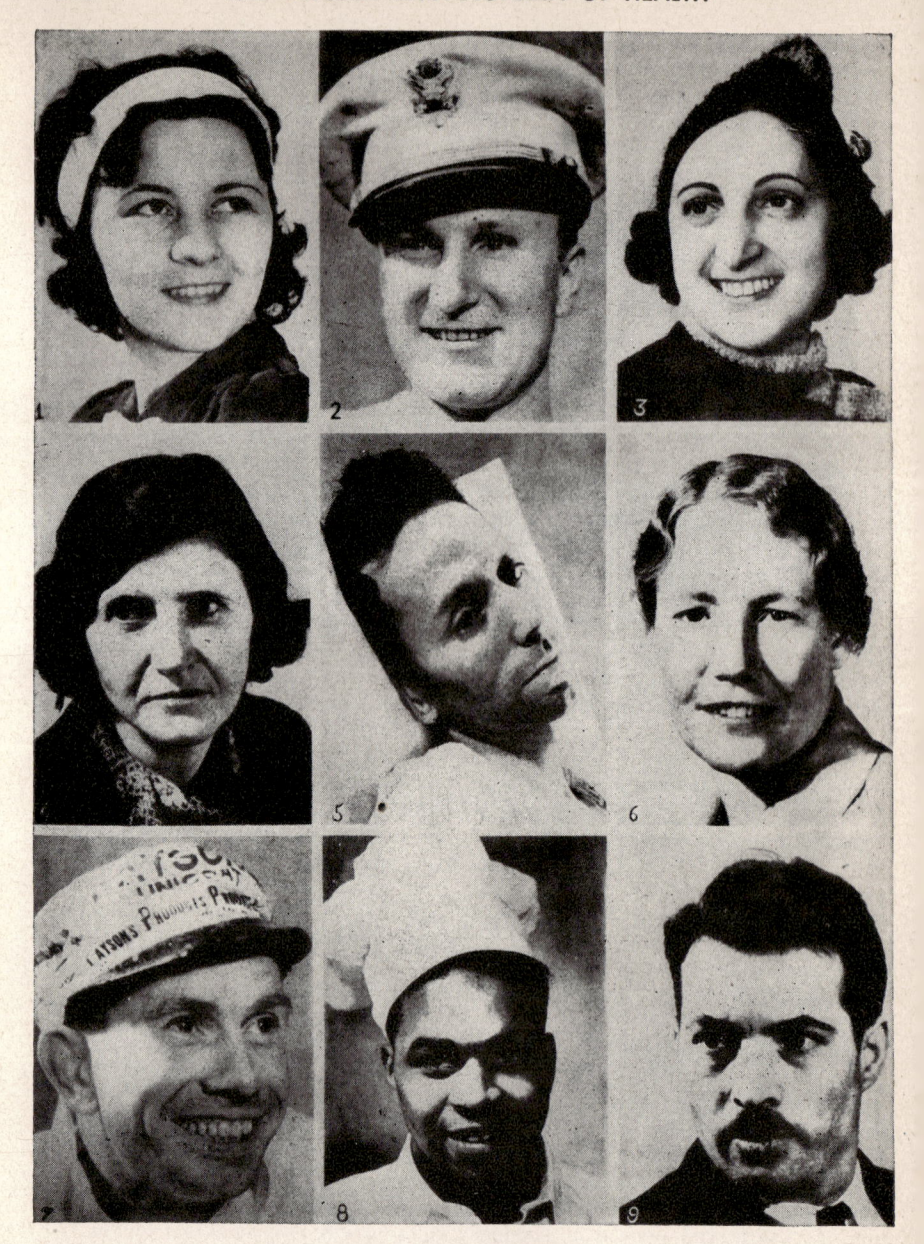

TUBERCULOSIS LIES HIDDEN

Three of these nine persons are free from tuberculosis; six have active cases. Try to identify them; then check with the correct information at the end of this caption. Regular physical examination and an alertness to suspect coughs and other respiratory troubles may be relied upon to detect the disease in time for rest and proper treatment to afford a good hope of cure. The uninfected persons in this group are No. 4, No. 6, and No. 9.

© *International News Photos*

ened, the power of reaction is to a great extent lost, and the tendency is for things to go from bad to worse.

The patient must be treated as recommended for bronchitis (page 1511). The bedroom must be well ventilated and kept fresh, but it is necessary to maintain it at a higher temperature than for pneumonia, and it should never be allowed to fall below 65° F. Greater care is also necessary to guard against drafts. The steam kettle should be used continuously. Hot linseed poultices or antiphlogistine applications are required. Stimulating liniments (turpentine or compound camphor) are useful, and should be rubbed on the chest and on the back energetically. Simple, nourishing food must be given.

In the later stages, especially if the breathing becomes more difficult, the complexion dusky, or the pulse very weak, alcohol is a good stimulant.

If the breathing is oppressed and the phlegm is accumulating in large quantities, much relief is obtained by an occasional emetic, although the danger of exhaustion brought about by the effort of vomiting must be borne in mind. A tablespoonful of tincture of ipecacuanha with one of water would be a suitable dose for this purpose. A large amount of phlegm is thus cleared off the chest, and as soon as the stomach will bear it some milk and brandy should be given. The inhalation of oxygen gas is also a most useful remedy in these cases.

In some cases a specific type of pneumococcus can be found by sputum examination. If the corresponding autiserum is available it will often be beneficial.

During convalescence great care is necessary to avoid a chill. Good nourishing food, a couple of glasses of good burgundy a day, a strong tonic, and cod-liver oil in as large doses as the stomach will bear, are to be advised. Change of air and rest of mind and body for a long period will be necessary before the health is fully restored.

The occurrence and treatment of bronchopneumonia in children is dealt with in the section on Diseases of Children.

CONSUMPTION OR TUBERCULOSIS OF THE LUNGS

Consumption is the name given to the condition of the lungs caused by the tubercle bacillus. Other names sometimes applied to the same disease are phthisis, decline, and pulmonary tuberculosis. As its name consumption implies, it is accompanied by a general wasting of the body. It is one of the oldest complaints known, and accounts of it can be found in early medical writings.

Causes. Consumption has a worldwide distribution, but is essentially a disease which has kept pace with civilization in its advance, and at the present time it constitutes one of the greatest blots upon social progress.

Climate is not an important factor in the incidence of consumption, although undoubtedly it plays a part in its treatment. The disease is less common at high altitudes. Dampness of the soil is a factor which is favorable for its appearance. It occurs with equal frequency both in the torrid and in the frigid zones.

Housing plays a very important part in the incidence of tuberculosis. It is a disease begotten of overcrowding and of slums, and thus is essentially a town disease, just as it is a disease of civilization. An insufficient supply of nourishing food, absence of fresh air, poor sanitation, dirt and dust, overwork and fatigue, all favor the development of the disease.

Consumption is also especially common in those whose work is accompanied by the inhalation of dust. This is well shown by the fact that workers in mines, except coal mines, have a high mortality rate.

Consumption is not common among children, although tuberculosis in other

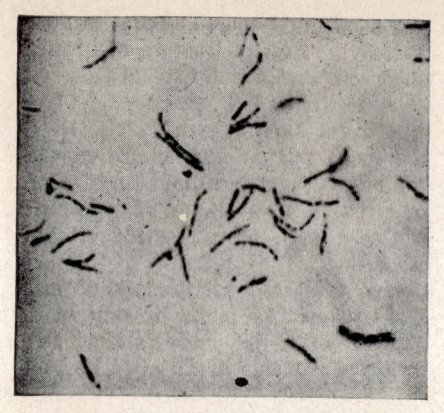

CAUSATIVE AGENT OF TUBERCULOSIS

The bacillus of tuberculosis discovered by Koch in 1882, as found in sections of diseased tissue or in secretions, is seen as a slender and often slightly curved rod.

Taken with the Davon Supermicroscope

parts of the body than the lung frequently occurs. The greatest number of cases of pulmonary tuberculosis are seen between the ages of fifteen and forty-five years. It is much more common among men than among women, but when it develops under the age of fifteen years it is more frequently met with in girls.

Though consumption is a very important disease, because of the number of deaths it causes each year, the death-rate is steadily falling. This is due to improvements which have taken place in general hygienic conditions, and in early diagnosis and treatment. Tuberculosis ranks seventh as a cause of death in New York state.

Consumption results from the entry of the tubercle bacillus into the lungs, and from no other cause. Outside the human body the tubercle bacillus is found in dust, in expectoration that has been coughed up by patients suffering from the disease, and in certain articles of food. Of the latter the most important is milk. Less important are cream, butter, and meat. The tubercle bacilli which are found in dust are derived from man; those present in the foodstuffs mentioned come from tuberculous cows. Contaminated milk is especially liable to be harmful in the early years of life, and it is only by boiling the milk that this danger can be averted.

The sufferer from tuberculosis is a source of danger to others if he coughs without putting a handkerchief in front of his mouth, and if he expectorates without receiving the sputum into a vessel containing a disinfectant fluid (see page 1080).

The open cough is dangerous because small particles of saliva are ejected from the mouth for some distance around. These may, and very often do, contain the living germs of consumption. If they fall into the air which someone else is breathing, that person runs the risk of developing consumption.

Sputum containing the tubercle bacilli, once it has settled out of the air, is dangerous only when it dries. As long as it is moist the tuberculosis germs remain in it. When, however, it dries they are liberated from the sputum and blow about in the air and dust. This explains how infection is often spread; thus a clerk working in the same office with a consumptive may breathe in dust which has been infected by the insanitary habit of expectorating on the floor or in the wastebasket, or even into the handkerchief, if the sputum dries upon it. The habit of moistening the fingers with saliva in turning over the pages of a book is also dangerous.

A number of contributing factors may be mentioned. Any intercurrent infection, but especially those of the respiratory tract can precipitate or aggravate tuberculous lesions. Pregnancy, lactation, or exhausting physical labor will bring about the same effect. Faulty hygiene and low standards of living are indirect but most important factors and are generally accepted as sufficient to account for the high incidence of tuberculosis among Negroes.

Tuberculosis frequently occurs in more than one member of a family the

DISEASES OF THE LUNGS

reason being that the risk of infection is very great if children are living in the same house where one member of the family is consumptive.

If the husband or wife is consumptive it does not follow that the mate is peculiarly prone to develop the disease; as the result of exposure to infection a certain degree of immunity appears to be produced. In most cases it will be found that a generally lowered condition of health has existed for some time before the onset of symptoms of consumption. This may have been due to some form of chronic toxemia or other depressant influence.

Onset and Symptoms. The symptoms may start with dramatic rapidity; nevertheless, it must be remembered that the germs of consumption have probably been firmly established in the lungs for some time before the first symptoms became manifest. The most dramatic of the acute forms of onset is the onset with the coughing up of blood, technically known as hemoptysis. The actual amount of blood thus expectorated may vary from a few streaks, small clots, or liquid blood up to half a pint or even more. It is most important to differentiate between blood which has come from the lungs (hemoptysis) and that derived from the stomach (hematemesis).

When blood comes from the lungs it is aerated or charged with an immense number of air bubbles and is bright red. Blood which is emitted from the stomach is brown and in appearance suggests coffee grounds.

It is found that hemoptysis is the first symptom in about 13 per cent of all cases of consumption, and further that the outlook for cases which commence

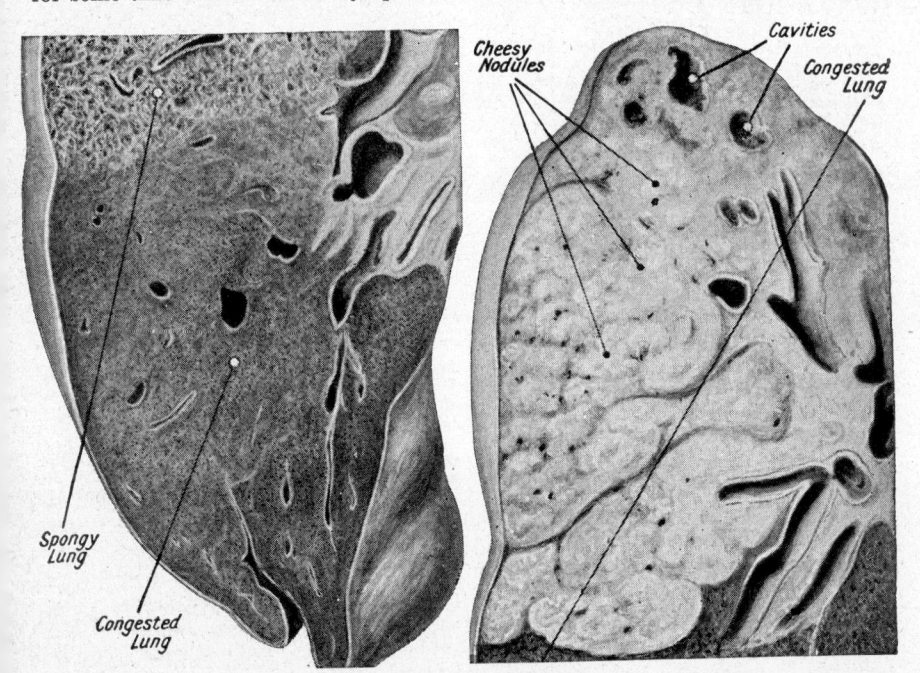

SIGNS OF TUBERCULAR DISEASE IN THE LUNG
Left, engorgement of the lung with blood in congestion encroaches on the air space in the tubes and air vesicles, thus impairing function. Right, the tiny masses of cells or tubercles in the lung in consumption tend to be altered into a cheesy substance. Here many tubercles have coalesced.

in this way is on the average better than for those with different modes of onset. This is probably because attention is drawn early to the fact that there is something amiss with the lungs, and efficient treatment is started before the

the pleural sac, give relief to the pain which is caused by these layers rubbing together.

Consumption at times begins in a manner in which the symptoms resemble those of an acute pneumonia or of

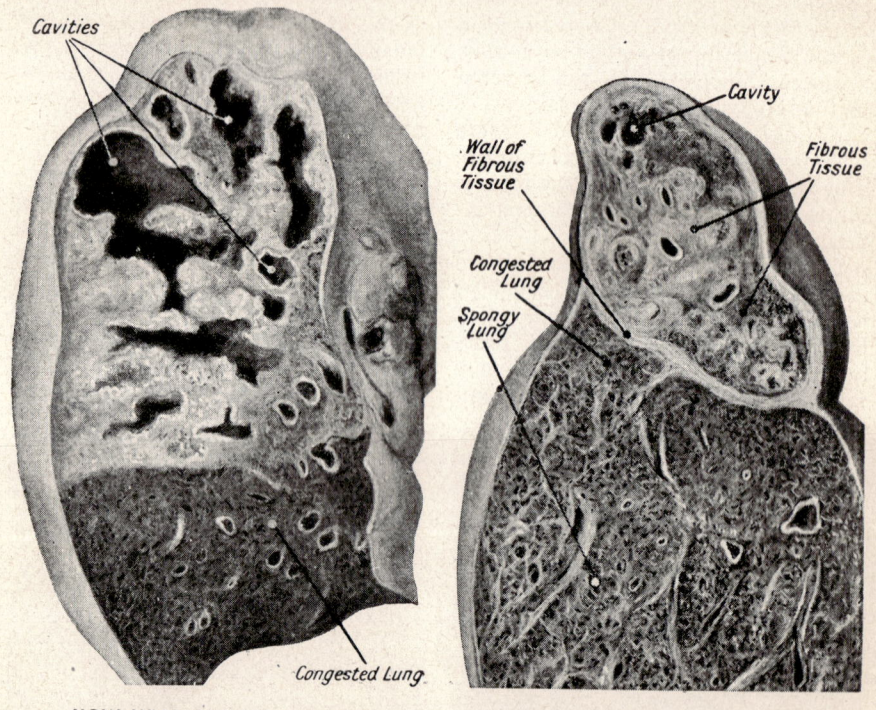

HOW LUNG CAVITIES ARE PRODUCED AND HEALING PROCESSES CARRIED OUT
Left, the cheesy substance may soften and be discharged through air tubes, thus leaving cavities, in the walls of which ulceration goes on. Right, the lung makes an effort to protect itself from the tuberculous infection by walling off diseased patches with fibrous tissues, often successfully.

disease has had time to spread extensively.

In about 10 per cent of cases of consumption the first symptom is an attack of pleurisy. This is characterized by a sharp, stabbing pain in the side of the chest, which is made much worse on drawing a breath, and is relieved by holding the breath. The pain is attended by a feeling of tiredness and general ill-health, and there is usually some fever. Fluid may form on the chest and, by separating the two inflamed layers of

bronchopneumonia. Examination of the expectoration shows the presence of tubercle bacilli. This is usually a very fatal form of consumption.

Consumption may begin acutely and pursue a very rapid and fatal course when it forms part of the variety of tuberculosis known as miliary (see page 1389). In this form the seeds of the disease are scattered all over the body in the various organs, and grow there. The lungs are nearly always involved, and death occurs in a few weeks.

In the acute forms of onset described above there is never any doubt that the patient is very ill and unfit for any work. When, however, consumption begins insidiously, as it does in the majority of instances, the initial symptoms are slight and very varied, and the sufferer often carries on with his work long before medical advice is sought.

The most frequent early symptoms of consumption are as follows:

A persistent cough, perhaps following on a severe cold or influenza. It may or may not be accompanied by some expectoration.

Lassitude, a very important symptom. Mental and physical exertion quickly cause fatigue.

A persistent loss of weight; the body weight forms a useful guide to the progress of the disease.

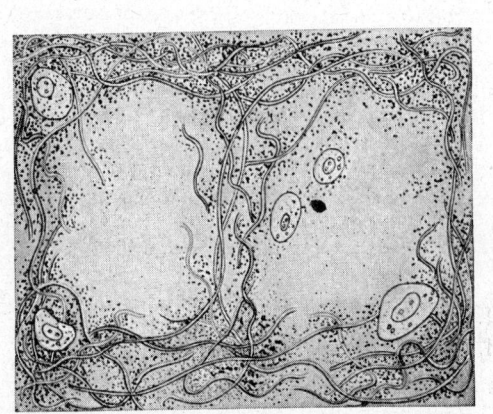

Loss of appetite, pains or discomfort after meals, or flatulence. In all such cases of indigestion a careful examination should be made of the chest.

Shortness of breath and palpitation.

Again, the nervous system may be markedly disturbed in the early stages. The patient lacks concentration and application, is easily exhausted, and may have groundless fears. In such a case neurasthenia may be diagnosed.

Periodical attacks of fever, with rise of temperature and shivering, may occur, or more often there is only a slight rise of temperature towards the end of the day. This may be followed by night sweats.

In women a cessation of the menstrual periods, a condition known as amenorrhea, may occur. Pain in the chest, apart from pleurisy, may develop insidiously and prove an early symptom of the disease.

Hoarseness is sometimes the first symptom that attracts attention, and from time to time patients are seen whose only complaint is of their voice, but in whom a chest examination reveals the presence of consumption.

FIBERS IN SPUTUM
The presence of elastic tissue in sputum, as shown by the microscope, indicates breaking down of lung tissue or ulceration of air tubes in advanced tuberculosis.

Early diagnosis by skilled medical examination is of vital importance and should be sought without delay. It is better to be needlessly alarmed than to lose precious time.

Consumption in the lungs may exist in various stages. Thus, in the early stage there is just a deposit of disease, usually in one lung near the top. As the disease progresses the deposits spread throughout the lungs, producing a state known as infiltration. The infected area may soften at some point, when caseation is said to have occurred; or the tissues soften and break down, leading to the formation of holes or cavities in the lungs, a state of excavation. Healing takes place in two ways, either by the production of scar tissue, which gradually contracts and causes a shrinking of the lung, a process called fibrosis, or else by fibrosis followed by the deposition of lime salts in the diseased spots, which are in this way dried up, and calcification results.

In cases of consumption in which extensive disease is present there is usually little difficulty in saying, after a careful examination, that tuberculosis is its cause. The diagnosis of early cases is, however, a matter usually of difficulty and requires expert skill. In addition to an inquiry into the history of the patient's illness and an examination of his chest by palpation, percussion and auscultation, certain other investigations should be carried out.

Of these the first is examination of the sputum, which must be tested for the presence of tubercle bacilli, the germs of consumption. Special methods of staining the germs by means of dyes are required for their identification under the microscope. Repeated examinations may be necessary. X-ray examination of the chest is another important aid in diagnosis. Infected patches of lung are more opaque to the rays and are seen as darker areas. Cases with no symptoms and no signs in the chest are sometimes picked up by X-ray examination alone.

Observation of the temperature and of the pulse is of great importance. The patient should be kept in bed for a few days, and records made of the temperature every four hours during the day. If consumption is present and the disease is active, it will be found that there is a rise in temperature above normal at some time during the day, usually about 6:00 p.m. In some cases, although there is not a rise above 99° F., there is a marked difference between the morning and the evening temperatures, the morning one being considerably below the normal average temperature of 98.6° F. If the temperature is satisfactory while the patient is in bed, the effect of exer-

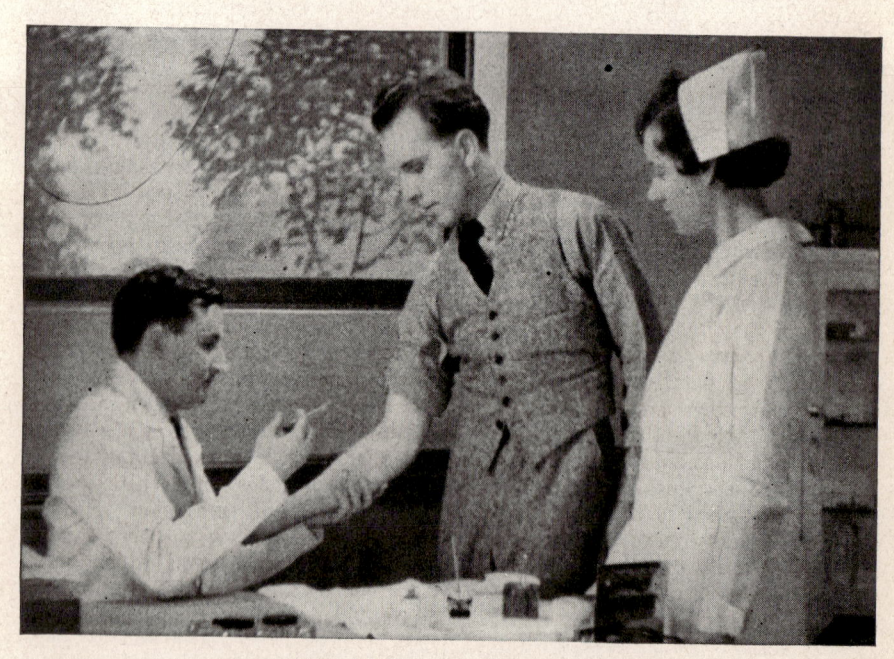

CASE FINDING IN TUBERCULOSIS

It has been more and more realized that much pulmonary and other tuberculosis arises and progresses without obvious symptoms being displayed, the patient being a menace to the health of those who associate with him. Public co-operation for check-ups has been sought and widely obtained; this young man is submitting to the skin test. In this test a minute quantity of tuberculin is placed in a small wound in the skin and the reaction enables the doctor to judge whether or not the subject is infected.

Courtesy of the National Tuberculosis Association

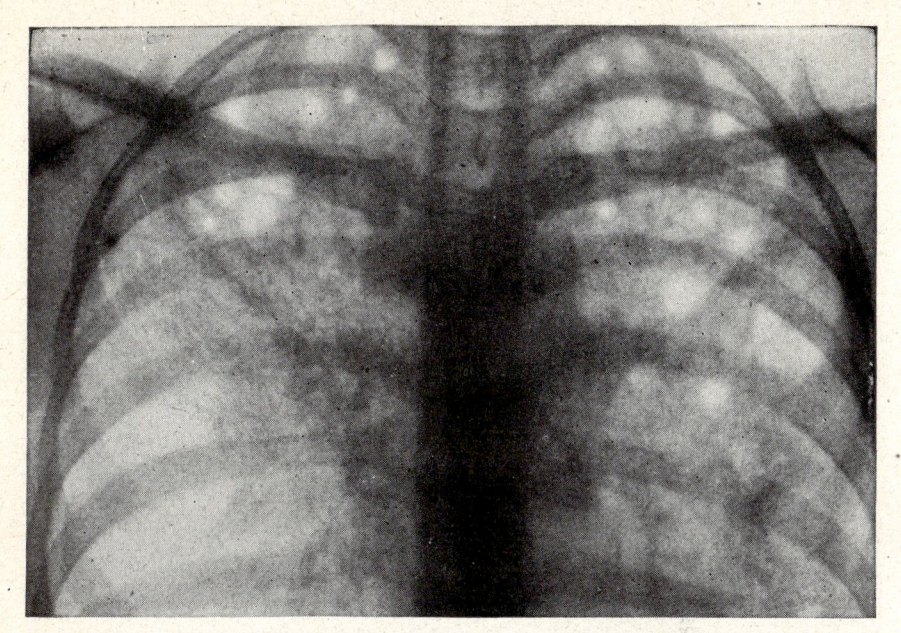

HOW AN X-RAY PHOTOGRAPH REVEALS TUBERCULOUS DISEASE OF THE LUNGS

In this X-ray photograph it will be noted that a number of more or less round, clear spaces appear in the upper part of each lung. These represent cavities produced by softening of collections of cheesy matter formed in the affected lung tissue. The walls of the cavities are thickened. These conditions are shown very clearly in the diagrams which appear on pages 1541 and 1542.

cise, such as walking for two or three miles, should be noted.

It is thus seen that in its early stages, when treatment will yield the best hopes of a cure, diagnosis is sometimes difficult and requires specialized knowledge.

Curative Treatment. Consumption is a disease in which prolonged treatment is required, usually over two or three years. It is essential to obtain co-operation between patient and doctor, and in order to do so it must be understood at the outset that there is no known drug which will act as a specific remedy, and that the treatment consists in a long-continued guidance of the patient in his fight against the disease.

The symptoms of the disease result from: (1) the local damage to the lung by the bacillus as it lives and multiplies in the lung tissue; (2) the absorption of the poisonous substances (toxins) produced by the bacillus and by the breaking down of the tissues.

On the other side there is the resistance of the body to the germs of consumption. Here, again, there are two main processes at work. First, in the lung the formation of scar tissue or the deposition of lime may completely shut off and surround the portion of lung in which the germs have settled down. They cannot then multiply or spread, and a healed tuberculous spot results. After death a large proportion of individuals, who have never, apparently, suffered from consumption show such healed spots in the lungs. The second line of bodily defense lies in the blood stream. Here antitoxins are formed which are able to neutralize the toxin produced by the germ of consumption. The white cells of the blood are also concerned with the destruction of tuberculosis germs.

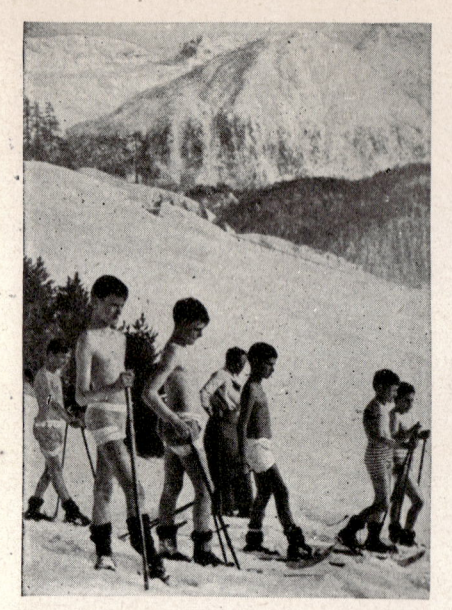

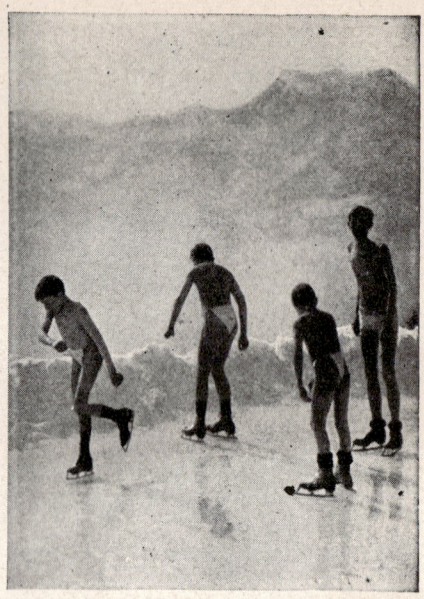

Early cases of tuberculosis in young and vigorous people benefit considerably from treatment at high altitudes. Exercise and sport of a not too strenuous nature is advocated.

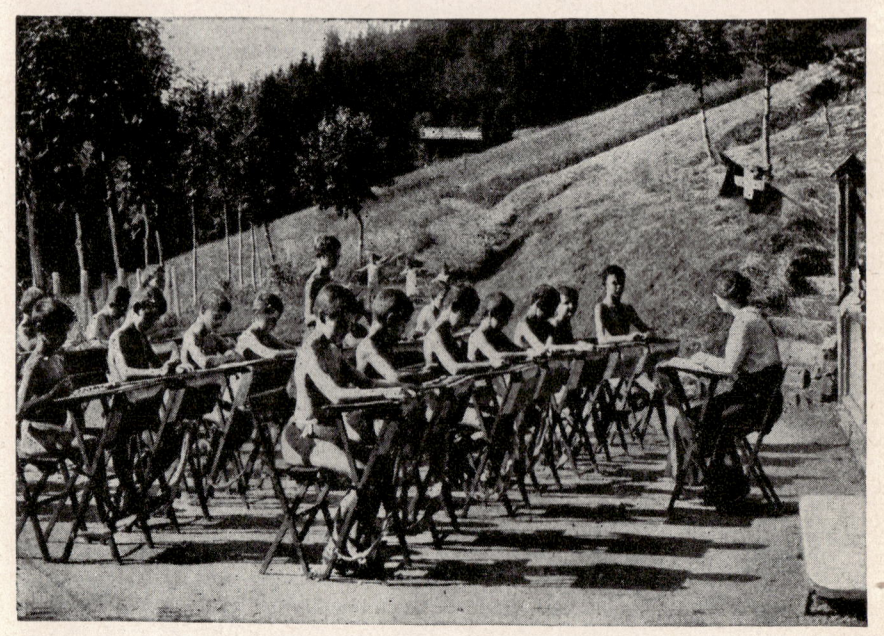

At Leysin, in the Alpes Vaudoises, Dr. A. Rollier instituted the treatment of pulmonary tuberculosis and other tuberculous diseases by means of direct sunlight. The patients spend as much time as possible in the open air, exposed to the rays of the sun.

FIGHTING TUBERCULOSIS WITH SUN AND AIR IN EUROPE

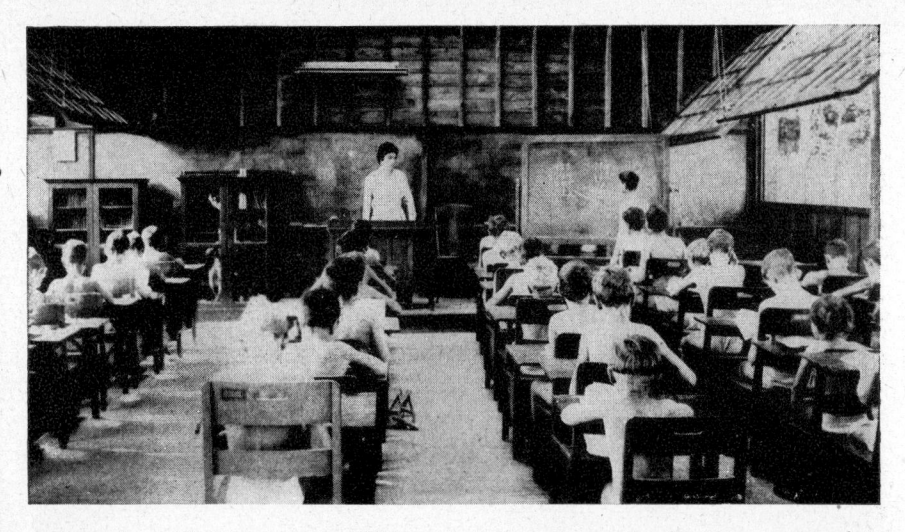

DISEASES OF THE LUNGS 1547

At Perrysburg, N. Y., tubercular children study in an open-air schoolroom, stripped to the waist.
© *Ewing Galloway*

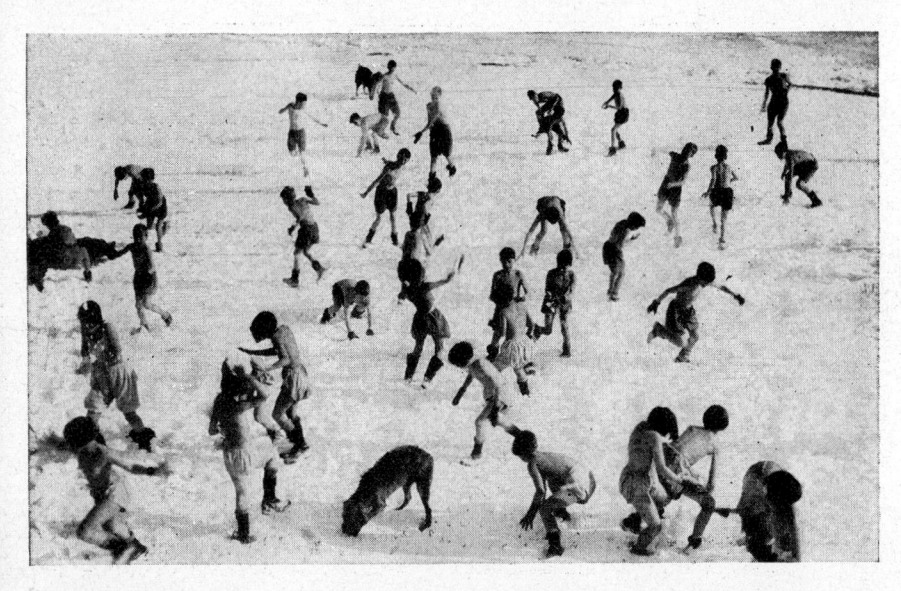

Outdoor air and sunlight, even in the New England winter, are part of the treatment for child tuberculosis patients of the Meriden State Tuberculosis Sanitarium, Meriden, Conn. It must not be supposed that this kind of sun-and-air treatment is applicable to all cases and types of tuberculosis. Above all, it is important to realize that delicate patients are never abruptly subjected to a drastic change in their mode of living. The exposure is begun gradually and after examination and authorization by a doctor. Patients are thereafter kept under observation to make sure that the effect of the exposure is to stimulate vital processes and increase metabolism, for the good result of the treatment depends on these responses. © *International News Photos*

FIGHTING TUBERCULOSIS WITH SUN AND AIR IN THE UNITED STATES

A successful fight against the disease calls for good resisting powers against the infection, both locally in the lung and generally in the blood stream. Every effort is directed to improving the patient's general well-being and to avoiding harmful influences.

Defective resistance is shown by continued loss of weight, fever, hemorrhages from the lung, increased cough and expectoration, and gradual loss of strength. The bacillus is in the ascendant and vigorous measures must be undertaken to combat it.

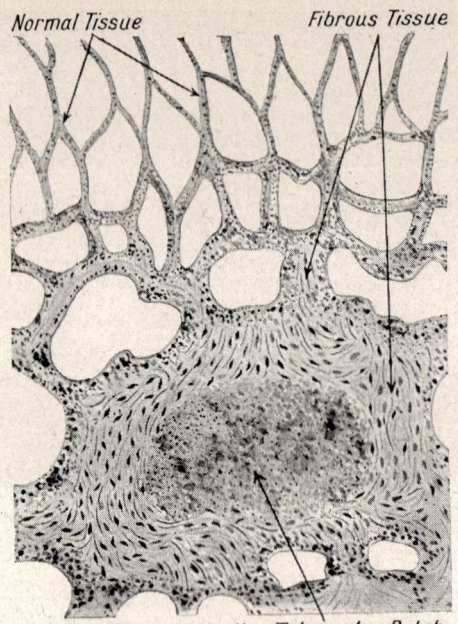

Aside from the specific surgical measures considered later on, the keystones of the treatment of tuberculous patients are three in number: fresh air, good food, and rest with graduated exercise.

Fresh Air and Climate. The value of fresh air in the treatment of consumption is now generally recognized. Open windows and open-air life are the sheet anchor in combating this most serious of all infectious diseases.

Sunlight and the graduated exposure of the body to the rays of the sun is a method of treatment which has been extensively practised at Leysin, in Switzerland, but while of special value in cases of glandular or abdominal tuberculosis, must be used with the greatest possible caution in the treatment of lung cases.

The role which altitude plays is uncertain, and it must be recognized that not all cases do well at altitudes of over 3000 feet.

At such heights the barometric pressure is considerably reduced, the atmosphere is still, the sun's rays have greater penetrating power and there is a freedom from dirt and pollution. The temperature is also lower than that experienced on the plains. The effect of these various conditions is to produce a stimulating and tonic effect upon all the vital processes of the body. Treatment at high altitudes is believed to be beneficial for early cases of consumption in young and vigorous individuals, but in older people, especially if there are complications such as disease of the heart or kidney or thickening of the arteries, the climate of elevated regions is often found to be unsuitable.

Other complications such as tuberculosis of the throat or the intestines and severe and repeated hemorrhages from the lungs are also conditions unsuited to mountain treatment.

Tuberculosis can be treated in any climate in the United States and it is not necessary to go to far-off sanatoria in preference to ones nearer home. Information as to the sanatorium nearest the patient's home can be obtained from a doctor or from any public-health officer or nurse or tuberculosis association. Damp, claylike soils are best avoided, and very wooded districts are unsuit-

HEALED TUBERCULOUS PATCH
In the piece of lung shown the darker portion consists of large round cells which destroy or wall up foci of disease; later they assume an elongated form, as seen in the periphery of the area.

DISEASES OF THE LUNGS

able in the autumn, when the leaves are rotting upon the ground.

Food in Consumption. This must be carefully adapted to the digestive powers and to the amount of exercise allowed, and it should include an abundance of foods rich in vitamins—dairy produce, green vegetables, fresh fruits, and whole cereals (see Chapters 34-40).

Alcohol is best omitted except perhaps in the convalescent stage. The bowels must be kept active and any source of focal infection in the teeth or tonsils or elsewhere attended to.

Rest and Exercise. These are very important factors in the treatment of consumption. As soon as the disease is diagnosed and irrespective of the temperature or pulse rate, the patient should be put to bed and kept there for at least a month. This early and prolonged rest will do much to expedite a cure, and the time thus spent will prove a most valuable investment. This is a point which at times is overlooked. If the temperature and pulse are then within normal limits, the patient may be allowed up and gradually increased amounts of exercise permitted.

If, on the other hand, after a few days in bed it is found that the temperature is above normal, or the pulse is unduly rapid, he must be kept at absolute rest. For this nurses are required who have been trained in the method. The patient lies quietly in bed and is not allowed to feed or wash himself, or to get out of bed for any purpose. He

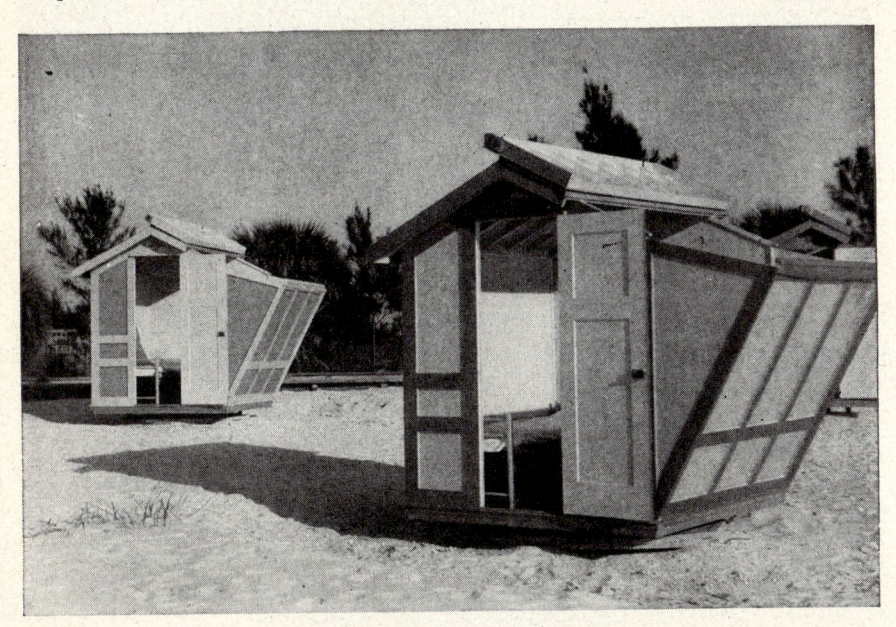

SUNLIGHT AND AIR WITH PRIVACY

Not every patient in the early and curable stages of tuberculosis can afford sanatorium treatment or a change of residence. But an outdoor sleeping shelter can be erected to meet the urgent need for fresh air, even in the back yard of a city home. Modern methods of treatment by fresh air require not only that the patient shall be subjected to sunlight during the day, but also that he shall sleep either outdoors or as nearly so as is possible. Such cabins as these meet the need. The hinged roof section and drop side admit maximum sun, and the building rotates on a circular track to follow the sun in its daily course or to shift the enclosed side toward an inclement wind. As here shown, the cabins are set up for sun-tan addicts at a beach, but they are obviously appropriate for tuberculosis treatment. © *Ewing Galloway*

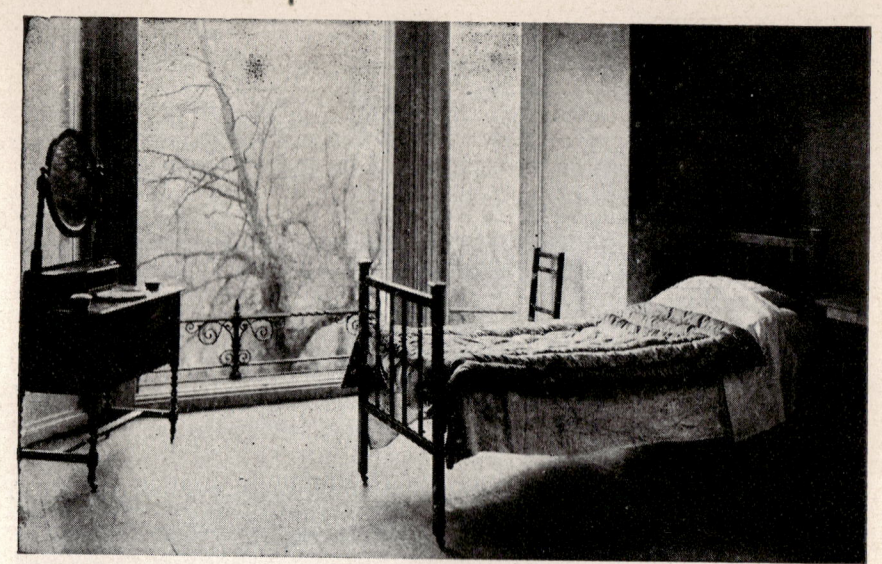

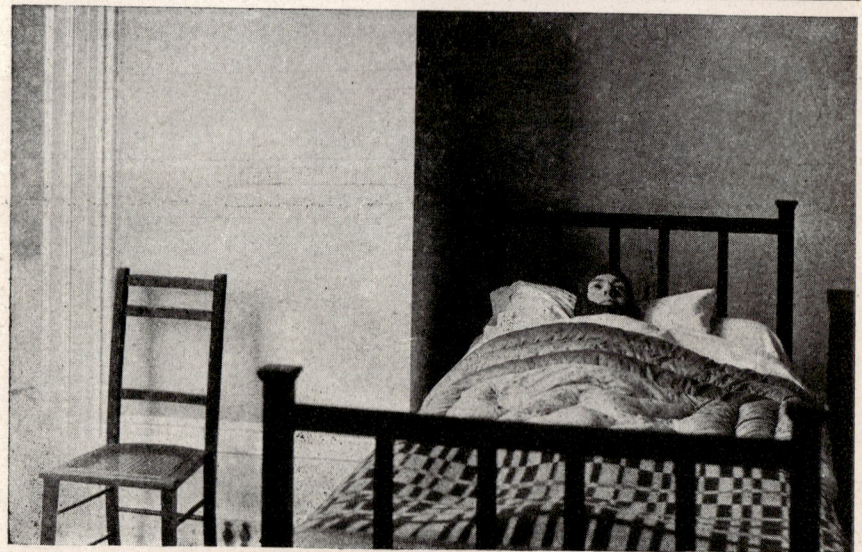

MAKING THE BEST OF INDOOR TREATMENT

When the provision of an outdoor shelter is, for some reason, impracticable, the most suitable room in the house must be adapted to the needs of the patient. One with a southerly aspect should be chosen, and the windows must be completely removed from their frames, so as to afford entrance to as much air and sun as possible. The sickroom must be furnished with the utmost sparseness, but since it is important that the patient should be kept warm, bedclothes must be adequate, and a knitted helmet should be worn to prevent the possibility of any chilliness. This arrangement, if the patient and his family observe the required routines and precautions, offers a good opportunity for recovery, although it contemplates perhaps the least favorable environment likely to be found in the United States outside city slums—a damp, cold winter in a neighborhood too closely built to permit porches or outdoor shelters

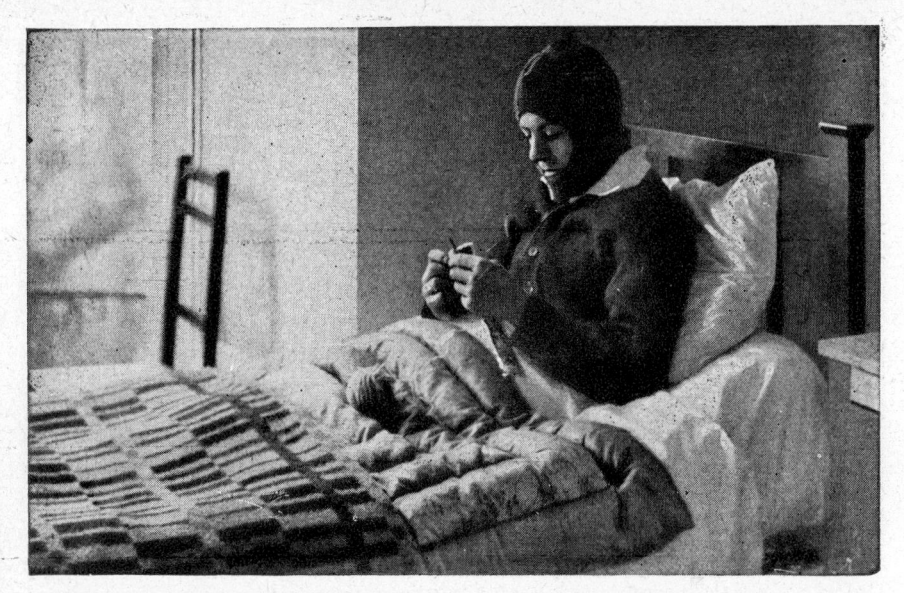

SUITABLE OCCUPATION FOR A MILD CASE OF TUBERCULOSIS
A consumptive patient who is kept continuously in bed should not be allowed to sleep during the day, or a restless night will ensue. Knitting and reading are both suitable daytime occupations provided the patient is well enough to sit up in bed.

must have sufficient bedclothes to prevent shivering. In the most strict regime he must be kept completely at rest, and is not even allowed to read. Absolute rest will often bring the temperature down to normal when ordinary rest has failed.

The stages through which a patient is allowed to pass, after satisfactory progress has been accomplished by rest in bed, are as follows. He first is allowed to spend two hours each day out of bed, but lying on a couch. This period may be increased to four hours a day if there is no renewed activity of the disease, as judged by temperature and pulse rate. After this he dresses and walks about for two hours a day, and this period is increased by two hours at a time until he is up eight hours a day. A short walk may then be taken of about a quarter of a mile. If no ill effects are observed the walking is gradually increased until six miles a day are accomplished. Light work out of doors may then be attempted, such as the various processes of gardening which require least effort. When the patient has improved to this extent he may be allowed to enjoy some kind of light game; clock golf, miniature golf, or croquet are most suitable.

In this way the resistance of the body is gradually built up. At all times during the period a careful watch is kept upon the pulse and temperature, and upon any sign or symptom of renewed activity of the disease.

Home Treatment. This includes, first, the actual care of the patient, and, secondly, the precautions necessary to prevent the spread of infection to others.

When bed treatment is indicated this should be carried out where possible in the open air. This involves the use of a shelter, ideally in the form of a revolving structure, which can be turned around to avoid rain and winds and to catch the rays of the sun. Or if a balcony is available, the bed may be placed there and sheltered from winds and rain by a waterproof sheet.

If this is not feasible the most suitable

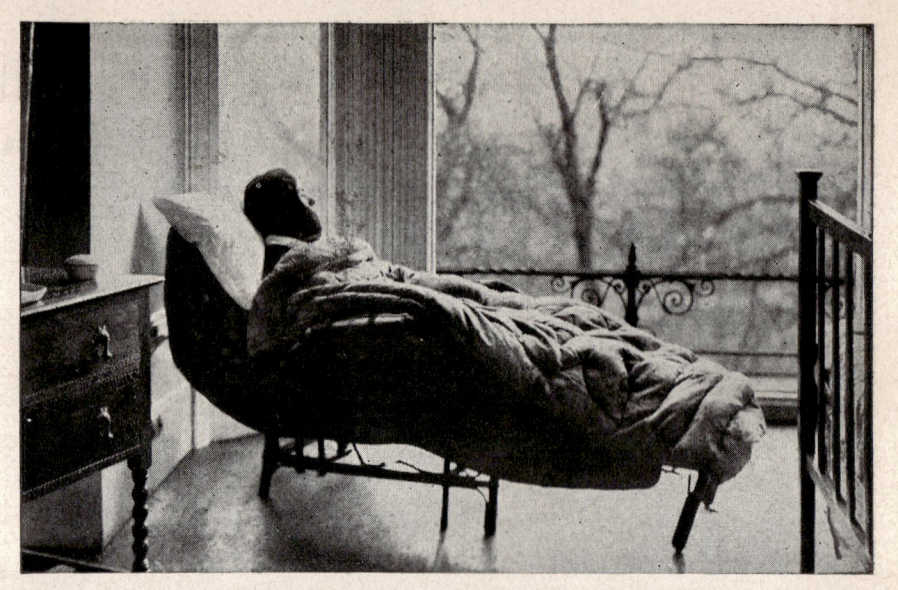

ON THE WAY TO CONVALESCENCE FROM TUBERCULOSIS

When the patient is at length allowed out of bed, he lies on the couch merely while the bed is being aired. This period is later increased to one or two hours, and so lengthened by gradual stages until he is allowed up for as much as eight hours a day.

room in the house must be given up to the patient. This should be as large as possible, with a capacity of at least 3000 cubic feet of air. The cubic space is calculated by multiplying the height, depth, and width of the room. Thus the room of minimum size is truly a large one: assuming ten-foot ceilings, it needs a floor dimension of fifteen feet by twenty, or the equivalent. It should face south or southwest. The window frames should be as large as possible, and the windows should be removed from the frames. An open-air apartment is thereby obtained. In many cases it will be less expensive to construct a porch, thus providing ventilation on two or three sides of the patient's bed and conserving heat in the house itself. The furniture in the room should be reduced to a minimum. Carpets, window, and bed curtains should be removed. The floors should be kept scrupulously clean, and dust removed by a damp cloth moistened in 1-in-100 phenol solution or in dilute lysol, one teaspoonful to the pint of water. All attempts at "hardening" by exposure cannot be too severely condemned, and it is therefore essential to see that the patient has an adequate amount of clothing and protection while in bed. Hot-water bottles should be used to keep the feet warm, if desired, and a woolen knitted helmet worn to protect the neck from draughts.

As long as he is running a temperature the patient must be washed in bed and must use a bedpan and urine bottle.

The question of food and activity of the bowels has already been referred to.

During the time that the patient is being kept at strict rest in bed he should be encouraged to breathe as slowly as possible. The normal rate of respiration is about twelve to fifteen times a minute while in bed. With practice it has been found that the respirations can be reduced to as low as seven or eight times a minute. The number of times the lungs have to expand and contract in the twenty-four hours is thus greatly reduced, and the rest thereby obtained is

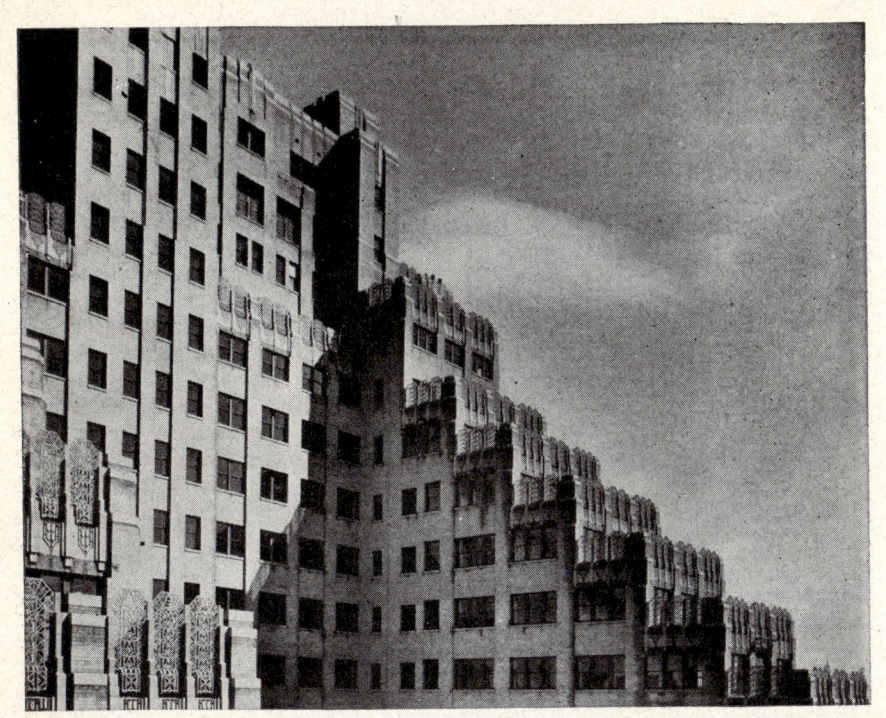

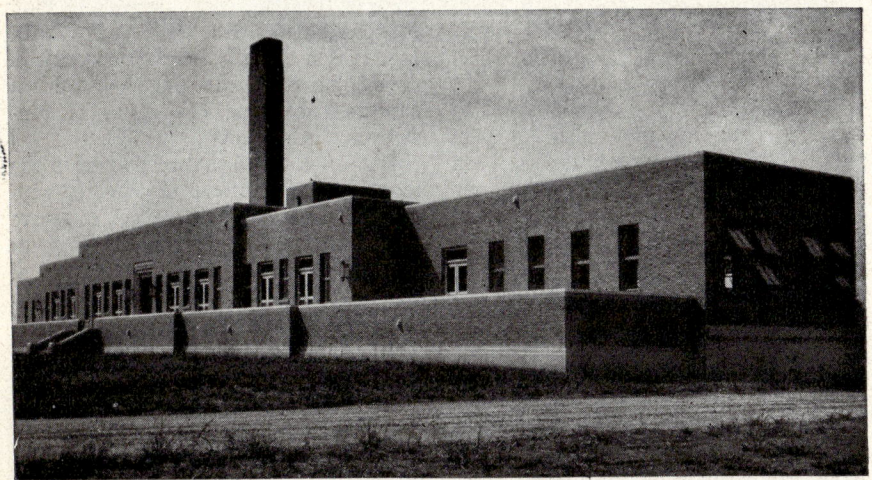

CITY CONGESTION AND OPEN SPACE

Tuberculosis can be treated successfully, in the light of modern understanding, almost anywhere. Here are shown the tuberculosis solaria on the stepped-back roofs of the Jersey City Medical Center in New Jersey, for comparison with the new building of the Tuberculosis Hospital at Roney's Point, W. Va., with its spacious terrace and single floor. The southern exposure, especially of the stepbacks, bathes the entire face of the buildings in sunlight during most of the day.

© *Harris & Ewing*

one of the best methods known for healing a tuberculous lesion.

The temperature should be recorded morning and evening. As it settles down the patient may be allowed restful occupations such as reading and knitting, and

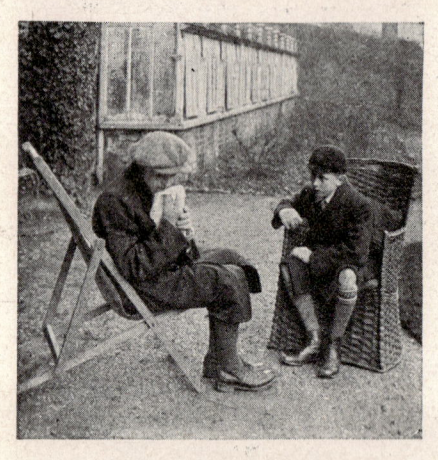

IMPORTANT PRECAUTIONS
When a tuberculosis patient coughs he should be particularly careful to hold his handkerchief before his mouth and to turn his head away from anyone near. It is best to use paper handkerchiefs, which can be destroyed after use.

occasional visitors may also be permitted. After the temperature has been normal throughout the twenty-four hours for a period of a week or, in early cases in which there has been little pyrexia, after the patient has been in bed from one to two months, he may be allowed up gradually by stages, as explained under the heading of Rest and Exercise on page 1549.

During these stages the patient should accustom himself to his rest hours. He should lie down for an hour before lunch and in the evening before dinner. During this time he must be kept absolutely still, and must not talk. When the patient is able to take short walking exercises he is ready for sanatorium treatment, if this is going to be adopted.

Smoking at all stages is best avoided; if the desire is very great it may be allowed in the open air. The patient must not inhale, and must not exhale smoke through the nose. He should smoke only a cigarette, in a holder at least four inches long.

Before passing to the consideration of the prevention of the spread of infection to others and of the sanatorium and its uses, the treatment of the most common symptoms and complications must be described.

Cough. In some cases the cough is dry, irritating and not accompanied by expectoration. It is then both ineffective and useless, and on account of the strain which it puts upon the lungs it may be dangerous. Such a cough should always be checked. Simple lozenges, such as those compounded of black currant and glycerine, should be slowly sucked. In other cases a throat paint will afford relief. A simple linctus made from lemon juice and honey will often stop a cough.

If the cough is accompanied by expectoration, medicines should be given to aid the patient to get rid of the sputum. On no account must he swallow his sputum. The danger of this lies in the fact that he runs a very serious risk of developing tuberculosis of the bowels if sputum containing the germs of consumption is swallowed.

It is often found that on waking in the morning there is a bout of coughing with expectoration, and this may be so severe as to lead to vomiting. A morning cup of weak tea or a glass of warm milk will generally help the patient to bring up easily the sputum which has accumulated during the night, and prevent vomiting. A simple medicine containing sodium bicarbonate and common salt in small doses, taken with a little warm water first thing in the morning, is very valuable.

Shortness of Breath. Rest in bed is the best means of overcoming this distressing symptom. In the more severe cases it is increased by weakness of the heart or by associated pleurisy. The inhalation of oxygen and the use of cardiac stimulants are then of value.

Fever. High temperatures are often met with in advanced cases of consumption. Absolute rest is the best method of treatment.

Night Sweats. This is often a very distressing symptom. Shortly after the patient has dropped off to sleep, he wakes up perspiring profusely, with his night garments soaked through. These should be changed immediately, and the patient sponged down with tepid water containing a little toilet vinegar. The occurrence of night sweats is often an indication either that there is an insufficient supply of fresh air in the room or that the bedclothes are too heavy. They are very much less frequent since the introduction of the open-air treatment. Drugs should not be used.

Spitting Blood. The occurrence of the spitting of blood, or hemoptysis, requires immediate treatment. If not in bed, the patient must at once lie down upon the bed, and he should lie on the right side if the right lung is affected, and upon his left if the left lung is diseased. If both lungs are consumptive, the doctor or nurse will know which lung

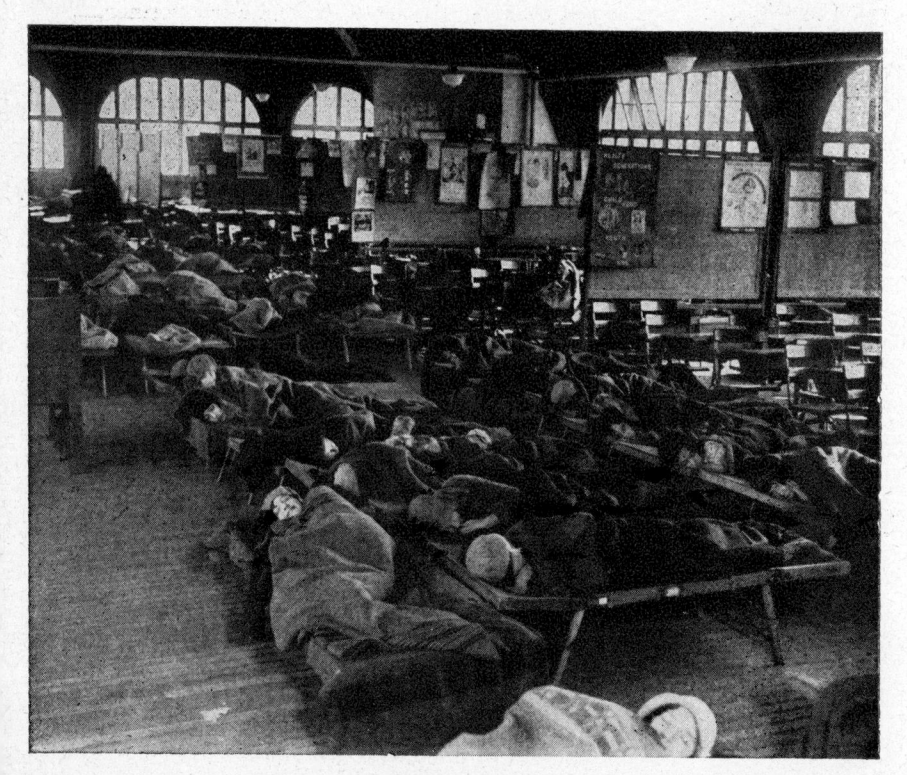

CARE FOR TUBERCULAR SCHOOL CHILDREN

It is unfortunate that in those social groups where tuberculosis most often occurs—that is, among the poor—it is often financially impossible to meet the expense of sending patients to resorts in particularly healthy climates. Good results are obtained with children even in large cities, however, by adapting the school routine to their special needs. As shown above, rest cots are part of the classroom furniture. The school is built over a pier and large windows provide light and air; the children are constantly impressed by posters, instruction, etc., with the importance of following hygienic routines for the improvement of their own health and the protection of others.

© *Ewing Galloway*

is more extensively diseased and the patient should lie upon that side. He should then be reassured that the bleeding does not mean that he is in any serious danger, thus allaying his fears. If ice is available a small quantity should be given to suck. The inhalation of turpentine is a simple remedy which is often effective; a few drops may be placed upon a mask or a handkerchief. A saline aperient should be administered.

All the food must be given cold, and it should consist of only very light articles, such as milk, custards, and thin bread and butter. An injection of morphine is of value in calming the patient and thus helping to arrest the bleeding. In those rare cases which do not respond to these measures, it may be necessary to collapse the lung by an artificial pneumothorax, a procedure which is described later in the special forms of treatment. Very slight degrees of blood spitting, in which the sputum is only colored or streaked with blood, do not require any special forms of treatment.

Pain. This is usually due to pleurisy. A shot bag may be applied to the chest, and the patient should be kept strictly at rest. If this does not afford relief the side of the chest should be strapped with adhesive plaster; should this cause shortness of breath it must immediately be removed.

Digestive Symptoms. Any tendency to failure of the appetite should be remedied. This is often very difficult to accomplish. Tonics, the use of insulin and other agents, are all of limited usefulness. Various digestive ferments may be given in the form of takadiastase, papain, pepsin, and malt extracts. Sodium bicarbonate, a teaspoonful in some warm water, is useful for relieving pain or flatulence after a meal.

Diarrhea. Occurrence of diarrhea does not necessarily mean that tuberculosis of the bowels is present. It should be treated by carefully scrutinizing the dietary and omitting all articles likely to leave a coarse residue, such as brown bread, oatmeal, stringy vegetables, and fruits. A mixture containing chalk and bismuth should be given.

Insomnia. There are various factors which tend to prevent a consumptive from sleeping well, especially if he is confined to bed. These have been mentioned above, and include sleeping by day, monotony of continuous confinement to bed, pain, cough, fever, and night sweats. The appropriate treatment for such conditions has been described above. A change of bed by day and by night often tends to promote sleep; a warm drink at night is also valuable. Hypnotic drugs are rarely required, but a dose of bromide may be given from time to time.

Laryngitis. Consumption affecting the throat is one of the most dreaded and painful complications of consumption of the lungs. On the slightest sign of weakness or huskiness of the voice, the throat must be examined. If a tuberculous spot is found, the essential of treatment consists in complete rest to the vocal cords. This is accomplished by forbidding the patient to speak, even in a whisper. Signs and writing must be used for communication. Such silence should be observed for at least six months. During this time a mask should be worn over the mouth almost continuously during the day, and from time to time moistened with a few drops of antiseptic solution. If the throat is painful it is usually found that only liquid food can be taken, but in severe cases the pain is so intense that even swallowing saliva causes great distress. There are three main methods by which pain can be alleviated so that the patient can take nourishment. An anesthetic powder may be inhaled through a glass tube (Leduc) which curves back over the tongue. A small quantity is inhaled just before a meal. Firm pressure with the palms of the hands over the patient's ears just as he swallows will sometimes enable him to do so without pain. If both these measures fail, the patient should lie on his face on the bed with his head over the side, and suck up his milk with a glass tube from a glass placed on the floor. This method will often enable a patient to take a glass of milk without pain, when he has been unable otherwise to feed without real agony.

Home Prevention of Infection. One of the most important points which have to be considered in the home nursing of a consumptive is the care necessary to prevent other members of the household from becoming infected.

The sputum is the main source of infection, as it often contains millions of the germs. The patient must expectorate into a metal sputum cup containing some disinfectant solution, such as one part of phenol in a hundred parts of water, or one teaspoonful of lysol to a pint of water. The sputum cup must have a lid, and this must always be kept closed when it is not actually being used. The contents of the sputum cup must be emptied every morning and evening and preferably burned. The cup should then be boiled in a saucepan especially kept for this purpose. Sputum cups with destructible paper liners are available and are much used; but if they are used the metal frame must be kept clean.

If the patient is up and about he must carry a sputum flask, made of glass with a metal cover. This contains a little antiseptic fluid, such as dilute lysol or phenol. The contents are emptied daily or oftener, and the flask is washed out with strong disinfectant, then boiled in water. If due care is taken over the disposal of sputum there is very little risk

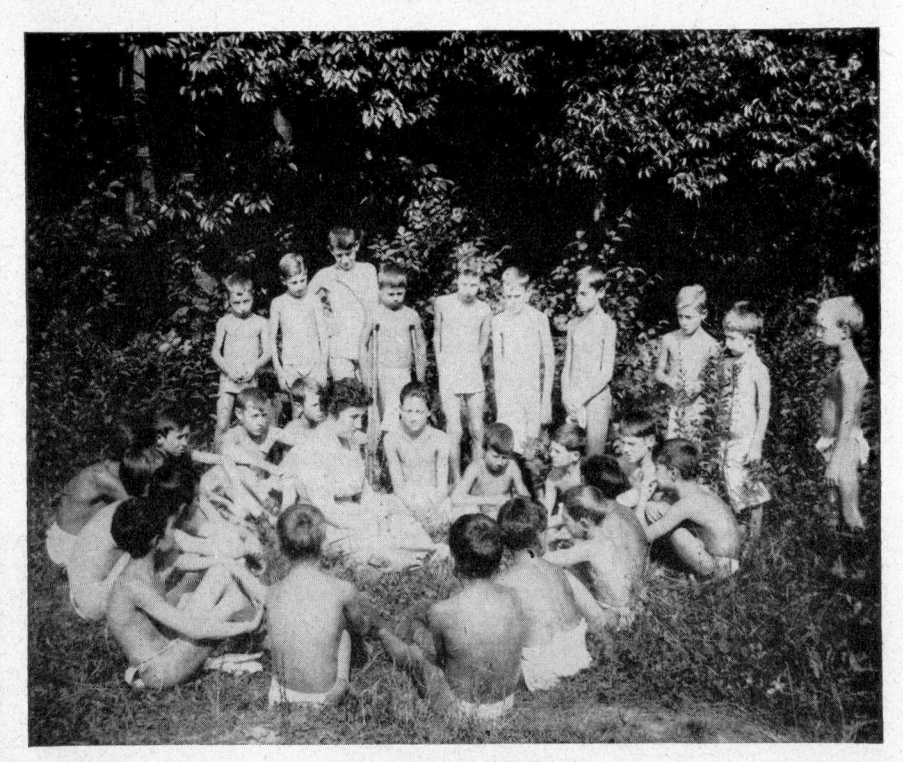

OPEN AIR AND SUNSHINE
Minimum clothing and maximum exposure to the sun contribute to improving the health of these tuberculous children at Perrysburg, New York. Outdoor classes and fresh air improve general health as well.
Photo from Ewing Galloway—C. P. Cushing

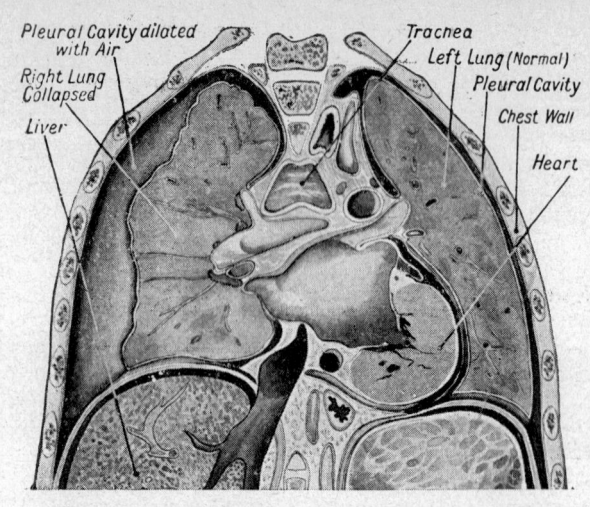

REST FOR TUBERCULOUS LUNG BY PNEUMOTHORAX
Here part of the right chest is occupied by gas, which is causing compression of the right lung. This condition may occur spontaneously from damage to air tubes or vesicles, but is now often produced deliberately in certain types of consumption. The effect is to rest the lung and thereby aid the cure of the disease.

of the disease spreading to others. If, however, an uncovered sputum cup is used, flies will have access to it and spread the germs about the house.

When a consumptive coughs he must always hold a handkerchief before his mouth and nose and turn his head away from anyone in close proximity. The consumptive should always use paper handkerchiefs, which should be burned after use. If linen ones are used, they should be placed in lysol at the end of the day and never be allowed to dry before being disinfected or washed. No consumptive should kiss another person. He should sleep in a separate bed, and preferably in a separate room. His room should be disinfected weekly by being washed over with a cloth dampened in a 1-in-100 solution of phenol. This cloth should then be disinfected by boiling before it is allowed to dry.

Those who are in attendance upon a consumptive must wash their hands immediately after leaving him, and the hands and face should be washed before every meal. The patient should have all his personal utensils, including knives and forks, plates, dishes, spoons, etc., kept separately for himself and washed separately. The books which he reads should be burned after use and should not be read by others. His soiled linen, etc., must be disinfected by boiling before sending to the laundry.

Sanatorium Treatment.
The most suitable cases for sanatorium treatment are those in whom the disease is of slight extent and in an early stage, and certain more chronic types of the disease. Very acute cases are unsuitable unless home conditions render it obligatory.

At the sanatorium the patient is instructed in that mode of living best suited for a person suffering from consumption in a quiescent or arrested stage. The basic principles of treatment are explained and inculcated and a regular routine of living is taught. The patient is kept under close and constant medical supervision, and the individual treatment is given best suited for each case. He is shown how to appreciate the indications that too much exercise or strain is being undertaken, and that a risk is being run of the disease becoming active again.

Exercise varying from graduated walks to heavy manual labor is prescribed under careful supervision.

For other cases suitable indoor and outdoor recreations are arranged so as to encourage mental and physical activity and prevent chronic invalidism. A patient should not expect cure by going to a sanatorium for three months. Even in the most favorable cases six months should be allowed, and in many two years are required.

Aftercare. The aftercare of patients with arrested tuberculosis is a very important problem. It is probably best that the consumptive throughout his treatment should look forward to returning to his former occupation, unless it be one of those in which tuberculosis is prone to occur. On return, however, he should take care to carry out the hygienic principles of living that he has learned. He must avoid stuffy atmospheres and must devote the week-ends to fresh air and rest. Open-air occupations are obviously the most suitable if not too strenuous. Weight should be watched carefully and kept a few pounds above normal.

At the sanatorium the patient learns many things which he must continue to do to stay well and to avoid having the disease become active again. Perhaps the most important consideration is the regulation of rest and exercise, with the accent strongly on rest. When the patient returns home, all the time spent moving about the house doing even slight household duties must be counted as exercise and the remainder of the day spent as rest.

Special Forms of Treatment. This study of pulmonary tuberculosis would not be complete without mentioning the important forms of special treatment of consumption, and considering briefly their indications and utility.

Tuberculins. Ever since the germ of consumption was discovered, in 1882, it has been hoped that this would lead to

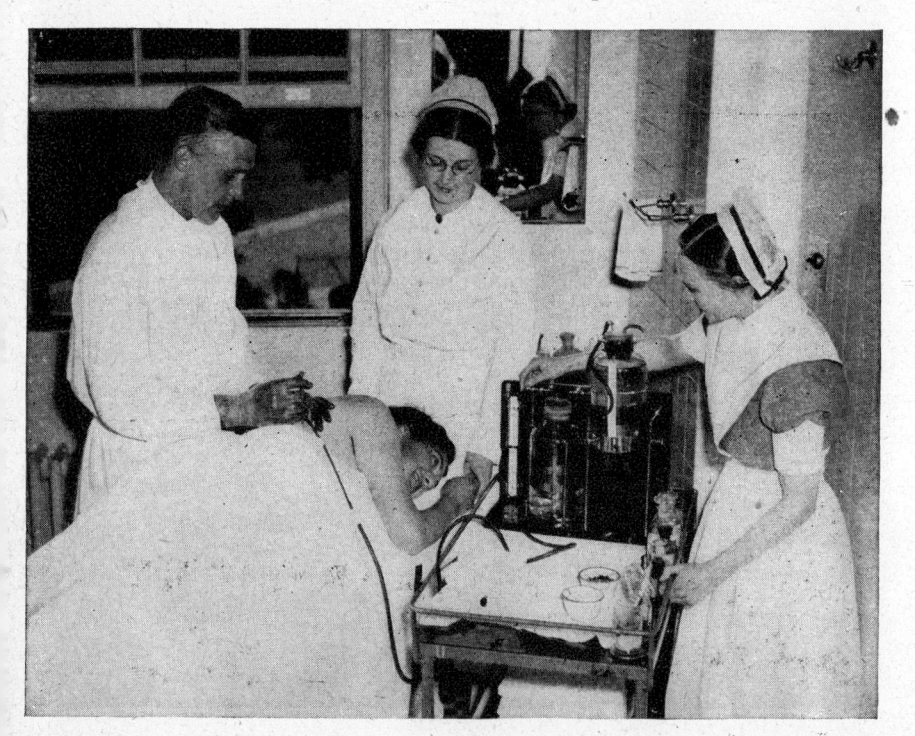

RESTING A TUBERCULAR LUNG
The injection of air into the chest cavity in order to collapse an infected lung is one method of putting that lung at rest in order to allow it to resist and overcome the tuberculosis. The operation is shown here; the doctor is attending to the needle while a nurse watches the pressure and functioning of the apparatus supplying the air.
Courtesy of the National Tuberculosis Association

a means of cure either by a vaccine prepared from the germ or by a serum produced by inoculating it into an animal. Unfortunately, neither of these hopes has been realized at present. The tuberculins are preparations made from dead tubercle bacilli, and there are at least eighty varieties of them. The results so far have proved disappointing.

Vaccines both for cattle and human beings are prepared, and it is claimed that cattle are rendered immune from bovine tuberculosis. If this claim were borne out in practice in large-scale use there is little doubt that the incidence of human consumption would be reduced to a very great extent. The value of the method in human tuberculosis, however, can be assessed only after a long period of experience in general use.

Drugs. Numerous drugs have from time to time been put forward as a cure for consumption, but none has proved of great value.

Cod-liver oil or halibut-liver oil may be given by the mouth, or injected under the skin in the form of sodium morrhuate. In some cases one or the other undoubtedly does good. Creosote may be taken by the mouth or used as an inhalation. Iodine and arsenic are occasionally useful in chronic cases. Treatment by injections of preparations of gold have given equivocal results.

Sunlight. The value of sunlight in the treatment of tuberculosis of the glands and bones has been mentioned already. We owe our knowledge of this method largely to Rollier of Leysin. It has been carried out in Switzerland, and good results obtained. The subject is dealt with in Chapter 42.

Artificial Pneumothorax. The most common of the surgical techniques employed is called artificial pneumothorax. This requires a simple operation whereby a hollow needle is pushed into the chest and air is injected into the pleural cavity, the membranous sac which separates the lung from the chest wall (described on page 1568). The affected lung is thus collapsed and air is prevented from entering it during breathing. In a few days the air is absorbed and the collapsed lung tends to expand again, and then it is necessary to repeat the operation for collapsing it. When healing is complete the lung is permitted to remain expanded and carry on its normal work. Artificial pneumothorax is the most effective way of resting the lung. It can only be used, however, in certain suitable types of cases; e.g., where adhesions exist collapse will not occur and if air is injected there is danger of rupturing the adhesions with resultant severe hemorrhage.

In such a case as this, where the lung is bound down to the chest wall, an extensive surgical operation is sometimes performed known as a thoracoplasty. In this operation a number of ribs are removed on the affected side so that the chest wall falls in and the lung is collapsed. The collapse is of course permanent, but when done by a skilled surgeon causes very little deformity and does not interfere with normal activity.

Another operation for resting the lung is performed by crushing or tearing the phrenic nerve in the neck. This results in paralysis of the diaphragm and consequent diminution in lung motion.

Public Prevention. This can be effected only by a combination of measures directed to public and personal hygiene. Among the former are health education, better housing, slum clearance, the reporting of all cases to health authorities, plentiful sanatoria, and the provision of a wholesome dietary at economic prices. Personal hygiene includes all the factors making for robust health, and of these proper food is the most important.

Spreading of the disease by infected persons must be prevented by isolation and by severe penalization of the spitting in public places which is still too prevalent. Tuberculous persons should marry only with medical permission. In any case the risk to possible children is considerable. Case-finding by means of tuberculin testing and X-ray examinations must be done on a large scale.

CHAPTER 111

DISEASES OF THE PLEURA

Pleurisy — Chronic Pleurisy — Pneumothorax — Artificial Pneumothorax.

THE pleural membranes are very important to the efficient function of the lungs. When there is disease of the pleurae, the organs contained by them are severely handicapped, just as the heart suffers from inflammation of the pericardium.

Pleurisy. Inflammation of the pleura is known as pleurisy. When the pleura is inflamed the first change in it is that it becomes swollen, dry, and very sensitive, and with each breath its two surfaces—that which covers the chest wall and that which covers the lung—rub against one another and cause the most acute pain, called a pleuritic stitch. The next change produced by inflammation is the oozing of watery fluid from the inflamed surface into the bag of the pleura, and as this collects it separates the sore surfaces, and the stitch disappears.

Fluid may contine to collect until the bag gets full and distended, and a pleural effusion is formed, or what is called "water on the chest." This fluid is the watery material of the blood, and as it collects it pushes the lung away from the chest wall. In extreme cases the lung may be pushed backwards against the spine, and the whole of that side of the chest be occupied with water. In such cases the compressed lung is quite put out of use, and no air enters it during the movements of respiration. If the fluid is allowed to remain a long time in this cavity the lung becomes fixed in its abnormal position, and will not expand again when the fluid disappears.

To avoid so serious a result it often becomes necessary for the doctor to remove the fluid. This is done with a hollow needle, which is passed through the soft part of the chest walls between the ribs, and is connected by a soft rubber tube with a bottle from which all the air has been withdrawn by an air-pump. When the tap on the tube is turned the water flows out of the chest into the bottle, to occupy the place of the pumped-out air. This instrument is called an aspirator. In most cases, when once the water has been drawn off it does not collect again, and if the operation has been done sufficiently early the air enters the lung, which expands and fills the chest, again coming into contact with the chest wall. The two surfaces of the pleura once more **touch one another,**

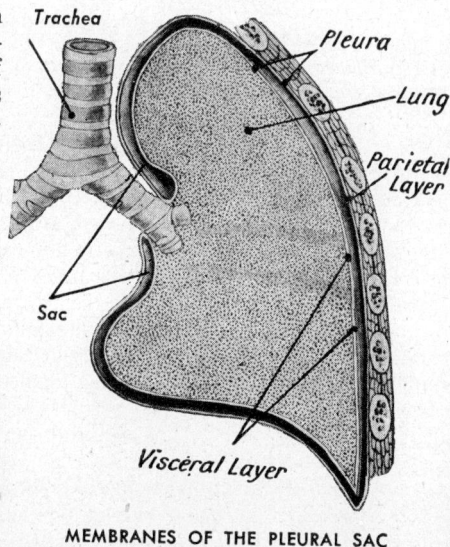

MEMBRANES OF THE PLEURAL SAC
The pleura is an example of a serous membrane and is shown here diagrammatically. One layer lines the chest cavity while the other covers the lung, but these are continuous and enclose a space, or sac.

(1563)

and in many cases the stitch returns, but in this instance the pain is a good sign as showing that water no longer separates the surfaces. The inflamed surfaces may not only touch one another, but may stick together and form bands or adhesions.

Sometimes an unfortunate complication occurs in pleurisy, and the watery fluid gradually becomes mixed with pus which is poured out from the inflamed surfaces; it then forms an empyema, or abscess of the chest. This is a serious condition. The pus may be removed by the aspirator, but it generally re-forms, and it is then necessary for the surgeon to make an opening into the chest between the ribs and allow the matter to run out through a tube as it is formed. For further information along this line read the explanations under the heading Drainage of Wounds, page 2113, and Tapping, page 2119.

Causes. We must now turn to the causes of pleurisy. The most common is cold, exposure to damp, or sitting in a draft. It may result from a blow or fall on the chest, or from the irritation of the pleura by a broken rib. It is a very common complication of disease of the lungs, the inflammation spreading in pneumonia or consumption from the lung to the pleura. Many attacks come on as part of a general disease, such as acute rheumatism, infectious fevers, or tuberculosis (consumption), but tuberculosis may cause pleurisy without other signs of its presence being evident.

All pleurisies which may arise spontaneously, *i.e.*, in the absence of other obvious causes, should be regarded as presumably tuberculous. Infection of the breathing organs and their annexes with tuberculosis is extremely common. Fortunately, in most of us defensive processes are adequate, and the disease obtains no foothold; at the most we suffer from a period of slightly lowered health, from which we recover without the true nature of the cause of the temporary departure from health being recognized. The usual seats of such an infection are the bronchial glands and the pleura. Small healed areas of tuberculosis are commonly found upon the pleural surface of the lung; fibrous adhesions between the pleural surfaces are extremely common findings in post-mortem examinations without the history of any lung disease being forthcoming; the majority of these are of tuberculous origin.

The signs and symptoms may be slight and vague. A painful catch in the breathing for a few weeks, a slight irregular rise of temperature over a period of weeks or months, a failure of appetite and energy or an ill-defined sense of fatigue, may be all that is noticed. Many cases clear up without treatment, leaving only a small localized scar, a chalky

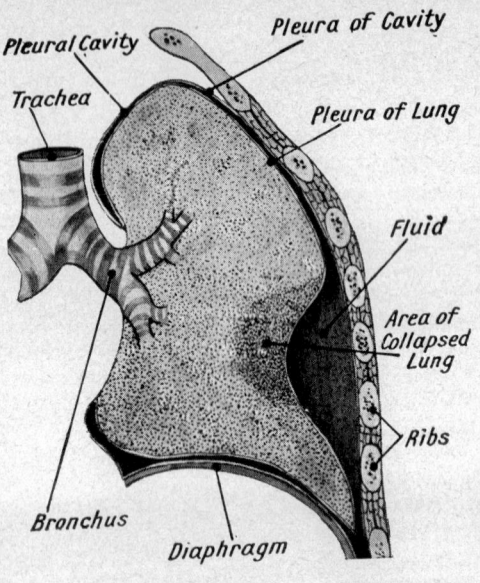

PLEURISY: COLLECTION OF FLUID
Here is shown the lung with a large collection of fluid between it and the chest wall. The lung compressed by the fluid is comparatively airless, a condition called collapse of the lung.

nodule, or a patch of adhesions. Others progress to the formation of an effusion (see below), often insidious in its collection and mild in its results.

The effused fluid under the microscope is seen to contain a large number of the special form of white blood corpuscles, known as small lymphocytes, which are such a characteristic feature of all tuberculous effusions in any region; occasionally there is evidence of old or recent bleeding into the fluid. In some cases the fluid is thick and purulent and partakes of the nature of an empyema.

Symptoms. One of the first symptoms of the disease is the sharp, stabbing pain in the side, which comes on with any movement of the body and with every deep breath. With the pain there is usually some fever and a feeling of chilliness or even shivering. Fever and stitch occurring together are enough to make us suspect pleurisy. The breathing is affected; it is short, jerky, and shallow, and, to avoid bringing on the pain, is much restrained. A slight cough comes on which is exceedingly painful, and is half-suppressed, dry, and ineffectual; there is either no expectoration or a little frothy fluid. The temperature is not usually very high; it may reach 104° F., but is much more frequently only 100° or 101° F. With the increase in temperature appear a hot skin, quickened pulse, impaired appetite, furred tongue, increased thirst, headache, and pain about the body.

This is the stage of dry pleurisy, which, if not checked by treatment, passes into a pleural effusion. The pain passes off, or, at any rate, is much less sharp, but the breathing grows more difficult and more rapid, and the slightest exertion puts the patient out of breath. In the majority of cases, at the end of a week the fluid has ceased to increase, and then in a day or two begins to grow less. The symptoms now subside, the breathing gets easier, fever disappears, and the patient gradually passes into convalescence by daily slight improvement, rather than by any definite sudden change in his condition. The alarming symptom of a return of pain need, as we have explained, cause no anxiety, but may be looked upon as a hopeful sign. If, however, the fluid continues to increase in amount the breathing becomes more impeded. When it is on the left side the heart is displaced. The general health suffers, and if the case should be neglected the fluid may, as we have seen, gradually become purulent. The pus will find its way to the surface, and discharge either through the lung by coughing, or through the chest wall.

Treatment. The treatment of pleurisy ought most certainly to be carried out under the orders of a doctor whenever possible. The patient must be put to bed and be kept on light simple food. A hot linseed poultice or antiphlogistine should be applied to the side to ease the pain, or a mustard leaf or a belladonna plaster.

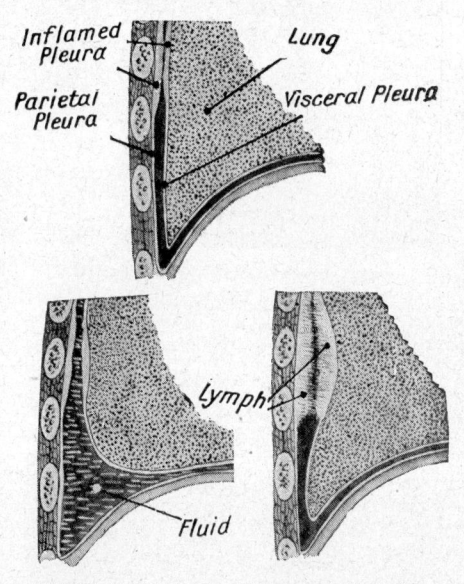

INFLAMMATION OF PLEURAL MEMBRANES
Diagrammatic views of the pleura: Above: opposing surfaces of pleura are inflamed and by rubbing together cause pain—dry pleurisy. Below, left: fluid has accumulated, separating the surfaces and preventing rubbing—wet pleurisy; Below, right: the fluid has been absorbed but lymph has been deposited on the inflamed areas.

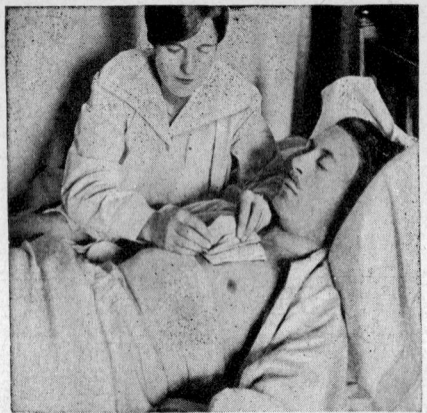

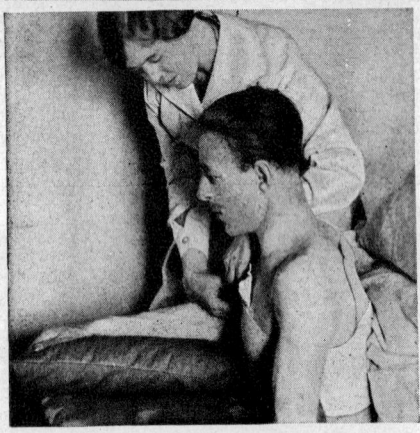

RELIEVING PAIN IN DRY PLEURISY

It is essential that the patient should be kept in bed. To relieve the pain the back and chest should have hot fomentations, and a bandage should be fixed round the body to hold them in position. A wide bandage should be used, and tied firmly, as shown below; this relieves pain by lessening movement.

If these measures are not effectual nothing is better than to strap up the painful side with plaster. To do this use adhesive plaster in strips about three inches wide and eighteen to twenty-four inches long. Six to eight strips will be needed. A strip should then be warmed in front of a fire or radiator, or against a vessel of hot water, and when it is quite moist and sticky the patient must empty his chest of air as completely as possible, and the strip of plaster is then applied to the lowest part of the chest, beginning at the spine, passing downwards and forwards in the direction of the ribs, and reaching just beyond the middle line in front. The next strip should be placed just below the first at the back, and cross it, passing forwards and upwards to the middle line in front. The third strip runs parallel with the first, overlapping it about an inch, the fourth parallel with the second, also overlapping it, and so on until the painful part has been well covered. Each strip is put on after the patient has well emptied his chest, for the object is to secure the ribs in this position and prevent their movements by the plaster.

If the pain is very severe and if the fever is high, ten grains of salicylate of soda may be given.

When the pain has disappeared the plaster may be taken off and the stickiness removed with some spirits of turpentine. The chest may then be painted daily over the lower half of the affected side with diluted tincture of iodine. The same effect may be obtained by substituting for the iodine either ointment of iodide of potash or ointment of oleate of mercury, which should be rubbed into the chest. Occasional doses of Epsom or Glauber's salts are necessary, as the bowels should be made to act rather freely.

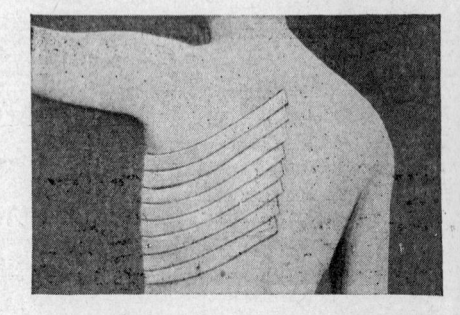

IMMOBILIZATION BY PLASTER

Strips of adhesive plaster are applied round the chest from below upwards and passing beyond the middle line both in front and behind. They are laid on in the direction of the ribs and applied during expiration.

Convalescence may be hastened by good food and tonics, but these must not be begun until all fever has disappeared. The complete recovery of the local condition is often very tardy, and always takes some time, and yet it is of the utmost importance to secure it if possible, for an incomplete cure is likely to be followed by a return of the disease, or even by some tuberculous trouble. Change of air, absence of worry and overwork, warm clothes, and hygienic surroundings are all useful auxiliaries in bringing about complete and speedy recovery.

Chronic Pleurisy. As a sequel of an acute tuberculous pleurisy, either of acute tuberculous pleurisy, either of the dry or moist form, a condition of chronic pleurisy may arise. This takes the form of a more or less localized thickening of the pleural membrane with adhesion of the opposed surfaces, and usually a gradual spread of fibrous tissue into the lung, producing shrinking of the lung and a falling in of the chest wall in the vicinity. This is extremely common in the region of the apex of the lung, often in association with underlying disease of the lung in the form of fibrosis or cavitation, but it may be more widely spread and productive of considerable deformity with gross shrinkage of lung, twisting of the thorax and curvature of the spine. This is the form which produces the drooped shoulder and the warped chest of the older man; it does not lend itself to treatment in most cases, though improvement may follow operation to divide adhesions or to strip thickened membrane from the lung surface.

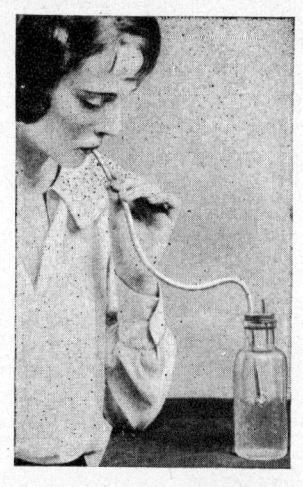

BREATHING EXERCISE
Expansion of a compressed lung can be assisted by blowing water out of a bottle through a rubber tube. Blowing up balloons is another aid to deep breathing and expansion of the lung.

PNEUMOTHORAX

A condition in which air or gas is present in the pleural cavity is known as pneumothorax. It may result from some disease or accident, when it is called spontaneous, or it may be produced by the physician introducing air as a special form of treatment, when it is called artificial (see illustration, page 1559).

The gas in spontaneous pneumothorax usually enters the pleural cavity from the lung, as the result of the rupture of some tuberculous spot near the surface which allows communication to take place between the air in a bronchus and the pleural sac. Rupture of a distended emphysematous vesicle is a less frequent cause. When pus is present in the pleural cavity, constituting an empyema, it may burst into the lung with the development of a pneumothorax.

In other cases a pneumothorax may be caused by external injury to the chest. In nearly 95 per cent of all cases of spontaneous pneumothorax, however, the underlying cause is tuberculosis of the lungs.

The onset of a pneumothorax is usually sudden, and may occur while the patient is at rest or while he is indulging in some violent form of exercise, such as running. He experiences a lancinating pain in the side of the chest, and the breathing is considerably embarrassed. This is due to the rupture of the lung and the tearing of the covering pleural membrane. The air then escapes into the pleural sac and causes the lung on

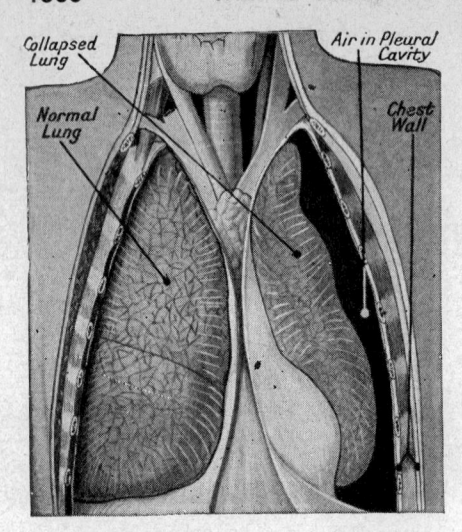

PNEUMOTHORAX: AIR IN PLEURAL CAVITY
The illustration shows the lungs with the pericardium between them. Air has leaked into the left pleural cavity, and the lung has thereupon collapsed. Ordinarily the lung is held against the chest wall by atmospheric pressure and by the absence of air pressure within the pleural cavity.

the same side to collapse, and the heart is displaced simultaneously and drawn to the sound side. The patient is not usually able to walk about, but suffers from profound shock, and on being placed in bed prefers to be propped up and leaning a little to the affected side.

In some varieties of spontaneous pneumothorax the hole connecting the lung with the pleural cavity remains open, so that the air whistles in and out as the patient breathes, and the pressure in the pleural sac is raised to that of the atmosphere. In other cases, however, the tear in the plural membrane acts as a flap valve, allowing air to escape from the lung into the pleural sac, but preventing its passage in the reverse direction. In a short time, therefore, the intrapleural pressure is raised considerably and is higher than that of the atmosphere. This causes great distress unless air is allowed to escape through a hollow needle inserted through the chest wall.

Artificial Pneumothorax. The establishment of an artificial pneumothorax is a form of treatment of certain cases of pulmonary tuberculosis. It is performed by inserting a hollow needle through the chest wall between two ribs into the pleural cavity. The end of the needle which projects from the chest is attached by a rubber tube to a series of two bottles containing some antiseptic fluid. By raising one of the bottles fluid will pass out of it into the other bottle, and in so doing will drive air along the rubber tube to the chest. The pressure in the pleural cavity is measured by means of a manometer. Only a small amount of air is injected at a time, the subsequent injections being known as refills. In this way the pleural space is gradually filled with air and the adjacent lung is collapsed. The lung is thus prevented from moving with respiration and put completely at rest, a condition which is most favorable for the repair of a tuberculous lesion in the lung tissue.